Intestinal Parasites - New Developments in Diagnosis, Treatment, Prevention and Future Directions

Edited by Nihal Dogan

Published in London, United Kingdom

Intestinal Parasites - New Developments in Diagnosis, Treatment, Prevention and Future Directions
http://dx.doi.org/10.5772/intechopen.1002145
Edited by Nihal Dogan

Contributors
Alka Sharma, Amandine Nachtergael, Amit Baliyan, André Pagnah Zoli, Anshu Chaudhary, Bindu Sharma, Brian S. Dorr, Chimezirim Ezeano, Claudia Muñoz Yañez, Cyril Blavo, Célestin Pongombo Shongo, Douglas Causey, Dumar A. Jaramillo-Hernández, Emmanuel Assana, Emmanuel Kokori, Gaël Nzuzi Mavungu, Gbolahan Olatunji, Hirut Tesfahun Alemu, Inderjeet Kaur, Ismaila Ajayi Yusuf, Janeth Oliva Guangorena-Gómez, Joshua Bernard, Jyotsna Chawla, Kate L. Sheehan, Km. Deepika, Muili Abdulbasit, Nicholas Aderinto, Nihal Dogan, Pierre Duez, Rachid Khatouf, Ram Gopal Nitharwal, Reena Negi, Ryan F. Hechinger, Said Dahani, Samatar Abshir Mahamed, Sarika Thakur, Sonja Barber, Taiwo Akinnubi, Timilehin Isarinade, Victor Okombe Embeya, Welcome Muyumba Nonga, Wilfred Ofosu, Wiwien S. Utami, Yohannis Derbew Molla

First published in London, United Kingdom, 2024 by IntechOpen
IntechOpen is the global imprint of INTECHOPEN LIMITED, registered in England and Wales, registration number: 11086078, 167-169 Great Portland Street, London, W1W 5PF, United Kingdom

British Library Cataloguing-in-Publication Data
A catalogue record for this book is available from the British Library

Additional hard and PDF copies can be obtained from orders@intechopen.com

Intestinal Parasites - New Developments in Diagnosis, Treatment, Prevention and Future Directions
Edited by Nihal Dogan
p. cm.

This title is part of the Infectious Diseases Book Series, Volume 31
Topic: Parasitic Infectious Diseases
Series Editor: Alfonso J. Rodriguez-Morales
Topic Editor: Amidou Samie

Print ISBN 978-0-85466-572-3
Online ISBN 978-0-85466-571-6
eBook (PDF) ISBN 978-0-85466-573-0
ISSN 2631-6188

IntechOpen Book Series

Infectious Diseases

Volume 31

Aims and Scope of the Series

This series will provide a comprehensive overview of recent research trends in various Infectious Diseases (as per the most recent Baltimore classification). Topics will include general overviews of infections, immunopathology, diagnosis, treatment, epidemiology, etiology, and current clinical recommendations for managing infectious diseases. Ongoing issues, recent advances, and future diagnostic approaches and therapeutic strategies will also be discussed. This book series will focus on various aspects and properties of infectious diseases whose deep understanding is essential for safeguarding the human race from losing resources and economies due to pathogens.

Meet the Series Editor

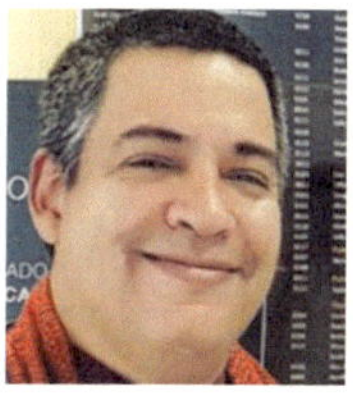

Dr. Rodriguez-Morales is an expert in tropical and emerging diseases, particularly zoonotic and vector-borne diseases (notably arboviral diseases), and more recently COVID-19 and Monkeypox. He is the president of the Publications and Research Committee of the Pan-American Infectious Diseases Association (API), as well as the president of the Colombian Association of Infectious Diseases (ACIN). He is a member of the Committee on Tropical Medicine, Zoonoses, and Travel Medicine of ACIN. Dr. Rodriguez-Morales is a vice-president of the Latin American Society for Travel Medicine (SLAMVI) and a member of the Council of the International Society for Infectious Diseases (ISID). Since 2014, he has been recognized as a senior researcher at the Ministry of Science of Colombia. He is a professor at the Faculty of Medicine of the Fundacion Universitaria Autonoma de las Americas, in Pereira, Risaralda, Colombia, and a professor, Master in Clinical Epidemiology and Biostatistics, at Universidad Científica del Sur, Lima, Peru. He is also a non-resident adjunct faculty member at the Gilbert and Rose-Marie Chagoury School of Medicine, Lebanese American University, Beirut, Lebanon, and an external professor, Master in Research on Tropical Medicine and International Health, at Universitat de Barcelona, Spain. Additionally, an invited professor, Master in Biomedicine, at Universidad Internacional SEK, Quito, Ecuador, and a visiting professor, Master Program of Epidemiology, at Diponegoro University, Indonesia. In 2021 he was awarded the "Raul Isturiz Award" Medal of the API and, the same year, the "Jose Felix Patiño" Asclepius Staff Medal of the Colombian Medical College due to his scientific contributions to the topic of COVID-19 during the pandemic. He is currently the Editor in Chief of the journal Travel Medicine and Infectious Diseases. His Scopus H index is 55 (Google Scholar H index 77) with a total of 725 publications indexed in Scopus.

Meet the Volume Editor

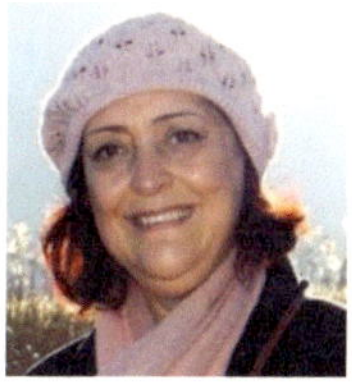

Prof. Dr Nihal Dogan has worked in the Department of Microbiology, Faculty of Medicine, Osmangazi University, Turkey, since 1986. Her master's and Ph.D. thesis focused on the diagnosis and sero-epidemiology of toxoplasmosis. She was a visiting researcher on the diagnosis of *Entamoeba histolytica* at the University of Virginia, USA, in 2003 and an observer researcher working on trypanosomes at the Faculty of Medicine, Universidad De Chile, in 2016. She was appointed a professor in 2008 and is the leading academic in the field of parasitology, with expertise in the epidemiology of parasitic diseases. Her research interests include medical ethics; seroepidemiological surveys; intestinal, blood, tissue, and ocular parasites; vector-borne diseases; and zoonotic parasites. Her research has been published in more than 40 national and international journals. She also made 85 poster presentations, plus many oral presentations and keynote speeches at international and national congresses. She has written numerous book chapters on infectious diseases, clinical parasitology, and clinical microbiology, as well as medical microbiology laboratory applications and manuals.

Contents

Preface

The history of intestinal parasites is as old as human history itself. Paleoparasitological data show that humans and their parasites have been co-evolving for centuries, with this relationship remaining as strong as it was 10,000 years ago. Since the 1970s, significant improvements in public health conditions have been reported in developing and developed countries. However, there has been no significant change in the number of new protozoan and helminth parasites emerging between 1940 and 2000. In today's modern world, parasitic infections are re-emerging on the infectious disease radar in the developed world. This resurgence is due to increasingly immunocompromised populations and longer life expectancy, even though the developed world seemed to have freed itself from intestinal parasites.

A wide variety of intestinal parasites are prevalent in different parts of the world. Among the major contributors to the global intestinal parasite disease burden are *Ascaris* sp., *Entamoeba* sp., *Cyclospora* sp., *Giardia* sp., and *Cryptosporidium* sp. However, parasites such as *Enterobius* are often overlooked, despite their ability to impair the growth and learning abilities of the younger population. These parasites can spread from endemic areas to different geographical areas due to globalization, global warming, wars, migrations, and touristic travels. This spread increases the burden of infectious diseases all over the world, especially in developing countries, and leads to significant economic losses. Epidemiologic data indicate that one-third of the world is affected by intestinal parasites, with the highest prevalence in Sub-Saharan Africa, Latin America, China, Asia, and India. Due to their high prevalence, wide geographical distribution, impact on the nutritional status and immunity, and the economic losses they cause, intestinal parasites remain a significant worldwide public health problem.

Today, about one-third of the population in cities in developing countries live in urban slums, and it is estimated that within a few years, this proportion may exceed 60%. The prevalence of infections caused by *Entamoeba histolytica* and *Giardia intestinalis*, as well as the prevalence and intensity of *Ascaris lumbricoides* and *Trichuris trichiura* infections, are increasing among rural populations migrating to these urban and suburban settings due to favorable transmission conditions. Therefore, there is an urgent need to improve sanitation in deprived urban areas and periodically treat these populations to reduce the worm burden, especially in school-age children.

While the majority of people worldwide live in tropical developing countries, the transmission or potential transmission of intestinal parasites in economically developed, temperate climates has emerged as a growing problem in recent years. In developed countries, protozoan parasites cause gastrointestinal infections more commonly than helminths. *Giardia intestinalis, Entamoeba histolytica, Cyclospora cayetanensis*, and *Cryptosporidium* sp. are among the most common protozoan infections causing diarrhea. Whereas protozoa can replicate in the human body, most soil-borne intestinal helminth infections do not replicate in the human body and remain in the same numbers as when they were acquired. The four most common species in humans—*Ascaris lumbricoides* (roundworms), *Trichiuris trichiuria* (whipworms), *Ancylostoma duodenale*, and *Necator americanicus* (hookworms)—continue to be a major cause of morbidity and mortality in tropical and subtropical areas without adequate water and sanitation. In addition to their impact on health, intestinal helminths also impair the physical and mental development of children, negatively affecting educational achievement and economic development.

Rapid and effective drug treatment of intestinal parasites is one of the most important factors that can reduce the incidence. Providing clean potable water and promoting handwashing habits are among the most important factors in prevention and control strategies. A global approach is needed to control intestinal parasites, which continue to be a global threat. To establish a global and sustainable control strategy, the fight must be carried out in many areas simultaneously. Hygiene education and the improvement of public health conditions will play a major role in the prevention and control of intestinal parasites.

In this book, studies on intestinal parasites affecting human health include historical perspectives, their place in taxonomy, epidemiological data, diagnosis, treatment (herbal and chemical), and prevention protocols from past to present. The book also covers the damage caused by tapeworms in the intestines and brain, the effects of protozoa and helminths on child development, and epidemiological data for specific populations. It delves into new developments in diagnosis and treatment, as well as the effects of zoonotic parasites on human health in animals consumed for nutritional purposes. Additionally, the book includes extensive and comprehensive epidemiological and experimental studies.

Nihal Dogan
Medical Faculty Microbiology Department,
Eskisehir Osmangazi University,
Eskisehir, Turkey

Chapter 1

Intestinal Parasites from Past to Present: Taxonomy, Paleoparasitology, Geographic Distribution, Prevention and Control Strategies

Nihal Dogan

Abstract

Intestinal parasites are among the oldest human infectious agents. Throughout history, many parasite species have continued to evolve with humans during migrations, hunting, and domestication. Intestinal parasites are still a major cause of morbidity and mortality in the world, especially among children in underdeveloped countries. In developing countries, helminth infections such as hookworms, Ascaris, whipworms and amoebiasis caused by *Entamoeba histolytica* are parasitic agents that cause significant mortality and growth retardation. Soil-transmitted helminths and intestinal parasites of zoonotic origin cause significant mental and physical developmental disorders in poor people in endemic areas. It is an important public health problem affecting a quarter of the world's population, increasing the global health burden and impairing quality of life. Intestinal protozoa are among the leading causes of diarrhea in developed and developing countries. In order to achieve success in prevention and control programs, it is necessary to identify people with parasites through community-based epidemiological studies and to carry out treatment and post-treatment controls. Although epidemiologic studies on intestinal parasites are mostly related to children, infants, pregnant women, and immunocompromised populations are at significant risk. Today, microscopy is still the gold standard for diagnosis, but serologic and molecular techniques have also been successfully applied.

Keywords: intestinal parasites, taxonomy, paleoparasitology, prevention, control, evolution, diagnosis, future prospects

1. Introduction

Intestinal parasites are the leading infectious agents among the causes of death in the world, especially in children. Diseases caused by *Ascaris lumbricoides, Ancylostoma duodenale, Necator americanus, Schistosoma* species, *Enterobius vermicularis, Giardia lamblia* and *Entamoeba histolytica* are intestinal parasites that cause significant morbidity and mortality in developing countries [1–6].

Although intestinal parasites do not have obvious clinical symptoms, abdominal pain, sleep disorders, nervous symptoms, growth and development disorders due to malabsorption are the most prominent symptoms, especially during childhood. The most important factor in the spread of intestinal parasites is people with parasites. Epidemiologic surveys with intermittent controls in societies can identify and treat many people infected with parasites. In this way, societies provide the necessary measures to prevent an important disease that will cause destruction in individuals and to prevent social destruction. From past to present, microscopic examination of stool samples taken on consecutive days for the presence of parasites (cysts, trophozoites, eggs and larvae) is an easy, cheap and gold standard method in diagnosis. It can be applied wherever a microscope is available, but requires experience [1–7].

Intestinal parasites are most common in tropical climates and in regions where the necessary infrastructure and sanitation conditions are not provided, and clean drinking water is not available. The best preventative measurements in a community are the provision of infrastructure and safe water supplies, as well as the identification and treatment of people with parasites. With regard to infectious diseases, people can be infected with a parasite throughout their lives without showing any symptoms. A slight change in the system host-parasite-environment relationship can shift the balance, and diseases can develop [4, 5, 8–10].

Gastrointestinal parasites have been described as the "infectious disease of poverty". Protozoa and helminths living in the human gastrointestinal tract are estimated to infect one-sixth of the global population. Children in sub-Saharan countries have the highest prevalence, followed by rural areas in Asia, Latin America and the Caribbean. It is estimated that 250 million people in sub-Saharan countries, mostly children, are infected with at least one type of intestinal parasite. Although developed donor countries and local communities are taking various initiatives, economic crisis, poor personal and environmental conditions for hygiene, lack of education, population growth, wars and migration as well as inadequate treatment facilities in these regions are causing the increase of new cases [1, 4, 8–10]. According to WHO reports, although safe and effective drugs have now been developed for the treatment of intestinal parasites, their availability in mass treatment programs and for individual treatment worldwide may be limited by economic resources, existing production and distribution networks and national regulations. Increasing population density, environmental pollution and global migration patterns will continue to encourage the transmission of human intestinal parasites in the future.

In the twenty-first century, malabsorption, diarrhea, blood loss, impaired work capacity and reduced growth rate due to intestinal parasitic infections continue to pose significant health and social problems in many countries. The success of prevention and control strategies depends on safe and effective treatments, improved diagnostic procedures and the availability of general health services. For successful control, it is necessary to know the history of parasites, their migration routes, old and new methods used in diagnosis, treatment protocols and most importantly prevention and control strategies. In this review article, the place of intestinal parasites in classification, history, epidemiology, diagnosis, treatment and prevention methods are discussed in a historical perspective from past to present.

2. Classification of intestinal parasites

Although common names are often used to describe parasitic organisms, these names may represent different parasites in different parts of the world. To avoid these problems, a binomial nomenclature system is used, where the scientific name consists of genus and species. As with all living things, intestinal parasites are classified according to certain rules. Today, this classification can be moved to different places and changed from time to time with the discovery of some biochemical and physiological features depending on phylogenetic studies. Based on phylogenetic classification, living organisms are divided into Prokaryotes and Eukaryotes according to the presence of a nuclear membrane. All parasites are in the Eukaryotes group and in the Animalia kingdom (**Figure 1**) [11, 12].

In addition to unicellular protozoan parasites, many species of parasites called helminths can be found in the human gastrointestinal tract. Intestinal parasites are among the most common gastrointestinal infections worldwide, especially in developing countries. They are also among the leading causes of child mortality in developing countries, especially in the tropics and subtropics [1, 4, 6, 8]. Intestinal parasites, which are still an important source of morbidity and mortality in the world, are divided into two important groups [11, 12].

2.1 Intestinal protozoa

Sarcomastigophora (Amoebae): Entamoeba histolytica, Entamoeba dispar, Entamoeba hartmanni, Entamoeba coli, Entamoeba polecki, Entamoeba moshkovskii, Entamoeba gingivalis, Endolimax nana Iodamoeba bütschlii and *Blastocystis hominis.* The place of some of these (*Blastocystis sp* etc.) in the classification and their pathogenicity are still controversial.

Mastigophora (flagellates): Giardia lamblia, Chilomastix mesnili, Dientamoeba fragilis, Pentatrichomonas hominis, Trichomonas hominis, Enteromonas hominis and *Retortomonas intestinalis*.

Coccidia: Cryptosporidium spp. Cyclospora cayetanensis, Isospora (Cystoisospora) belli, Sarcocystis hominis, Sarcocystis suihominis and *Sarcocystis bovihominis.*

Ciliata (cilia): Balantidium coli.

Microsporidia: Enterocytozoon bieneusi and *Encephalitozoon (Septata) intestinalis.*

2.2 Intestinal helminths

Nematodes: Ascaris lumbricoides, Ascaris suum, Enterobius vermicularis, Ancylostoma duodenale, Necator americanus, Strongyloides stercoralis, Strongyloides fuelleborni, Trichostrongylus spp. Trichuris trichiura, Capillaria philippinensis, Oesophagostomum spp. and *Ternidens deminutus.*

Cestodes: Diphyllobothrium latum (broad, fish tapeworm), Dipylidium caninum (dog tapeworm), Hymenolepis (Rodentolepis) nana (dwarf tapeworm), Hymenolepis diminuta (rat tapeworm), Taenia solium (pork tapeworm), Taenia saginata (beef tapeworm) and *Taenia asiatica (Taiwanese variant of T. saginata).*

Trematodes: Fasciolopsis buski (giant intestinal fluke), Echinostoma ilocanum, Eurytrema pancreaticum, Heterophyes heterophyes, Metagonimus yokogawai and *Alaria spp.*

In addition to these, species of the *Annelida* and *Acanthacephala*, which are less common in the world, can also parasitize. These are not normally human-specific parasites and are known as "unusual parasites" that can be found in sporadic cases.

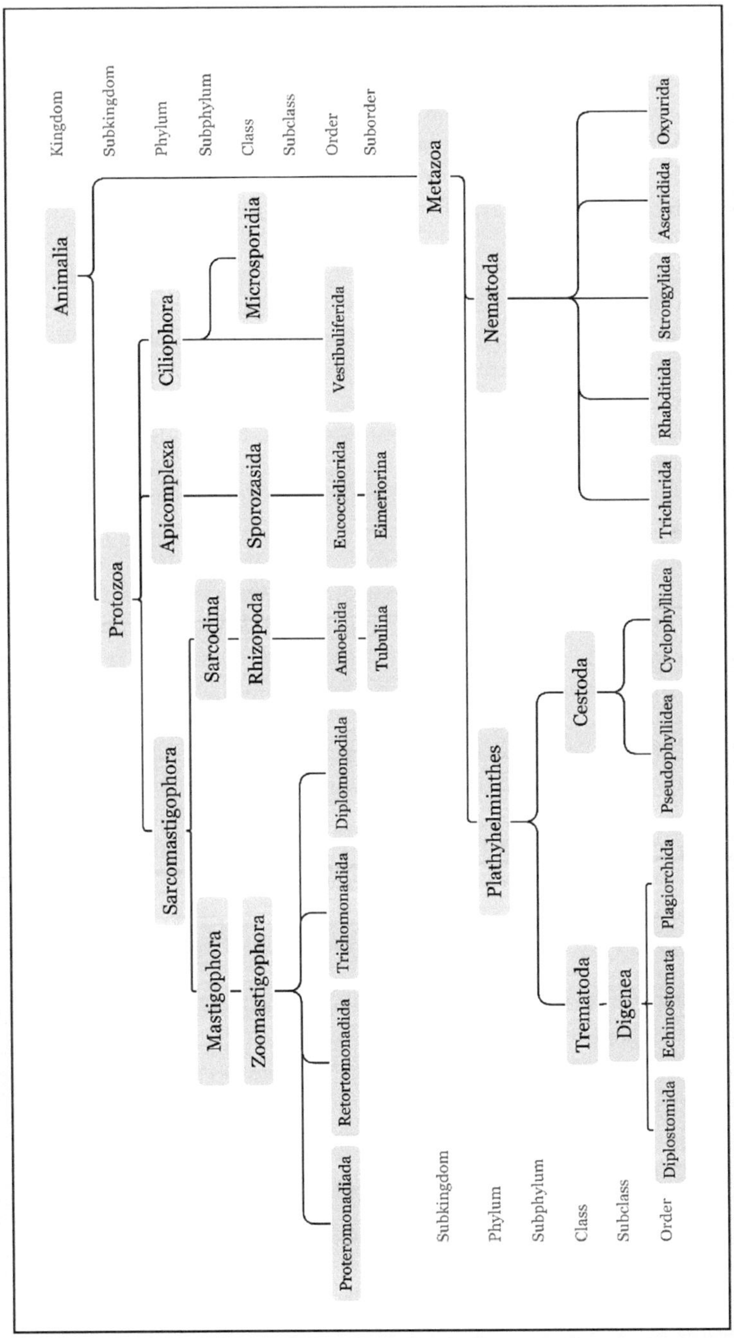

Figure 1.
Taxonomy and classification of human parasitic protozoa and helminths.

The evolution of a small number of species of *Acanthocephala* has been elucidated, as they have a complex evolutionary history, changing many hosts during their evolution. The three most common species implicated in human disease, *M. hirudinaceus, M. ingens* and *M. moniliformis*, use pigs, raccoons and rodents, respectively, as their primary definitive hosts, but other carnivores can also function as definitive hosts. *Acanthocephaliasis* may be an ancient disease of humans. Analysis of fossilized feces from prehistoric humans in Utah revealed *Moniliformis sp.* eggs, but it is not known whether this represents real or spurious infections. Of the few cases described today, most have been identified in diapers of children under 2 years of age. It is thought to be caused by infants ingesting a cockchafer (*Melolontha melolontha*) in their environment. The larvae cause mild to severe reactions in the gastrointestinal tract and are usually diagnosed incidentally [11, 12].

3. Intestinal parasites in historical process and paleoparasitology

In the 1990s, standard scientific analyses of parasitology were carried out from the perspective of a new discipline, anthropology of knowledge. With this period, studies on the historical and sociocultural development, limitations, relations with other disciplines and social needs were initiated within the science of parasitology. There are certain periods in parasitological history that are characteristic of all emerging disciplines of the natural sciences. The first systematic description of natural phenomena and their interpretation began in the sixteenth century and continued until the mid-eighteenth century. During these periods, many of the correct facts were not adequately explained and were based on different natural phenomena and religious rituals, many of which were not accepted by Western scholars. Natural sciences gained momentum in the late eighteenth century, and most of the parasites were systematized in this period. Population growth, intensified urbanization, wars and the rapid increase in infectious diseases among humans played an important role in these developments. In the nineteenth century Europe, different theorems due to scientific competition in different countries continued until World War I. Parasitology emerged as a separate discipline in this period. Due to wars and many tropical diseases such as malaria that emerged in colonized countries, European settlers established tropical institutes in various regions. Not satisfied with this, sub-disciplines of Parasitology were established and financially supported by European and American supporters in colonial and developing countries. After the Second World War, parasitology departments were established in universities in many places. Many specialists were trained and specialized diagnostic and treatment stations for parasitic diseases, and their vectors were established in both developed and developing countries [13–15].

The concept of Paleoparasitology has been formed by bringing together studies in different disciplines that have been carried out for 30 years. Paleoparasitology, which is also interpreted as the study of the presence of parasites in the remains of ancient times, is a field of parasitology that has developed as a research field combining archaeology, anthropology, biology and health sciences. Paleoparasitology aims to detect traces of parasites in prehistoric times and to study the evolution of parasitism over time and space and is the study of parasites in archeological remains of humans and animals [13–17].

It has long been hypothesized that the ancient ancestors of humans hosted various species of parasites, especially large worms, but until recently, there has been no direct evidence to support such an assumption. However, studies of archeological artifacts, such as the presence of helminth eggs or protozoan cysts in coprolites and preserved bodies, are now providing researchers with information about parasitic diseases of the past [17–20].

Throughout history, humans have encountered and been infected with more than 400 parasite species through the evolution process and migrations. Most of these were acquired from animals they came into contact with in their immediate environment or through nutrition. However, they were most exposed to parasites in the process of domesticating various animals in their immediate environment. Most of the domestication process took place in Asia. It can also be said that examples of this are still going on in nomadic communities to this day [15, 16].

Humans first appeared on the African continent, and when they started to migrate, they carried their dietary habits and parasites with them to the new areas they explored. According to previous knowledge, most researchers blame the Portuguese and Spanish sailors and their slave trade in the tenth and eleventh centuries for the spread of parasites around the world, but paleoparasitological studies reveal that the situation was different [14–16].

Luiz Fernando Ferreira from the Oswaldo Cruz Institute in Brazil was one of the first to pioneer paleoparasitological studies. The studies that started with the identification of *Schistosoma* eggs in the kidney tissue of Egyptian mummies were followed by two bodies found in a swamp in Prussia: *Ascaris lumbricoides, Trichuris trichiura* and *Diphyllobothrium latum* in two bodies found in a swamp in Prussia. In the following years, paleoparasitological studies have continued, and many data on the relationship between humans and parasites and their evolution have been obtained. Today, with the use of molecular tests in paleoparasitology, protozoan parasites can be identified in coprolites. In 2009, the Journal of Parasitology published a large special issue under the title "Paleoparasitology" [15, 16].

Paleoparasitological research began with *Schistosoma haematobium* eggs identified in the kidney tissues of Egyptian mummies, followed by Professor Szidat's publication of notes on three different helminth eggs identified in two corpses from the fifth century in a swamp in East Prussia. Around this time, Taylor described helminth eggs in Roman remains in England. During this period, the first paleoparasitological publications in the New World were made by Professor Pizzi from the University of Chile, who reported *Trichirus trichiura* eggs together with *Entamoeba coli* cysts in an Inca mummy [21]. This study was the first detection of protozoa in coprolites and paved the way for the forthcoming assumptions on the identification of different protozoan species in the future. Prof. Camerun also identified *Diphyllobothrium sp*. eggs in coprolites from the prehistoric inhabitants of Huaca Prieta on the Peruvian coast [15, 16, 19, 22].

Parasite eggs and cysts found in coprolites, mummies and other human remains tell us little about parasitic infections and diseases of the past, which is why most historians prefer to rely more on written records. The first such records belong to a period of Egyptian medicine between 3000 and 400 BC, notably the Ebers papyrus of about 1500 BC, which mentions worms clearly identifiable as roundworms (*Ascaris lumbricoides*), threadworms (*Enterobius vermicularis*) and Guinea worms (*Dracunculus medinensis*). Of all the diseases caused by parasitic worms, the best documented since ancient times is dracunculiasis caused by the Guinea worm *D. medinensis* [19, 20, 22, 23].

Few parasitic infections cause specific and clear signs and symptoms, but references to some of them, notably dracunculiasis, hookworm disease, elephantiasis, schistosomiasis, malaria and amoebiasis, often appear in early literature.

The concept of parasitism consists of three subsystems:

1. Parasite

2. Host

3. Environment.

With the emergence of life on the Earth, parasites began to evolve along with their hosts and the environment. Their diversity, which may have been minimal at the beginning, is constantly changing due to biodiversity and climatic factors. Population density, people's constant mobility, new technologies, agriculture, migrations, domestication of animals and climatic changes have led to a rapid expansion of their global distribution. When early humans lived among small groups of hunter-gatherers on the African savannah, only some parasite species were able to infect these nomadic hosts without establishing themselves in a permanent habitat. Two parasite species can be used here as examples: Nematodes, *Enterobius vermicularis*, and Arthropods, the head louse, *Pediculus humanus*. Closely related species of these parasites are found in hosts closely related to humans, such as chimpanzees and gorillas, indicating that they have a common host ancestor. The direct transmission and migratory dispersal of these two parasites is due to the fact that they did not evolve in the soil. They are not affected by environmental changes and can migrate anywhere with humans [19, 20, 22, 23].

Paleoparasitological studies also define the geography of distribution of helminths and protozoa. For example, it has been easy to identify and protect helminth eggs from external conditions due to their 30–160 micron-sized structures and multi-layered eggs that are highly resistant to external conditions. However, protozoan cysts cannot withstand environmental conditions for a long time due to their 4–40 micron-sized cyst forms and delicate structures, and the possibilities of identification by standard diagnostic methods are limited. For these reasons, protozoa have only been identified by immunologic molecular methods in the last 10 years. While the first identified helminth egg was *Schistosoma haematobium* seen in the kidneys of an Egyptian mummy at the beginning of the twentieth century, recently the presence of *Entamoeba histolytica* was identified in coprolites from a cave in the USA by radiocarbon and ELISA tests. The selection of the appropriate material and method is of particular importance in identification. Extraction of helminth eggs requires three consecutive steps: rehydration, homogenization and filtration/sieving. Antigen research can be performed on samples prepared following the standard method described previously. However, the use of additional solutions (e.g., formalin) for sample preservation and storage can be problematic. For this reason, the identification of protozoan parasites due to the use of the wrong method in the early years of paleoparasitological diagnosis has only now been possible [14–20, 22, 23].

Coproparasitological examinations are carried out through various extraction stages according to the residue material examined. Coprolite, sediment or textile-like samples are usually taken for microscopic examination after rehydration, homogenization and sieving/filtering. The amount of residues is very important for parasitological investigations. Recently, parasites identified in coprolites have provided information about the migration routes and climatic conditions of humans in prehistoric times. Some parasites require special environmental conditions to complete their life cycle. For example, hookworms and *Trichuris trichiura* are two intestinal parasites that probably originated from African human ancestors. They are transmitted from one host to another after maturing in soil under limited climatic conditions. Eggs or larvae passed in host feces need pH, moisture and a temperature close to 22°C in the soil to reach the infective stage and infect another individual. In this way, the journey that started from the African continent has shown that especially geo-helminths cannot withstand cold climatic conditions and cannot reach the Americas [14, 17, 18, 22, 24, 25].

Recent discoveries have shown that parasites were also prevalent in the Americas in prehistoric times. However, the fact that the number of eggs found was lower than in Africa is an indication that the prevalence was lower in these regions. In addition, the fact that there were more hunter-gatherer nomadic groups during these periods is also a significant factor. When European colonizers set foot on the continent, they came with various diseases, built villages and enslaved the indigenous people. Later, they brought slaves from Africa and spread new diseases to Americas. The global spread of parasites is indisputably linked to human activity. Migration, in all its different forms, played an important role in introducing parasites into new areas. In ancient times, mass migrations were the main causes of the spread of parasites, while in the recent past and today, migration, immigration, relocation, internal and external migration and labor migration are the causes of the spread of parasites. With the advent of offshore vessels, long-distance trade has become another important route for the spread of parasites. This article summarizes the spread of parasites using remarkable examples. Different hypotheses explaining the arrival of *Plasmodium vivax* and soil-transmitted helminths in pre-Columbian America are also discussed [15–17, 22, 23, 26].

According to phylogeographic studies, a new field, the distribution of human parasites can be categorized into three groups.

1. Out-of-Africa

2. Domestication

3. Globalization

According to these three main hypotheses, new zoonotic parasites were added to the parasites that migrated with African people, domesticated in new places and during the transition to sedentary life, or during nutrition. These numbers have reached approximately 400 species. The species, which spread to other regions and continents with the first human migration, have reached a global scale due to human activities such as trade, migration, wars and travel. Since domestication took place mostly in Asia, paleoparasitological and phylogenetic studies show the highest species diversity in the Middle East and Asia [22, 23, 27–29].

In studies on the Asian continent, seven species of intestinal parasites have been identified in evidence from Neolithic Qing Dynasty mummies, ancient toilets and soil from the pelvic region of bodies in tombs. These are *Ascaris lumbricoides, Trichuris trichiura*, Chinese liver fluke, *Schistosoma sp., Enterobius vermicularis, Taenia sp*. and *Fasciolopsis buski*. In the past, the roundworm, whipworm and Chinese liver fluke were much more common than other species. While the roundworm and whipworm remained widespread until the late twentieth century, a marked decline in the incidence of the Chinese liver fluke has been reported over time [16, 21, 30–32].

The Silk Road may have played an important role in the distribution of ancient diseases. On this route, *Fasciolopsis buski*, which is found in endemic areas of China, was reported to have been carried 1500 km by traders following this route [33].

Today, with the addition of various sub-disciplines to the research, paleoparasitology studies continue with more than 50 scientists and more than 500 scientific publications.

Parasite cysts and eggs identified in paleoparasitological studies provide information on the evolutionary dimensions of the human-parasite relationship, as well as the hygiene and health habits of prehistoric human communities. Paleoparasitology is advancing by interpreting the findings and drawing inferences about the impact of parasitic diseases among prehistoric populations. Hunter-gatherers were found to be less infected by helminths, while agricultural groups had a relatively higher prevalence of intestinal parasites at archeological sites in the United States [23, 26, 31, 34–36].

Although parasitism can occur in all living organisms, paleoparasitology has focused more on species living in the intestines of humans and animals. These studies have yielded information on diet and lifestyle, habits, culture, organic waste and hygiene habits. For example, as intestinal parasites are ingested orally, parasite biodiversity has undergone many variations over the centuries. For example, fish parasites in coprolites indicate that people were fishing and feeding on fish in the 3400 s BC; later, a variety of animal helminths were identified in the Old World and New World due to their diet of land creatures; and during the migration of humans from Siberia to the Americas, soil-borne helminth infections disappeared due to cold climatic conditions. For this reason, helminth infections were not found in those who migrated to the North American continent, while helminths were found in those who reached North and South America by different routes. Paleoparasitological studies have also facilitated the study of the transmission cycles of different species infecting humans and animals [36–40].

In medieval Europe during this period, coprolites and mummies were full of intestinal worms, and geo-helminth infections took over large parts of the population due to poor sanitation and overcrowding. However, due to strict religious beliefs during this period, written records are almost non-existent. Epidemiologic information from a large-scale survey of intestinal helminths in medieval Europe was obtained by analyzing 589 samples of grave remains from seven different regions in Europe between 680 and 1700 AD. The most common helminths found in the soil samples were *Ascaris lumbricoides, Trichuris trichiura, Diphylobothrium latum* and *Taenia sp.* These studies show that especially soil-transmitted helminths were very common in medieval Europe [41–45].

The coastal city of Acre in present-day Israel dates back to 3000 BC. Under the control of the Ottoman Empire between 1516 and 1517, and the city was a commercial port city that controlled a large part of Southeastern Europe, the Near East and the North African coast. During this period, the diversity of parasites in the region increased due to the large number of livestock products being shipped. Since the majority of the people were Muslims and Jews, it is estimated that parasites of animal origin such as liver fluke, tapeworms, whipworms and protozoa such as Giardia and entamoeba, which had not been seen in the region before, entered the region through ship trade. This research shows how cultural and dietary habits of societies influence transmission [46].

The nineteenth century can be considered the golden age of parasitology because it was during this century that most of the life cycles of parasites were elucidated and the various discoveries of previous centuries were brought together into coherent stories. It was also a period dominated by some of the biggest names in parasitology, all of whom made many contributions, often in different fields [47].

The twentieth century was not only a period of adding the finishing touches to what was known but also of defining the cause-and-effects of the blood and tissue parasites now called Chagas disease. In the early years and towards the end of the century, a number of opportunistic parasitic infections in immunocompromised patients, particularly those with AIDS, came to the fore [31, 47–53]. During this period, efforts were focused on control and eradication of many parasites due to the elucidation of their evolution. As a result of the elimination of copepod intermediate hosts from water sources, the Guinea worm is now almost completely eradicated, and *Onchocerciasis* continues to be eradicated through measures against housefly larvae, together with the availability of cheap and effective drugs [51–53].

Scientific debate on the mechanisms and migratory pathways that facilitate the spread of the major helminth species infecting human populations in the western hemisphere will continue into the twenty first century. From the 1990s to the present day, paleoparasitology has benefited from the creativity and productivity of its researchers. The accumulated results from decades of analyses of thousands of specimens have provided a database for framing research questions addressing the transmission and distribution of parasites as a function of epidemiological and evolutionary processes. Increased communication through the Internet has created more opportunities for collaboration and standardization of methods among researchers worldwide. This in turn has led to greater interest in paleoparasitology, as reflected in the number of publications submitted by researchers to various journals and the establishment of laboratories and postgraduate training programs identified with the sub-discipline [8, 17, 26, 47, 48, 51–53].

With the advent of ships sailing on the high seas, long-distance trade became an important route for the spread of parasites. The presence of parasites is the result of different lifestyles, habits or behaviors. Paleoparasitology provides information about ancient populations, cultures and environments. Funeral practices, cultural changes, organic waste management and hygiene are potential topics of such studies. In the case of intestinal parasites, since the route of contamination is mainly oral, some conclusions can be drawn about some aspects of ancient nutrition. For example, whipworms, tapeworms, giant kidney worms and liver flukes have been identified in the remains of human communities living by lakes between 3900 and 2900 BC in the northern Alpine region. The changing diversity of the parasites identified here over the years has been attributed to dietary, cultural and climatic changes. When parasite biodiversity is sufficient, it is possible to hypothesize about the biological origin of these specimens and/or the function of certain archeological structures by associating or considering parasites with a specific host spectrum [49, 52, 53].

Paleoparasitological studies have been carried out for many years and continue to make many contributions to science on evolution-migration and host-parasite relationships. Today, with the contribution of technological progress, microscopic and molecular methods can open new horizons and make new contributions. However, studies are still limited to certain regions. For example, paleoparasitological studies in West and Southern Africa, Eastern and Central Europe and Asia, which are very important in terms of early human density, will provide comprehensive information in understanding the global history and evolution of gastrointestinal parasites.

4. Intestinal parasites in evolution and geographic studies

Throughout history, people have been infected with various parasites due to cultural and behavioral changes. Domestication of animals, wildlife and climate change have increased the chance of contracting zoonotic and foodborne parasites. In fact, there is no organism that can resist parasites.

4.1 Intestinal nematodes

4.1.1 Trematoda (flukes)

The first trematode identified in paleoparasitological studies was *Schistosoma* from Egyptian mummies. Molecular data show that, unlike other parasites, they did not originate from the African continent, but were parasites of other mammals (monkeys) in Asia, and spread first to Egypt and then to West-Central and South Africa via their definitive and intermediate hosts (snails) via the slave trade with ships. Among these, it can be said that *Schistosoma mansoni* was brought to Latin America with enslaved Africans in the post-Columbian period. To give an example from recent history; during the establishment of the State of Israel in 1948, in a town built by the river by 500 thousand migrants from endemic areas, about 10% of school children swimming in the river were infected with Schistosomas. An example of parasite introduction by migrant workers is the spread of *S. mansoni* in the Wonji Sugar Estate in the upper Awash valley of Ethiopia. Initially, every effort was made to ensure that migrant workers were not infected, but by 1964, 10 years after the sugar factory was established, *S. mansoni* infection among workers exceeded 20%. In the 1980s, *S. mansoni* rates of 80% were reported in children playing on the sugar platform [15, 17, 19, 23, 27, 30, 37, 54].

A recent example is the outbreak of *Schistosoma haematobium* that infected more than 120 people swimming in the river Chavu on the island of Corsica in 2013. Another trematode that spreads through migration is *Opisthorchis viverrini*. In the 1950s, this parasite was found only in the north of Thailand, where almost the entire population was infected, but it has now spread throughout Thailand, with infected people moving to other parts of the country through labor migration. Liver parasites (fasciolids) are parasites of herbivores, but can also cause disease in humans. Molecular phylogenetic analysis shows that fasciolids spread from elephants in Africa to herbivores in Asia. The most common liver fluke, *Fasciola hepatica*, originated in Eurasia, where it spread to other continents through the ship trade of livestock. It was also taken to South America by Spanish sailors [54, 55].

4.1.2 Cestodes (tapeworms)

Data on tapeworm eggs from past periods are very rare. Cysticercus was found in Egyptian mummies dating back to 200–100 years BC. Julius Caesar, who lived between 100 and 400 BC, is thought to have died of neurocysticercus. Although not fully elucidated by paleoparasitological studies, phylogenetic analyses show that *Taenia solium* and *Taenia saginata* were present before the domestication of pigs and cattle. An interesting example of its geographical distribution is the pig tapeworm *T. solium*. In 1973–1976, indigenous people living in the highlands of New Guinea were repeatedly admitted to hospital with burns. After long investigations, it was revealed that the burns were caused by people falling asleep at night and falling into the fire, and that this was due to "neurocysticercus" caused by the larvae of the pork tapeworm *T. solium* settling in the brain. It was found that there were no pigs in the area before, and that the disease had spread from infected pigs sent to suppress the rebellion on the island a few years earlier [19, 23, 26, 56].

4.1.3 Nematodes (roundworms)

Nematode eggs isolated from archeological remains or from coprolites in mummies are the most important documents of the dietary habits of humans in the past.

Dating back 10 thousand years, lizard parasites in human coprolites are the most obvious example of the use of lizards as a source of protein. Among nematodes, *Ascaris lumbricoides*, hookworms and *Trichuris trichura* are nematodes originating from the African human ancestors of *Homo sapiens*, dating back 30 thousand years. However, geohelminths such as these did not reach other continents during the first human migrations, as they had to spend a period in warm and moist soil. However, it is thought that the geohelminths detected in the Americas and Europe during molecular research may have been brought to the continent by immigrants reaching the continent through different migration routes in later periods. On the other hand, directly transmitted nematodes such as *Enterobius vermicularis* are known to have reached other continents with the first migrations [13, 15–17, 21, 23, 24, 27, 30, 35, 36].

Soil-transmitted hookworm infections were thought to have been taken first to India and then to other continents by coastal migration in the 12th century BC. Even in recent history, hookworms have been recognized as an industrial occupational hazard thanks to migration and nomadic workers. Brought to the Americas by slaves brought from Africa during the Columbian era, hookworms spread to large areas as a miner's disease in many parts of Europe in the 1870s, causing significant morbidity and mortality [22, 23, 27].

New findings require a reassessment of old ones. For example, while hookworms, a geohelminth, were known to have entered the Americas with African slaves brought over during the Columbian era, the identification of hookworms in a Peruvian mummy showed that the parasite had been present here before [27, 35, 48].

Other nematodes brought to the Americas with infected African slaves during the Columbian era include *Onchocerca volvulus, Wuchereria bancrofti, Mansonella perstans* and *Loa loa*, known as "filarial nematodes". These vector-borne nematode diseases have found suitable vectors in the Americas, but have remained sporadic in certain regions. In fact, lymphatic filariasis, such as *Wuchereria banchrofti*, was reported to have originated in Asia 50,000 years ago, from where it spread to Madagascar and Africa 1500 years ago. The largest epidemiologic spread of this parasite was in hemp field workers in the Philippines between 1903 and 1937. Large numbers of people were infected due to stagnant water suitable for the development of vectors. *Dracunculus medinensis*, known as the guinea worm, is another nematode that came to the Americas with African slaves. However, this nematode could not spread here because it requires special conditions and intermediate hosts [23, 27, 30, 54]. In addition to a 10,000-year-old *Enterobius vermicularis* egg found in a coprolite sample, several trematode eggs are the oldest remains identified in coprolites [25].

4.1.4 Intestinal protozoa

Due to their sensitive nature, the history of protozoa has been limited to recent times, that is, to the period when molecular and immunologic methods were used. They collected historical data on amoebic dysentery and estimated that *Entamoeba histolytica* has been present in Western Europe since the Neolithic Age and spread to other countries with the crusades. In the data from the New World, molecular analyses have shown that it was present in the Caribbean and the Americas in the pre-Columbian period. Before paleoparasitological research, the history of amoebiasis caused by *Entamoeba histolytica* begins in 1859 when they saw amoebae in the feces of a patient with dysentery, but 10 years before that, a doctor named Lösh, who injected a fecal sample taken from a patient who died of dysentery in Russia into dogs and named the amoeba that caused ulcers in them "Amoeba coli". The parasite was shown to cause lysis by Shaudin in 1903. In 1913, the first experimental human studies were conducted on 20 volunteer prisoners. Diamond performed in vitro axenic culture of trophozoites in 1978. Diagnostic methods, pathogenesis and vaccine studies on amoeba have been carried out for the last 30 years. However, there are still some parts of the pathogenesis that remain to be understood [25, 26, 39, 48, 57].

Amoebiasis, of which many mechanisms have been elucidated today, is a parasitic disease caused by *Entamoeba histolytica*, an extracellular enteric protozoan. This infection mainly affects people in developing countries with limited hygiene conditions, where it is endemic. The parasite has different mechanisms of pathogenicity, adhering to the intestinal epithelium and degrading extracellular matrix proteins, producing tissue lesions, particularly in the large intestine, which progress to abscesses and an acute inflammatory response of the host. The World Health Organization (WHO) has reported that 500 million people worldwide may be infected with *Entamoeba sp*.; 10% of these individuals are likely to be infected with *E. histolytica* and the rest with other non-pathogenic species. Amoebiasis causes 40,000–100,000 deaths annually and is the fourth leading cause of death due to protozoan infection. *Blastocystis sp*. is an anaerobic intestinal parasite of humans and animals In numerous epidemiological studies conducted in different countries, *Blastocystis sp.* is the most common eukaryotic parasite reported in human fecal samples, but its pathogenicity is still controversial [8, 57–59].

More than 100 years have passed since Tyzzer described his first observations of the genus *Cryptosporidium* in 1907. Until the 80s, the parasite was considered an insignificant organism that occasionally caused disease in the intestines of vertebrates. With HIV, it has been named as an opportunistic parasitic infection with high morbidity and mortality and has been the subject of numerous studies. It causes waterborne outbreaks in developed and developing countries and has more than 40 species [60–62].

4.2 Geographical studies

The disease burden associated with intestinal parasites is considerable, threatening approximately 4.5 billion people worldwide. According to WHO data, 300 million people are affected by intestinal parasites. Regarding soil-borne helminths; 800–1000 million Ascaris lumbricoides, 700–900 million hookworm, 500 million *Trichuris trichiura*, 200 million *Giardia lamblia*, 500 million *Entamoeba histolytica/dispar* cases are reported. It is also estimated that around 39 million disabilities and life years are lost due to these infections. An important disadvantage is that 90% of cases are asymptomatic and therefore the spread of parasites continues [9].

Intestinal parasites are more prevalent in developing countries, especially in the tropics and subtropics. In these countries, their infectivity becomes more dominant with the effect of climate and socioeconomic conditions. It is generally believed that helminths are more prevalent in developing countries while protozoan intestinal parasites are more common in developed countries. Soil-borne helminths are endemic in countries with poor sanitation conditions and insufficient clean water. It is estimated that *Ascaris lumbricoides* still infects 1 billion people, *Trichuris trichiura* 800 million and hookworms 750 thousand. The weight of the parasite load, inadequate food and water supply, physical and mental developmental delays, as well as additional chronic diseases, make losses inevitable [50–53, 63, 64].

In addition to helminths, diarrhea caused by protozoa such as *Giardia lamblia*, *Entamoeba histolytica, Cryptosporidium* and *Cyclospora* is the third leading cause of death in these regions, especially in children. WHO reported that 50 million people are infected with invasive amobiasis each year and 40–100 thousand of them are fatal. Giardia and cryptosporidium and microsporidia are among the most important causes of diarrhea in developed countries. Intestinal parasites are particularly prevalent in developing countries and in growing children. The most important factor is the lack of clean water and inadequate personal and environmental hygiene conditions. However, there are some special groups in which the prevalence of intestinal parasites is higher than in the normal population. Among these, individuals with intellectual disabilities with low capacity for learning and understanding are at significant risk. In studies conducted in 10 different provinces of Iran in mentally disabled individuals, intestinal parasites were found to be considerably higher than in the normal population [8, 50–53, 63, 64].

Antiparasitic drugs, taken once or twice a year in endemic areas, are a low-cost solution. In this way, by preventing the treatment and spread of parasites in children, it will support their school success and healthy and productive living in the future. These studies are currently being carried out in certain areas, albeit limited [65, 66].

Intestinal parasites have also been suggested to play a potential role in or predispose to various metabolic diseases, for example, diabetes mellitus. There is also a large number of studies suggesting that intestinal parasites may coexist with different infectious diseases. Tuberculosis (TB) and intestinal parasites are two important infections affecting mostly poor people and are important risk factors for one another. In a meta-analysis study conducted in Ethiopia, where both infectious agents are common, 414 articles on the subject were reviewed from scientific databases, and in 11 articles involving a total of 3158 TB patients, one third of the patients were found to be infected with intestinal parasites, and the most common intestinal parasites were; *Ascaris lumbricoides* 10.5% (95% CI: 6.0, 17.5), hookworm 9.5% (95% CI: 6.10, 14.4), *Giardia lamblia* 5.7% (95% CI: 2.90, 10.9) and *Strongyloides sterocoralis* 5.6% (95% CI: 3.3, 9.5). In the study, there was no significant difference between protozoa and TB compared to the normal population, while the association of helminth infections and TB was higher than in the normal population [67].

Intestinal parasites continue to be a public health problem among patients with HIV. Rapid and effective antiretroviral therapy is needed to reduce parasite density [68].

Nomadic and pastoral communities have become geographical areas where many parasitic diseases of zoonotic origin are more intense. The most important risk factors are close contact with animals, inadequate hygiene conditions, lack of access to drinking water and food. Global health efforts are also insufficient in these groups [69]. In nomadic communities in the mountainous areas of Asia and in the highlands of Ecuador, where heat and poverty prevail, about 90% of children are reported to be infected with one or more intestinal parasites [70].

Zoonotic enteric parasites (ZEP), which can infect animals and humans, are transmitted through contact, contaminated water and food. Multicellular ZEPs, commonly called worms, are members of three taxonomic groups belonging to the Helminths group (Cestodes (tapeworms), Nematodes (*Ascaris sp.*, *Strongyloides spp.*, *Toxocara sp.* and *Trichinella sp.*) and Trematodes (*Fasciola spp., Clonorchissp.* and *Pentastomida sp.*). Most intestinal protozoa are human-specific and are usually transmitted through water and food. In nomadic communities, where ZEPs are most common, the major risk factors for transmission include contact with animals, nutritional habits, difficulties in obtaining clean water and inappropriate living conditions. Unfortunately, ZEPs are still not prevented today due to lack of education and low socio-economic status [69, 70].

Zoonotic enteric parasites that use humans or animals as hosts, like other enteric parasites, are transmitted through contaminated soil, water and food. Cystic echinococcosis, the larval stage of the canine cestode, Fasciola sp., the ruminant liver fluke, *Clonorchis* and *Pentastomids* are important helminths. However, zoonotic protozoa are a more common group that can occur anywhere in the world. They are microscopic and occasionally cause water and foodborne epidemics. *Cryptosporidium sp. Babesia sp.* and *Microsporidia sp.* are among the most common species. Enteric protozoa are easily transmitted through food products, contact with infected meat and meat products, and exposure to contaminated water [63, 70, 71].

Intestinal parasites, like many enteric pathogens, are also spread through people working in the food industry, as they cause foodborne infections. There are numerous papers showing that protozoa, especially protozoa such as amoeba, giardia, cryptosporidium species, as well as some soil-evolved helminths, tapeworms, *Enterobius vermicularis* are transmitted in this way [69, 70, 72].

According to the global disease burden concept first defined in 1993, the global burden of soil nematodes such as *Ascaris*, *trichuris* and hookworms has not fallen below 10%. *Entamoeba, Toxoplasma, Cyclospora, Giardia* and *Cryptosporidium* are among the major contributors to the global intestinal parasitic disease burden. The fact that intestinal parasites are generally not fatal and that they persist more frequently in developing countries and are not under control is largely due to the inattention of developed countries. Especially prevention and control strategies and treatment protocols are unfortunately inadequate in countries struggling with economic problems. Intestinal parasites are a major cause of morbidity and mortality, especially in sub-Saharan Africa, India and some Asian countries where access to food is difficult. They bring different co-infections with them. With the effect of heat and poor sanitation conditions, excreted cysts and eggs maintain their viability and infectivity in the environment for a long time. Considering that about half of the intestinal parasites are transmitted by fecal oral route, the prevalence increases with the effect of factors such as poor sanitation, suitable climatic conditions and lack of education. Studies have shown that the rates can be halved by hand washing, use of footwear, washing and cooking of food. Parasites not only take up certain vitamins in humans but also cause changes in the immune system due to the metabolites they produce [60, 65, 67–69, 73].

5. Diagnostic methods in intestinal parasites from past to present

Intestinal parasites continue to have a devastating impact from past to present. In recent years, they have been considered as an infectious agent only seen in developing countries, but nowadays, due to increased migration, international travel, wars and global warming, they have started to increase their effectiveness all over the world. One of the most important problems in this context has been the delay in diagnosis and treatment because intestinal parasites are not recognized outside endemic areas. Sometimes this leads to fatal outcomes in organ or blood transplants. Even today, when there are still major problems in antiparasitic treatment, the most effective method is the development of accurate and rapid diagnostic methods. Since the discovery of the microscope, microscopy has been the gold standard for parasitological diagnosis, especially for protozoan parasites. It is low-cost and is still successfully used in routine diagnosis, especially in epidemiologic studies, especially in countries with high parasite load. However, it is time-consuming and requires experienced personnel in large-scale epidemiologic studies. In addition, due to the fact that parasites are not always present in feces, diagnostic errors may occur. Today, various serologic and molecular methods are being developed for large-scale epidemiologic studies and more descriptive diagnosis. This enables faster and more accurate diagnosis. The microscopic examination method, which is inadequate to distinguish between amoebic dysentery and other amoebas and to prevent unnecessary treatment, can be prevented by serologic and molecular diagnostics used in diagnosis today. Again, it is almost impossible to distinguish helminths from each other by microscopic examination, especially in their larval stages. Today, with the use of serological and molecular techniques, a significant progress has been made in paleoparasitological diagnosis [7, 74–76].

Since 1908, qualitative research has been carried out in the parasitological diagnosis of stool samples. Initially applied to increase the chances of visualization, methods for removing residues and concentrating parasite cysts and eggs have continued with the identification of suitable solutions and dyes. Samples prepared by enrichment methods with the use of various equipment are examined by microscopic examination. However, Sporozoa group parasites such as *Microsporidium spp*. (1–2.5 microns), *Cryptosporidium spp.* (4–6 microns), *Cyclospora spp.* (6–8 microns), *Cystoisospora spp.* (20–30 microns), which are frequently encountered in immunocompromised patients today, cannot be seen under the microscope with routine parasitological examinations. They need to be examined with special staining methods and immersion objective. In the 1940s, Ritchie and Teleman offered new alternatives to parasitological examinations, and in 1970, they introduced the technique of sedimentation with the addition of ethyl-ether to break down stool artifacts. In the 1980s, the semi-automated commercial paratest method was used in fecal examinations. Today, sedimentation, flotation and Kato-Katz methods are still successfully used in routine diagnosis to increase the detection rate of cysts and eggs in stool, the only disadvantage being the need for experienced personnel/specialists. Baerman and Harada-Mori methods are used for identification of nematode larvae. Today, the search for fast, easy, inexpensive and accurate diagnostics for large-scale and routine research continues [74–77].

5.1 Microscopic diagnosis

The use of microscopy in biological specimens is a simple, inexpensive and often gold standard method of morphologic diagnosis of the parasitic agent. It requires a good microscope and an experienced microscopist. With this method, the appropriate sample (blood, urine, stool, vaginal swab, abscess material, duodenal aspirate and tissue biopsy) is examined under a light or fluorescence microscope using appropriate solutions (saline, lugol, various parasite dyes, calcoflour, etc.) using various lenses of the microscope. All protozoan parasites can be diagnosed by this method. For *Cryptosporidium sp*, *Cyclospora* and *Isospora*, microscopic examination is also performed with fluorescent stains as well as Ziehl-Nelsen and Kinyon stains. Microscopic diagnosis can also be used to identify the eggs or larvae of helminths. Microscopic examination has always been the gold standard in parasitologic diagnosis, but it requires a high level of parasitologic experience. It is labor-intensive and time-consuming and occasionally leads to inaccuracies in cases of poor excretion of parasites. In addition, it is microscopically almost impossible to differentiate pathogen from apathogen, especially for amoeba species. The diagnosis requires a high parasite load of protozoa or helminths in stool [7, 74–76].

5.2 Serologic tests

Unfortunately, the few serologic tests used in parasitologic diagnosis can only be used for the routine diagnosis of a limited number of blood and tissue parasites. There are no serologic tests routinely used for gastrointestinal parasites. Specificity and sensitivity are low compared to molecular tests. Cross-reactions can be seen due to the common antigenic structure of helminths [74–78].

5.3 Immunochromatographic tests

Based on the simple principle of reading the markings on the membrane of specific biomarkers in the material under study. They are commercial tests. The infrastructure conditions in the laboratory must be appropriate. Widely used in the diagnosis of blood and tissue parasites. It is used in the diagnosis of intestinal protozoa. It is easily used in large-scale serologic investigations as it does not require experience and time. However, special equipment and proper sample handling are required [74–76].

5.4 Multiplex PCR

As in many infectious diseases, molecular testing has ushered in a new era in parasitologic diagnosis. This method allows simultaneous analysis of multiple pathogens and resistance genes. It is easy to identify the parasite and its strains, to follow the treatment and control process, as well as in large-scale epidemiological and surveillance studies. Compared to microscopic examination, the detection rate of parasite infections is considerably higher when targets are included in multiplex PCR. Detection and quantification of parasite-specific DNA in stool is highly sensitive and specific. Numerous studies using various nucleic acid-based techniques have contributed to the genetic diversity, epidemiology and clinical significance of intestinal parasites. For evident reasons, in a routine setting, standardization and harmonization of protocols are essential for the cost-effective implementation of these new techniques. Gastrointestinal Multiplex molecular panels, unlike conventional tests, allow the identification of multiple pathogens in a single material (stool). They also contribute to diagnosis and treatment by determining the intensity of infection and demographic characteristics of the infection. They require appropriate laboratory equipment and are costly [77, 78].

Serologic and molecular tests are costly tests and unfortunately cannot be applied in poor communities where the burden of parasitic infections is high. Although the process of developing appropriate and rapid diagnostic methods against common infections in the world continues rapidly, unfortunately, there is not much progress on tests for parasitic diseases, which are seen as a problem in developed countries. However, it is limited to large-scale epidemiological studies of developed countries. Updates for these tests are ongoing. Gastrointestinal parasite panels are still limited to a small number of species. Diagnosis is difficult due to the nature of helminths. In addition to new specific markers, there is a need to improve specificity and sensitivity, to measure parasite load and to meet affordability requirements [74–78].

Delays in the accurate diagnosis of parasitic diseases lead to delays in treatment and control strategies, facilitating the spread of causative pathogens. Provided by developed countries, the use of affordable and reliable tests in endemic regions; training of specialists to work in these regions, as well as hygiene education of the public and provision of clean water, are important factors for the future of undeveloped countries regarding prevention of the spread of parasitic diseases.

5.5 Parasite cultivation

Although not all parasites can be cultivated, it is possible to produce a limited number of protozoa and larval stages of some helminths in cultivation. These are planned not only for diagnostic purposes but also for studies on parasite evolution, biochemistry, physiology and various invitro studies. Intestinal parasites can be grown in xenic, monoxenic and axenic cultivation, but are demanding due to contamination [76].

6. Prevention and control strategies

Intestinal parasites place an additional burden on people in poor and developing countries where they are endemic. Developed countries have been able to eradicate many soil-borne nematodes through clean water supply, education, sanitation and treatment of infected people. In these regions, protozoan outbreaks of protozoa from vegetables and fruits eaten raw or zoonotic origin can be seen occasionally. The most successful methods in the fight against intestinal parasites are as follows:

6.1 Hand hygiene

The most important method for all fecal-oral infections. The habit of washing hands with soap and similar products after toilet and before meals destroys the effect of eggs and cysts. The importance of hand hygiene in the prevention of infectious diseases has been proven in many epidemiologic studies.

6.2 Food and water

The most important source of intestinal parasites is contaminated food and water.

In developing countries, inadequate sewerage and the spread of human feces in the environment and food cause both the formation of endemic areas and the outbreaks of gastroenteritis in countries that trade with these countries. Areas where wastewater is used in agriculture are the most important factor in the spread of many helminths and protozoa. They are resistant to washing as well as cooking. In this way, imported fruits and vegetables cause outbreaks in developed countries. Street vendors are also among the most important sources of foodborne transmission. The main cause of large-scale epidemics in endemic areas is contaminated food and water. Lack of drinking and utiliary water also affects hand hygiene [1, 4, 5, 8, 58, 60, 64, 66, 69].

6.3 Chemotherapy

Treating infected people is one of the most important control strategies. This will break the chain of transmission. In developed countries, antihelminthic treatment has been effective in the elimination of soil-borne helminths for many years. In recent years, in project supported studies, it has been reported that the rate of parasites in patients and soil has decreased by more than half with antiparasitic treatment given 1 or 2 times a year in endemic areas. The biggest problem in these studies is the increasing resistance to antiparasitic drugs, which are already in short supply. The most successful study example came from South Korea. Between 1969 and 1995, the rate of intestinal parasites was reduced from 84 to 3% with antiparasitic treatment administered to primary school children. Chemotherapy as a fast-acting intervention is a good strategy to immediately improve the lives of poor populations in developing countries. However, such a practice is currently not possible in nomadic communities in poor countries. Chemotherapy is very important in reducing the prevalence of intestinal parasites. Chemotherapeutics developed for protozoa and helminths were originally intended for veterinary use, but were later developed and used in humans. In the late 1970s, they began to be given to children and adults with symptoms of parasites, especially helminth infections, all over the world. In the 1980s, Bundy and Stephenson led studies in children in which antiparasitic treatment was given to all children and a significant reduction in parasite load was observed in endemic areas.

The identification and treatment of infected people through epidemiologic studies is one of the most important factors in reducing the incidence. Reduction or termination of excretion, especially helminth infections, with treatment will prevent soil and water contamination. Antihelminthic chemoterpine has an important role in the fact that soil helminths are no longer seen in many parts of the world. In the southern Curry, a chemotherapy program in primary school children from 1969 to 1995 reduced the incidence of helminths from 90–3%. Economic progress, education and environmental regulation have all contributed to this. Chemotherapy alone cannot be successful where the necessary regulations are not in place [79, 80].

In 2001, Resolution 54.19 of the World Health Assembly (WHA) encouraged all member states endemic for schistosomiasis and nematodiasis to achieve "a minimum target of regular chemotherapy for at least 75% and up to 100% of all school-age children at risk of disease by 2010". Praziquantel has assumed important roles in anthelmintic treatment and control programs. Similar concerns have been shown for other therapeutic drugs commonly used to control hookworm infections, such as mebendazole and pyrantel. Various drug stewardship strategies (cyclical use of drugs) have been proposed to address these issues; however, if drug resistance trends continue, global efforts to control parasitic diseases using drugs may come to an end, a well-known phenomenon in the use of antibiotic/antiviral drugs [8, 58, 59, 79, 80].

Benzimidazole group of drugs used as antihelmintics are also used in cancer treatment. The mechanism of action of these drugs is to cause cell death by blocking the microtubule systems of parasite and mammalian cells. They also cause ovicidal, vermicidal, larvicidal and cell death of the parasite. Albendazole, ornidazole and mebandazole are used not only in the treatment of intestinal helminths and protozoon, but also in the treatment of tissue and reticuloendothelial nematodes. Ivermectin in combination with diethylcarbamazine is also used in the treatment of lymphatic filarial nematodes. Although these drugs are safe, liver toxicity and various side effects as well as resistance problems may develop [79].

7. Recent developments and future directions

Although more than 160 years have passed since the first identification of intestinal parasites, they are still an important cause of morbidity and mortality in developing countries, especially in children. In various immunosuppressive diseases that have been on the rise in the last 20 years, many chronic protozoa have emerged as important causes of mortality.

Today, amoebiasis caused by *Entamoeba histolytica* continues to be an important problem, especially in endemic areas. One of the most important problems of the parasite is the large number of asymptomatic infected people in the communities. Another problem is that traveling people returning home from endemic regions are often undiagnosed, leading to deaths and economic losses. The fecal-oral parasite causes no symptoms in some people, but sometimes causes tumor-like formations, especially in the colon mucosa, and fatal amoebiasis that can reach the brain. Today, epidemiologic diagnostic problems persist in many geographical areas and adequate and effective treatment cannot be provided due to economic problems. Although intestinal parasites, which have weakened and exhausted people's strength since prehistoric times, have become uncommon with education and treatment in some countries, they have increased again with the effect of growing migration, urban slum systems, poverty and global warming. It is one of the leading causes of child mortality and physical and mental retardation in developing countries. Due to increased migration from endemic areas, there are problems in the population control of countries and consequently, adequate health services cannot be provided. The lack of clean drinking water and sanitation in newly established urban slums causes the parasite to move from endemic areas to different regions. Conducting large-scale epidemiologic studies in areas of migration is one of the most important control strategies. The development of new and appropriate treatments to make treatment cheaper and widespread, and supporting R&D studies to develop appropriate vaccines for endemic areas will be the most effective methods to reduce the global parasite load. For sustainable and effective prevention, it is essential to develop global strategies rather than isolated or country-specific approaches. Mass hygiene education should be provided all over the world with appropriate funders. Countries should improve private and public health conditions and continue campaigns to combat parasitic diseases. In this way, the fight against other infectious agents will also be realized.

Author details

Nihal Dogan
Department of Microbiology/Parasitology, Eskişehir Osmangazi University Faculty of Medicine, Eskisehir, Turkey

*Address all correspondence to: nihaldogan42@gmail.com

References

[1] Harhay MO, Horton J, Olliaro PL. Epidemiology and control of human gastrointestinal parasites in children. Expert Review of Anti-infective Therapy. 2010;**8**(2):219-234

[2] Eyayu T, Kiros T, Workineh L, Sema M, Damtie S, Hailemichael W, et al. Prevalence of intestinal parasitic infections and associated factors among patients attending at Sanja primary hospital, Northwest Ethiopia: An institutional-based cross-sectional study. PLoS One. 2021;**16**(2):e0247075

[3] Beck DL, Doğan N, Maro V, Sam NE, Shao J, Houpt ER. High prevalence of Entamoeba moshkovskii in a Tanzanian HIV population. Acta Tropica. 2008;**107**(1):48-49

[4] Karagiannis-Voules DA, Biedermann P, Ekpo UF, Garba A, Langer E, Mathieu E, et al. Spatial and temporal distribution of soil-transmitted helminth infection in sub-Saharan Africa: A systematic review and geostatistical meta-analysis. The Lancet Infectious Diseases. 2015;**15**(1):74-84

[5] Majid MF, Kang SJ, Hotez PJ. Resolving "worm wars": An extended comparison review of findings from key economics and epidemiological studies. PLoS Neglected Tropical Diseases. 2019;**13**(3):e0006940

[6] Hotez PJ, Brindley PJ, Bethony JM, King CH, Pearce EJ, Jacobson J. Helminth infections: The great neglected tropical diseases. The Journal of Clinical Investigation. 2008;**118**(4):1311-1321

[7] Dogan N, Oz Y, Kocman NU, Nursal AF. Comparison of individual differences in the direct microscopic examination in the diagnosis of intestinal parasites. Türkiye Parazitolojii Dergisi. 2013;**36**(4):211-214

[8] World Health Organization. Prevention and Control of Intestinal Parasitic Infections: Report of a WHO Expert Committee. Geneva: WHO; 1987. 86 p (Technical Report Series/World Health Organization). ISBN 978-92-4-120749-2

[9] Soil-transmitted helminth infections [Internet]. Available from: https://www.who.int/news-room/fact-sheets/detail/soil-transmitted-helminth-infections [Accessed: March 3, 2024]

[10] Zuzarte-Luís V, Mota MM. Parasite sensing of host nutrients and environmental cues. Cell Host & Microbe. 2018;**23**(6):749-758

[11] Cox FEG. Taxonomy and classification of human parasitic protozoa and helminths. In: Jorgensen JH, Carroll KC, Funke G, Pfaller MA, Landry ML, Richter SS, et al., editors. Manual of Clinical Microbiology [Internet]. Washington, DC, USA: ASM Press; 2015. pp. 2282-2292. DOI: 10.1128/9781555817381.ch132 [Accessed: March 3, 2024]

[12] Garcia LS. Classification of human parasites, vectors, and similar organisms. Clinical Infectious Diseases. 1999;**29**(4):734-736

[13] Lonc E, Płonka-Syroka B. Scientific standards in parasitology in historical perspective. Wiadomości Parazytologiczne. 2005;**51**(3):197-207

[14] Ferreira LF, Reinhard KJ, Araújo A, editors. Foundations of Paleoparasitology [Internet]. Rio de Janeiro RJ/Brazil: Editora Fiocruz; 2014. Available from:

http://books.scielo.org/id/zngnn [Accessed: March 3, 2024]

[15] Araujo A, Reinhard K, Ferreira LF, Pucu E, Chieffi PP. Paleoparasitology: The origin of human parasites. Arq Neuro-Psiquiatr. 2013;**71**(9B):722-726

[16] Cox FEG. History of human parasitic diseases. Infectious Disease Clinics of North America. 2004;**18**(2):171-188

[17] Gonçalves MLC, Araújo A, Ferreira LF. Human intestinal parasites in the past: New findings and a review. Memórias do Instituto Oswaldo Cruz. 2003;**98**(Suppl. 1):103-118

[18] Argüello MRH. New paleoparasitological techniques. Journal of Archaeological Science. 2006;**33**(3):372-377

[19] Araújo A, Jansen AM, Bouchet F, Reinhard K, Ferreira LF. Parasitism, the diversity of life, and paleoparasitology. Memórias do Instituto Oswaldo Cruz. 2003;**98**(Suppl. 1):5-11

[20] Araújo A, Ferreira LF. Paleoparasitology and the antiquity of human host-parasite relationships. Memórias do Instituto Oswaldo Cruz. 2000;**95**(Suppl. 1):89-93

[21] Pizzi T, Schenone H. Discovery of eggs of Trichuris trichiura in the contents of the intestines of an Inca archeological body. Boletín Chileno de Parasitología. 1954;**9**(3):73-75

[22] Cockburn A. Where did our infectious diseases come from?: The evolution of infectious disease. In: Elliott K, Whelan J, editors. Novartis Foundation Symposia [Internet]. 1st ed. Basel, Switzerland: Wiley; 1977. pp. 103-113. Available from: https://onlinelibrary.wiley.com/doi/10.1002/9780470715406.ch6 [Accessed: March 4, 2024]

[23] Araujo A, Reinhard KJ, Ferreira LF, Gardner SL. Parasites as probes for prehistoric human migrations? Trends in Parasitology. 2008;**24**(3):112-115

[24] Araújo AJGD, Ferreira LF, Confalonieri UEC, Nuñez L, Ribeiro Filho BM. The finding of enterobius vermicularis eggs in pré-Columbian human coprolites. Memórias do Instituto Oswaldo Cruz. 1985;**80**(2):141-143

[25] Camacho M, Iñiguez AM, Reinhard KJ. Taphonomic considerations on pinworm prevalence in three ancestral Puebloan latrines. Journal of Archaeological Science: Reports. 2018;**20**:791-798

[26] Reinhard KJ, Ferreira LF, Bouchet F, Sianto L, Dutra JMF, Iniguez A, et al. Food, parasites, and epidemiological transitions: A broad perspective. International Journal of Paleopathology. 2013;**3**(3):150-157

[27] Chai JY, Seo M, Shin DH. Paleoparasitology research on ancient helminth eggs and larvae in the Republic of Korea. Parasites, Hosts and Diseases. 2023;**61**(4):345-387

[28] Jiménez FA, Gardner SL, Araújo A, Fugassa M, Brooks RH, Racz E, et al. Zoonotic and human parasites of inhabitants of Cueva de los Muertos Chiquitos, Rio Zape Valley, Durango, Mexico. The Journal of Parasitology. 2012;**98**(2):304-309

[29] Søe MJ, Nejsum P, Seersholm FV, Fredensborg BL, Habraken R, Haase K, et al. Ancient DNA from latrines in Northern Europe and the Middle East (500 BC–1700 AD) reveals past parasites and diet. PLoS One. 2018;**13**(4):e0195481

[30] Ruffer MA. Note on the presence of "Bilharzia Haematobia" in Egyptian

mummies of the twentieth dynasty [1250-1000 B.C.]. British Medical Journal. 1910;**1**(2557):16

[31] Faulkner CT, Reinhard KJ. A retrospective examination of paleoparasitology and its establishment in the journal of parasitology. The Journal of Parasitology. 2014;**100**(3):253-259

[32] Yeh H-Y, Mitchell PD. Ancient human parasites in ethnic Chinese populations. The Korean Journal of Parasitology. 2016;**54**(5):565-572. Available from: https://www.ncbi.nlm.nih.gov/pmc/articles/PMC5127531/

[33] Mitchell PD, Yeh HY. Intestinal parasites at the Xuanquanzhi Relay Station on the silk road 2000 years ago. In: Mehlhorn H, Wu X, Wu Z, editors. Infectious Diseases along the Silk Roads Parasitology Research Monographs. Vol. 17. Cham: Springer International Publishing; 2023. pp. 131-139. Available from: https://link.springer.com/10.1007/978- 3-031-35275-1_9. [Accessed: March 4, 2024]

[34] Chaves SADM, Reinhard KJ. Critical analysis of coprolite evidence of medicinal plant use, Piauí, Brazil. Palaeogeography, Palaeoclimatology, Palaeoecology. 2006;**237**(1):110-118

[35] Reinhard K. Reestablishing rigor in archaeological parasitology. International Journal of Paleopathology. 2017;**19**:124-134

[36] Bouchet F, Guidon N, Dittmar K, Harter S, Ferreira LF, Chaves SM, et al. Parasite remains in archaeological sites. Memórias do Instituto Oswaldo Cruz. 2003;**98**(Suppl. 1):47-52

[37] Araújo A, Reinhard K, Ferreira LF, Pucu E, Chieffi PP. Paleoparasitology: The origin of human parasites. Arquivos de Neuro-Psiquiatria. 2013;**71**(9B):722-726

[38] Faulkner CT, Patton S, Johnson SS. Prehistoric parasitism in Tennessee: Evidence from the analysis of desiccated Fecal material collected from big bone cave, Van Buren County, Tennessee. The Journal of Parasitology. 1989;**75**(3):461

[39] Le Bailly M, Gonçalves ML, Lefèvre C, Roper DC, Pye JW, Araujo A, et al. Parasitism in Kansas in the 1800s: A glimpse to the past through the analysis of grave sediments from meadowlark cemetery. Memórias do Instituto Oswaldo Cruz. 2006;**101** (Suppl. 2):53-56

[40] Dutour O. Paleoparasitology and paleopathology. Synergies for reconstructing the past of human infectious diseases and their pathocenosis. International Journal of Paleopathology. 2013;**3**(3):145-149

[41] Herrmann B. Parasite remains from mediaeval latrine deposits: An epidemiologic and ecologic approach. Note et Monographie Technique. 1988;**24**:135-142

[42] Aspöck H, Auer H, Picher O. Parasites and parasitic diseases in prehistoric human populations in Central Europe. Helminthologia. 1999;**36**:139-145

[43] Bouchet F, Bentrad S. Recovery of equine helminth eggs in a medieval lacustrine settlement. The Veterinary Record. 1997;**141**(23):601-602

[44] Flammer PG, Ryan H, Preston SG, Warren S, Přichystalová R, Weiss R, et al. Epidemiological insights from a large-scale investigation of intestinal helminths in medieval Europe. PLoS Neglected Tropical Diseases. 2020;**14**(8):e0008600. Available from: https://journals.plos.org/plosntds/article?id=10.1371/journal.pntd.0008600

[45] Mitchell PD. Parasites in Past Civilizations and their Impact upon Health. Cambridge New York: Cambridge University Press; 2023

[46] Eskew WH, Ledger ML, Lloyd A, Pyles G, Gosker J, Mitchell PD. Intestinal parasites in an ottoman period latrine from acre (Israel) dating to the early 1800s CE. The Korean Journal of Parasitology. 2019;**57**(6):575-580

[47] Cox FEG. The Golden Age of parasitology-1875-1925: The Scottish contributions. Parasitology. 2017;**144**(12):1567-1581

[48] Côté NML, Daligault J, Pruvost M, Bennett EA, Gorgé O, Guimaraes S, et al. A new high-throughput approach to genotype ancient human gastrointestinal parasites. PLoS One. 2016;**11**(1):e0146230

[49] Dittmar K, Araujo A, Reinhard KJ. The study of parasites through time: Archaeoparasitology and Paleoparasitology. In: Grauer AL, editor. A Companion to Paleopathology. Chichester, West Sussex; Malden, MA: Wiley-Blackwell; 2012

[50] Chan MS, Medley GF, Jamison D, Bundy DA. The evaluation of potential global morbidity attributable to intestinal nematode infections. Parasitology. 1994;**109**(Pt. 3):373-387

[51] Horton J. Human gastrointestinal helminth infections: Are they now neglected diseases? Trends in Parasitology. 2003;**19**(11):527-531

[52] Carrero JC, Reyes-López M, Serrano-Luna J, Shibayama M, Unzueta J, León-SicairosN,et al.Intestinalamoebiasis: 160 years of its first detection and still remains as a health problem in developing countries. International Journal of Medical Microbiology. 2020;**310**(1):151358

[53] Chen KT. Emerging infectious diseases and one health: Implication for public health. International Journal of Environmental Research and Public Health. 2022;**19**(15):9081

[54] Parija SC. Paleoparasitology and human evolution. Tropical Parasitology. 2023;**13**(1):1-2

[55] Rothe C, Zimmer T, Schunk M, Wallrauch C, Helfrich K, Gültekin F, et al. Developing endemicity of Schistosomiasis, Corsica, France. Emerging Infectious Diseases. 2021;**27**(1):319-321

[56] Bruschi F. Was Julius Caesar's epilepsy due to neurocysticercosis? Trends in Parasitology. 2011;**27**(9):373-374

[57] Pinilla AE, López MC, Viasus DF. History of the Entamoeba histolytica protozoan. Revista Médica de Chile. 2008;**136**(1):118-124

[58] World Health Organization. WHO patient safety. In: WHO & WHO Patient Safety. WHO Guidelines on Hand Hygiene in Health Care. Geneva, Switzerland; 2009; p. 262 (WHO/IER/PSP/2009/01). ISBN: 9789241597906

[59] Haque R. Human intestinal parasites. Journal of Health, Population, and Nutrition. 2007;**25**(4):387-391

[60] Hart BL, Hart LA. How mammals stay healthy in nature: The evolution of behaviours to avoid parasites and pathogens. Philosophical Transactions of the Royal Society B. 2018;**373**(1751):20170205

[61] Verweij JJ, Stensvold CR. Molecular testing for clinical diagnosis and epidemiological investigations of intestinal parasitic infections. Clinical Microbiology Reviews. 2014;**27**(2):371-418

[62] Dogan N, Aydin M, Tuzemen NU, Dinleyici EC, Oguz I, Dogruman-Al F. Subtype distribution of Blastocystis spp. isolated from children in Eskisehir, Turkey. Parasitology International. 2017;**66**(1):948-951

[63] Prevention CC for DC and CDC - Soil-transmitted Helminths [Internet]. 2022. Available from: https://www.cdc.gov/parasites/sth/index.html [Accessed: March 5, 2024]

[64] Tegen D, Damtie D, Hailegebriel T. Prevalence and associated risk factors of human intestinal protozoan parasitic infections in Ethiopia: A systematic review and meta-analysis. Journal of Parasitology Research. 2020;**2020**:1-15

[65] Taylor-Robinson DC, Maayan N, Soares-Weiser K, Donegan S, Garner P. Deworming drugs for soil-transmitted intestinal worms in children: Effects on nutritional indicators, haemoglobin, and school performance. Cochrane Database of Systematic Reviews. 2015;**2015**(7):CD000371

[66] Bockarie MJ, Kelly-Hope LA, Rebollo M, Molyneux DH. Preventive chemotherapy as a strategy for elimination of neglected tropical parasitic diseases: Endgame challenges. Philosophical Transactions of the Royal Society B. 2013;**368**(1623):20120144

[67] Alemu A, Bitew ZW, Worku T. Intestinal parasites co-infection among tuberculosis patients in Ethiopia: A systematic review and meta-analysis. BMC Infectious Diseases. 2020;**20**(1):510

[68] Ntonifor NH, Tamufor ASW, Abongwa LE. Prevalence of intestinal parasites and associated risk factors in HIV positive and negative patients in northwest region, Cameroon. Scientific Reports. 2022;**12**(1):16747

[69] Barnes AN, Davaasuren A, Baasandagva U, Gray GC. A systematic review of zoonotic enteric parasitic diseases among nomadic and pastoral people. PLoS One. 2017;**12**(11):e01888

[70] Lowenstein C, Vasco K, Sarzosa S, Salinas L, Torres A, Perry MJ, et al. Determinants of childhood zoonotic enteric infections in a semirural Community of Quito, Ecuador. The American Journal of Tropical Medicine and Hygiene. 2020;**102**(6):1269-1278

[71] Mendoza-de Gives P, López-Arellano ME, Olmedo-Juárez A, Higuera-Pierdrahita RI, von Son-de FE. Recent advances in the control of endoparasites in ruminants from a sustainable perspective. Pathogens. 2023;**12**(9):1121

[72] Girma A, Aemiro A. Prevalence and associated risk factors of intestinal parasites and enteric bacterial infections among selected region food handlers of Ethiopia during 2014-2022: A systematic review and meta-analysis. The Scientific World Journal. 2022;**2022**:1-14

[73] Brooker S. Estimating the global distribution and disease burden of intestinal nematode infections: Adding up the numbers–A review. International Journal for Parasitology. 2010;**40**(10):1137-1144

[74] Garcia LS, Arrowood M, Kokoskin E, Paltridge GP, Pillai DR, Procop GW, et al. Practical guidance for clinical microbiology laboratories: Laboratory diagnosis of parasites from the gastrointestinal tract. Clinical Microbiology Reviews. 2018;**31**(1):e00025-e00017

[75] Momčilović S, Cantacessi C, Arsić-Arsenijević V, Otranto D, Tasić-Otašević S. Rapid diagnosis of parasitic diseases: Current scenario and

future needs. Clinical Microbiology and Infection. 2019;**25**(3):290-309

[76] Anantrasirichai N, Chalidabhongse TH, Palasuwan D, Naruenatthanaset K, Kobchaisawat T, Nunthanasup N, et al. ICIP 2022 challenge on parasitic egg detection and classification in microscopic images: Dataset, methods and results. In: 2022 IEEE International Conference on Image Processing (ICIP) [Internet]. Bordeaux, France: IEEE; 2022. pp. 4306-4310. Available from: https://ieeexplore.ieee.org/document/9897267/ [Accessed: March 4, 2024]

[77] Weiss JB. DNA probes and PCR for diagnosis of parasitic infections. Clinical Microbiology Reviews. 1995;**8**(1):113-130

[78] Demeler J, Ramünke S, Wolken S, Ianiello D, Rinaldi L, Gahutu JB, et al. Discrimination of gastrointestinal nematode eggs from crude fecal egg preparations by inhibitor-resistant conventional and real-time PCR. PLoS One. 2013;**8**(4):e61285

[79] Chai JY, Jung BK, Hong SJ. Albendazole and Mebendazole as anti-parasitic and anti-cancer agents: An update. The Korean Journal of Parasitology. 2021;**59**(3):189-225

[80] Hotez PJ, Bottazzi ME, Franco-Paredes C, Ault SK, Periago MR. The neglected tropical diseases of Latin America and the Caribbean: A review of disease burden and distribution and a roadmap for control and elimination. PLoS Neglected Tropical Diseases. 2008;**2**(9):e300

Chapter 2

Navigating the Intestinal Parasite Landscape

Jyotsna Chawla, Joshua Bernard and Cyril Blavo

Abstract

Intestinal parasitic infections afflict over 3.5 billion individuals globally, leading to an estimated 200,000 deaths annually. Acknowledging variations in susceptibility and outcomes across diverse demographic groups is essential for effective intervention. This chapter provides an in-depth examination of medically significant intestinal parasites, including three protozoa, two nematodes, two cestodes, and one trematode, selected specifically for their primary pathogenesis within the intestines. We offer comprehensive insights into their morphology, pathogenesis mechanisms, and current and emerging diagnostic and therapeutic modalities. By fostering a deeper understanding of intestinal parasitic diseases, this work aims to contribute to the formulation of targeted intervention strategies, ultimately reducing morbidity and mortality associated with these widespread infections.

Keywords: parasitic infections, intestinal parasites, diarrhea, diagnosis, treatments, pathogenesis, tropical medicine, medically significant parasites

1. Introduction

Intestinal parasites have been a persistent companion of humans since prehistoric times, evolving side-by-side with us and maintaining a strong association that dates back over 10,000 years [1]. These intestinal parasites present a formidable global health challenge, with an estimated 3.5 billion people affected worldwide [2]. As many as 450 million individuals are known to suffer from symptomatic infections, and more than 200,000 deaths are reported annually. The impact of these infections is profound, with one-fourth of known human infectious diseases attributed to the protozoan-helminth group [3].

Intestinal parasite infections are classified among the neglected tropical diseases (NID), a status that reflects the challenges faced in managing them effectively, particularly in resource-limited nations [4]. Factors such as inadequate environmental and personal hygiene, malnutrition, overcrowding, and erratic climatic conditions create ideal environments for the transmission of these parasites [5–7]. Most of these infections have been controlled effectively in resource-abundant and developed nations; however, it is noteworthy that parasitic infections are resurging in these nations, a trend that may be linked to the growing number of immunocompromised individuals and increased life expectancy [1, 8].

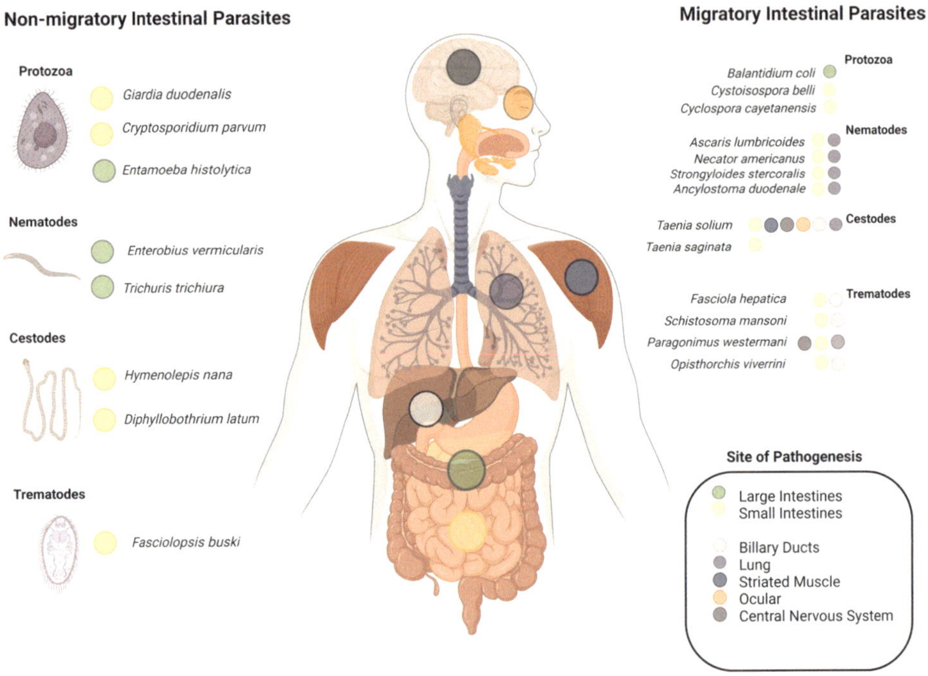

Figure 1.
Overview of Clinically Significant Intestinal Parasites. Medically relevant intestinal parasites are classified according to the site of pathogenesis. Non-migratory intestinal parasites reside primarily within the intestines, causing localized intestinal illness. In contrast, migratory intestinal parasites travel beyond the intestines, establishing themselves in other organs or tissues and causing disease. The figure was generated with BioRender.com.

This chapter primarily investigates a specific group of medically important intestinal parasites: three protozoan and six helminth species with established intestinal tropism and pathogenic potential (**Figure 1**). While the focus remains on these key players, the chapter acknowledges the presence of other intestinal parasites that may traverse or temporarily inhabit the intestinal tract during their life cycles. Details regarding these additional parasites will be provided in dedicated sections. The fundamental objective of this chapter is to emphasize the significant burden posed by these intestinal parasites on a global scale, elucidate their role in intestinal pathophysiology, and contribute to the development of targeted interventions designed to reduce morbidity and mortality associated with these infections.

2. Clinically significant intestinal protozoan parasites

2.1 Giardia duodenalis (Giardia lamblia)

Giardia duodenalis, formerly known as *Giardia lamblia*, causes Giardiasis, one of the most common parasitic intestinal infections worldwide [9]. Giardia is a causative agent for endemic and epidemic diarrhea, mainly in tropical and subtropical settings. It is the third most prevalent cause of diarrheal illness in children under the age of five globally, with over 300 million cases recorded each year [10]. Giardiasis is a substantial contributor to gastrointestinal disease in locations with poor sanitary conditions and to epidemics in daycare centers and among travelers [11, 12].

2.1.1 Morphology of Giardia duodenalis

Giardia duodenalis is a protozoan parasite that completes its life cycle within a single host [13]. *G. duodenalis* exists in two forms: the trophozoite (the metabolically active and vegetative form) and the cyst (the dormant and environmentally stable form) [14]. The trophozoites exhibit a distinct pyriform structure that closely resembles the shape of a tennis racket [13]. They typically measure 10–20 μm and may show two large nuclei. In addition, four pairs of flagellae provide falling leaf-like motility to facilitate trophozoite movement [15–17]. The cysts exhibit an oval to ellipsoid shape and measure approximately 8–19 μm [18, 19]. The cyst wall is lined with hyaline which protects the parasite from the environment. Mature cysts typically contain four nuclei, whereas immature cysts contain two [20]. Within 30 minutes of entry, two trophozoites are released from each cyst (excystation) in the duodenum [21, 22]. The trophozoites then multiply in the small intestine and adhere to the upper jejunal mucosa, causing inflammatory damage to the villi. Gradually, the trophozoites pass through the large intestine, where encystation begins, and the cysts are excreted in the stool [13].

2.1.2 Pathogenesis of Giardia duodenalis

G. duodenalis primarily inhabits the duodenum and upper jejunum of the small intestine [23–26]. Transmission occurs through ingestion of food and water contaminated with mature cysts. Although less common, infection can also be acquired through sexual transmission [27]. The infective dose of *Giardia duodenalis* is low, with as few as 10–25 cysts capable of initiating the infection process [28]. Attachment of *Giardia duodenalis* to the intestinal mucosal epithelium relies on the ventral disk, which plays a critical role in the colonization and establishment of infection.

Giardia duodenalis invades enterocytes, inflicting substantial damage and eroding the brush border of intestinal epithelial cells. This insult compromises intestinal absorptive capacity by triggering microvillous atrophy and epithelial barrier dysfunction [26]. Malabsorption is particularly pronounced in fats, leading to the hallmark symptom of steatorrhea: foul-smelling, profuse, frothy diarrhea [27, 28]. The malabsorption may extend to lactose and xylose, resulting in disaccharide intolerance [29, 30]. Recent studies shed light on Giardia's cysteine proteases potentially disrupting goblet cell function in the intestine. This disruption could lead to decreased protective mucus production and changes in its composition, leaving the host more vulnerable to pathogens [31]. Understanding the molecular mechanisms of giardiasis is crucial for comprehending disease pathogenesis and devising effective therapeutic approaches.

2.1.3 Clinical manifestations of Giardia duodenalis

The clinical course of Giardia infection includes asymptomatic carriage, acute giardiasis, and chronic giardiasis. Acute giardiasis develops after an incubation period of 1 to 14 days (average of 7 days) and usually lasts 1 to 3 weeks [32, 33]. In chronic giardiasis, the symptoms are recurrent and may cause malabsorption and debilitation. The clinical manifestations of giardiasis include fatty or greasy diarrhea (steatorrhea), dull epigastric pain, bloating of the abdomen, and foul-smelling flatulence. Occasionally, nausea, vomiting, fever, rashes, or constipation may occur [13, 34]. Extraintestinal manifestations are rare. They include conditions such as urticaria, erythema multiforme, bronchospasm, reactive arthritis, and biliary tract disease [9]. In HIV patients with compromised immune function, giardia infection becomes a more likely culprit for persistent diarrhea, highlighting the need for its inclusion in the diagnostic workup.

2.1.4 Diagnosis and treatment strategies for Giardia duodenalis

The diagnostic approach for *G. duodenalis* is stool examination for the presence of cysts and trophozoites [35]. The CDC recommends collecting three patient stool specimens over several days to enhance accuracy. Several methods for analyzing stool samples include wet mount, trichrome stain, direct fluorescent antibody (DFA) assay, and enzyme immunoassay (EIA). However, microscopy with DFA is considered the gold standard due to its increased sensitivity compared to non-fluorescent microscopy techniques [36]. Additionally, guidelines from the Infectious Disease Society of America (IDSA) suggest utilizing duodenal aspirate microscopy when stool studies yield inconclusive results, but suspicion of Giardia remains high. Duodenal aspirate microscopy is deemed sensitive because trophozoites are abundant in the proximal small bowel and can be promptly recognized due to their motility [37]. Moreover, recent research suggests that utilizing Giardia microRNA (miR5) as a marker for Giardia infection in duodenal biopsies may offer a promising new diagnostic method for giardiasis, demonstrating greater sensitivity compared to histological diagnosis [38].

Metronidazole has served as the mainstay treatment for human giardiasis since 1959. However, concerns regarding its efficacy are escalating due to rising therapeutic failure rates and the emergence of Giardia resistance to the nitroimidazole class of drugs [39]. Alternative treatment options include tinidazole, nitazoxanide, and even metronidazole in some cases. While a 5–7 day course of metronidazole typically achieves cure rates exceeding 90%, single-dose regimens of tinidazole or ornidazole offer comparable effectiveness [33].

Although no recent clinical trials or drug approvals for *Giardia duodenalis* have occurred in humans, research suggests promising alternatives. Studies have explored robenidine, a commercially available anticoccidial drug since the 1970s, as a potential lead compound for developing new antigiardial drugs [40]. In vitro studies demonstrate that robenidine exhibits potent and rapid activity against *G. duodenalis*, particularly during the trophozoite stage, exceeding the efficacy of metronidazole.

2.2 Cryptosporidium parvum

The microscopic parasite *Cryptosporidium parvum* triggers cryptosporidiosis, a widespread diarrheal illness [41]. The intracellular protozoan parasite colonizes human intestinal epithelia and is found throughout the world, with the highest prevalence in low- and middle-income countries [42]. Estimates suggest that cryptosporidiosis affects a significant number of people in the United States, with around 823,000 cases occurring annually [43]. While swimming pools, unpasteurized beverages, and contact with animal care have been linked to outbreaks in the United States, the parasite predominantly thrives in areas with inadequate water treatment and sanitation. *C. parvum* is best known for causing self-limiting watery diarrhea, but it can lead to severe and chronic cryptosporidiosis in immunocompromised individuals [44]. In immunocompetent individuals, the prevalence of infection ranges from 2.4–15% in developing countries and 1.4–6% in developed countries.

In immunocompromised hosts, the prevalence is significantly higher, ranging from 12 to 46% in developing countries and 7–21% in developed countries [22].

2.2.1 Morphology of Cryptosporidium parvum

Cryptosporidium parvum, exists as a small oocyst, measuring 4–6 μm in diameter, with a thick, resistant wall containing four sporozoites. Once inside the host, the parasite undergoes various developmental stages, beginning with invasive sporozoites and progressing to reproductive stages within the host's intestinal epithelial cells. During sexual reproduction, zygotes are formed, giving rise to two types of oocysts: thick-walled and thin-walled oocysts. The host excretes thick-walled oocysts, which possess two electrodense cyst walls. An outer thick coarse layer and an inner fine granular layered wall with a suture point at one pole. The thin-walled oocysts are enveloped by a single-layered membrane and are often involved in internal autoinfection and are therefore, they are not typically discharged in stool [22, 45]. The infected host excretes sporulated oocysts through their feces. The most common modes of transmission include ingestion feces-contaminated water or food, as well as through direct contact. Upon ingestion, excystation occurs in the small intestines, releasing four sporozoites from each oocyst to parasitize epithelial cells in the gastrointestinal tract and begin a new cycle of infection [45, 46].

2.2.2 Pathogenesis of Cryptosporidium parvum

C. parvum is known for its wide host range, capable of infecting various mammalian species including humans, suggesting the presence of diverse isolate types even from the same host species [47]. The principal method of *C. parvum* transmission to hosts is via the fecal-oral route, typically through the ingestion of contaminated food or water in its oocyst form. A relatively low infective dose (10–100 oocysts) combined with its ability to evade host immune response, contribute significantly to the pathogenicity of *C. parvum* [48, 49]. Furthermore, the infective form of Cryptosporidium is highly resistant to most environmental factors, including routine chlorination and other disinfectants [50, 51].

Sporozoites of *C. parvum* commonly target the epithelial cells at the ileocecal junction of the small intestine, where they complete their life cycle. An important virulence factor of Cryptosporidium is the CP47 protein, which facilitates the attachment of sporozoites to the brush border epithelium of the small intestines [52]. The parasite does not typically elicit systemic inflammation or penetrate deep tissues. Instead, it stays localized on the apical surface of the intestinal epithelium within its membrane-bound compartments [53]. When penetration does occur, the parasite can trigger host cell kinase signaling pathways, leading to the local induction of a pro-inflammatory host response. This response includes the production of TNF-alpha, IL-8, and prostaglandins, which can result in intestinal mucosal inflammation and diarrhea [22, 54]. While *C. parvum* primarily targets the intestines, rare cases like pulmonary infection highlight the need for further research on its pathogenesis for broader disease management [55].

2.2.3 Clinical manifestations of Cryptosporidium parvum

Symptoms of cryptosporidiosis include watery diarrhea and stomach cramps, accompanied by fever, nausea, vomiting, and loss of appetite in some cases. The onset of symptoms usually occurs within 1–12 days after infection, with most individuals experiencing symptoms around 7 days post-infection. The watery diarrhea associated with cryptosporidiosis is self-limiting and usually resolves within 2–3 weeks. Though very rare, pulmonary and tracheal cryptosporidiosis may cause coughing and fever [55, 56]. In immunocompromised individuals such as those with HIV/AIDS, diarrhea can worsen to uncontrollable levels, resulting in severe dehydration and potentially life-threatening consequences [57].

2.2.4 Diagnosis and treatment strategies for Cryptosporidium parvum

The oocyst of *C.parvum*, which is excreted in human host feces, functions as both the infective and diagnostic form of the organism [58]. Consequently, routine diagnosis of cryptosporidiosis hinges on the examination of stool samples. The challenge in diagnosing oocysts primarily stems from their diminutive size, ranging from 4 to 6 μm [59, 60].

Clinical laboratories employ acid-fast staining to visualize and diagnose *C.parvum* oocysts by staining their cell walls [61]. Immunofluorescence microscopy is favored for its superior specificity and sensitivity, followed by enzyme immunoassays (EIA). Molecular methods are utilized for species-level identification of Cryptosporidium. ELISA assays have been developed to detect *C. parvum*-specific coproantigen in stool samples, showing sensitivity ranging from 66 to 100% and very high specificity. Additionally, *C. parvum*-specific antibody testing and PCR may be utilized to identify specific *C. parvum* genes in both clinical and environmental samples [22].

Most immunocompetent individuals recover from cryptosporidiosis without treatment. Adequate oral fluid intake manages diarrhea. For more severe cases, nitazoxanide is approved by the FDA as a treatment. However, its efficacy in immunocompromised patients such as those with HIV/AIDS is yet to be demonstrated [62, 63]. In such cases, antiviral therapy may decrease or eliminate symptoms of cryptosporidiosis [64]. Even though the symptoms of cryptosporidiosis may diminish on their own, the infection is often not considered curable. This is because the parasite Cryptosporidium has a complex life cycle that allows it to persist and cause symptoms to recur if the host's immune system is not robust. Furthermore, the parasite's remarkable resilience against numerous disinfection techniques hinders complete eradication efforts.

Another limiting factor in managing Cryptosporidium has been the difficulty of propagating the parasite in vitro for therapeutic research. Conventional intestinal cell line models poorly mimic the complex human gut environment, hindering parasite infection and observation of the complete life cycle [65]. However, a recent breakthrough in CRISPR/Cas9-mediated transfection of *C. parvum* sporozoites offers promise for generating genetically modified parasites and propelling treatment research forward [66].

2.3 Entamoeba histolytica

Entamoeba histolytica is a parasitic amoeba that primarily inhabits the large intestines of humans and other animals. It is considered the third leading cause of parasitic death worldwide, following malaria and schistosomiasis [67]. The World Health Organization (WHO) estimates there are approximately 50 million cases of *E. histolytica* with 110,000 deaths annually [68]. Amoebiasis, the disease caused by

Entamoeba histolytica, represents a substantial public health burden, particularly in resource-limited regions with warm climates, including China, Central and South America, and the Indian subcontinent [69]. Transmission of *E. histolytica* occurs primarily through ingestion of contaminated food or water or through direct contact with fecal matter. *E. histolytica* infection in the United States is more frequent among individuals with limited sanitation infrastructure and travelers returning from endemic areas. A less common mode of transmission involves exposure to cysts and trophozoites in fecal matter during sexual contact [70]. Amoebiasis is estimated to affect about 10% of the world's population.

2.3.1 Morphology of Entamoeba histolytica

Entamoeba histolytica, an anaerobic protozoan, completes its life cycle within a single host, typically a human. This life cycle consists of three stages: trophozoite, precyst, and cyst [22]. Infection typically begins with the ingestion of mature, quadrinucleate cysts from fecally contaminated food, water, or hands [71]. The cysts of Entamoeba histolytica are spherical and measure between 10 to 20 μm in diameter. A mature cyst contains four nuclei, while immature cysts have one to three nuclei [72]. Following ingestion, excystation occurs in the small intestine, releasing trophozoites that migrate to the large intestine. Trophozoites are typically larger, measuring between 10 to 60 μm, with an average size of 15 to 20 μm [73]. They have a single nucleus with evenly arranged chromatin on the nuclear membrane and a small, centrally located karyosome [74]. Trophozoites exhibit active, directional movement facilitated by pseudopodia. The precyst phase is an intermediate stage between the trophozoite and cyst stages, where the organism is smaller than the trophozoite but larger than the cyst [75]. During this stage, the organism loses its pseudopodia and prepares to encyst.

2.3.2 Pathogenesis of Entamoeba histolytica

Following ingestion of mature *E. histolytica* cysts, excystation occurs in the small intestine, triggered by exposure to the host's digestive enzymes and the alkaline environment [71]. This process releases trophozoites, the active form of the parasite, which then migrate to the large intestine and colonize the lumen. Colon colonization is facilitated by the ability of the trophozoites to adhere to the colonic mucus and epithelial cells via lectin-mediated binding. The galactose/N-acetylgalactosamine (Gal/GalNAc) lectin is a key molecule in this adhesion process, allowing the parasite to attach firmly to the host cells [74]. The trophozoites penetrate the intestinal mucosa primarily through the action of cytolytic and proteolytic enzymes such as cysteine proteinases and glycosidases [76]. Glycosidases, particularly β-N-acetyl-D-glucosaminidase, aid in degrading the glycoproteins of the mucosal layer, further facilitating tissue invasion [77]. Secretion of amoebapores by Entamoeba histolytica facilitates tissue damage through host cell lysis. [78]. Trophozoites induce significant damage to the intestinal mucosa through contact-dependent mechanisms, including apoptosis and necrosis [79]. As the trophozoites invade the intestinal mucosa, they trigger a local inflammatory response, leading to the destruction of the epithelial layer and the formation of characteristic flask-shaped ulcers in the colonic epithelium [80].

While trophozoites and cysts are excreted in feces, cysts are typically found in well-formed stool, and trophozoites are found in diarrheal stool. Cysts, the infectious form, can survive for days to weeks due to their protective walls. On average, a carrier *E. histolytica* excretes around 45 million cysts daily, with an infectious dose of approximately 1000 cysts [81]. Amoebiasis patients may also pass trophozoites and immature cysts in their stool, which are destroyed outside the host.

2.3.3 Clinical manifestations of Entamoeba histolytica

Entamoeba histolytica infection exhibits a spectrum of presentations, ranging from asymptomatic carriage with cyst shedding to invasive intestinal amebiasis [82]. The latter can manifest as amebic dysentery (bloody diarrhea, abdominal pain, fever, mucus in stool) or non-dysenteric colitis (intermittent watery diarrhea, abdominal pain, weight loss, fatigue) [83].

Chronic intestinal amebiasis is characterized by recurrent episodes of diarrhea, abdominal pain, and weight loss. Entamoeba histolytica infection can also progress to extraintestinal amebiasis, a severe complication where the parasite spreads beyond the intestines. A common manifestation of this is amebic liver abscess, caused by trophozoites reaching the liver through the portal vein [84]. Symptoms include right upper quadrant abdominal pain, fever, hepatomegaly, and occasionally jaundice. Pulmonary amebiasis can develop through direct extension from the liver or hematogenous spread [85]. Although less frequent, severe complications such as cerebral and genitourinary amebiasis may arise [86, 87]. Cutaneous amebiasis can also occur, often stemming from underlying infections or post-surgery [88]. Timely diagnosis and treatment are essential for managing *E. histolytica* infection and averting potential complications.

2.3.4 Diagnosis and treatment strategies for Entamoeba histolytica

The common method for diagnosing *E. histolytica* is the microscopic identification of cysts and trophozoites in stool samples. This can be achieved by using fresh stool or concentrates derived from fresh stool. A key diagnostic feature of pathogenic *E. histolytica* is the presence of red blood cells within the cytoplasm of the trophozoites [72]. *E. histolytica* trophozoites phagocytize red blood cells to obtain essential nutrients and iron from hemoglobin [89]. Direct visualization of trophozoites is achievable through examination of aspirate or biopsy specimens procured during colonoscopic or surgical procedures. The sensitivity of Entamoeba histolytica detection is enhanced by analyzing three consecutive stool samples collected within a ten-day interval [90]. Microscopic examination is limited in definitively distinguishing *Entamoeba histolytica*, from morphologically identical and non-pathogenic species such as *E. bangladeshi*, *E. dispar*, and *E. moshkovskii*. Therefore, confirmatory molecular diagnostic methods like PCR are essential for accurate species identification [91]. Antibody detection is useful when organisms are not generally found in stool examinations, as seen in patients with extraintestinal disease. The routine serodiagnosis of amebiasis now utilizes commercially available enzyme immunoassay (EIA) instead of the indirect hemagglutination (IHA) test, which detects antibodies against *E. histolytica* [90].

Current treatment guidelines recommend immediate administration of antiparasitic medications, such as metronidazole or tinidazole, for individuals with symptomatic intestinal infections or extraintestinal complications caused by

Entamoeba histolytica. This initial therapy targets and eliminates the motile trophozoite stage of the parasite. However, following this with a luminal agent like paromomycin or iodoquinol is crucial. These medications eradicate the encysted stage of the parasite, preventing potential relapse and further transmission [92]. Asymptomatic individuals are also advised to undergo treatment with paromomycin or iodoquinol due to their potential to unknowingly transmit the parasite. Additionally, research suggests that a significant portion (4–10%) of untreated asymptomatic cases may progress to symptomatic disease within a year [93].

Metronidazole remains the mainstay of amebiasis treatment due to its affordability and availability. However, concerns regarding potential genotoxic and neurotoxic side effects, coupled with the looming threat of resistance, necessitate the exploration of alternative therapies. While a vaccine is not available, promising results from rodent and non-human primate models suggest progress toward preventative measures (**Box 1**) [71].

- *Balantidium coli (Balantidiasis)*

Largest protozoan (40 μm to 200 μm in length) and the only ciliated parasite known to infect humans.
Host: Primary –Pig, *Secondary* –Humans.
Transmission: Ingestion of cysts through contaminated food/water.
Pathogenesis: Trophozoites cause inflammation and colonic mucosal ulcers, most of which are mild or asymptomatic but can be severe in immunocompromised.
Clinical Manifestations: Persistent diarrhea (watery or bloody stools), abdominal pain, weight loss, nausea, and vomiting.
Diagnosis: Detection of trophozoites with a bean-shaped macronucleus from stool samples.
Drug of Choice: Tetracycline and metronidazole

- *Cystoisospora belli (Cystoisosporiasis)*

Opportunistic coccidian parasite.
Host: Primary – Humans; *Secondary* – None.
Transmission: Ingestion of sporulated cysts in contaminated food or water.
Pathogenesis: Sporulated oocysts release sporozoites in the small intestine, infecting the epithelial cells. Fertilized oocysts are shed in stool.
Clinical manifestations: Acute onset of watery diarrhea, fever, abdominal pain, and malabsorption.
Diagnosis: Repeated stool examinations to detect large, typical ellipsoidal-shaped oocysts (25–30 μm).
Drug of Choice: Trimethoprim-sulfamethoxazole (TMP-SMX).
Opportunistic coccidian parasite

- *Cyclospora cayetanensis (Cyclosporiasis)*

Opportunistic coccidian parasite.
Host: Primary – Humans; *Secondary* – None.
Transmission: Ingestion of sporulated cysts in contaminated food (Cilantro, Raspberries, Basil) or contaminated water.
Pathogenesis: Sporulated oocysts release sporozoites in the gastrointestinal tract, invading tire small intestine epithelium.
Clinical manifestations: Watery diarrhea, abdominal pain, low-grade fever; prolonged and chronic symptoms with potential weight loss, especially in immunocompromised individuals.
Diagnosis: Stool examination; small oocysts (8–10 μm), autofluoresce under UV, appearing blue/green.
Drug of Choice: Trimethoprim-sulfamethoxazole (TMP-SMX).

Box 1.
Additional Clinically Relevant Intestinal Parasitic Infections: Protozoa [94–99].

3. Clinically significant helminthic intestinal parasites - nematodes

3.1 Enterobius vermicularis

Enterobius vermicularis, is an intestinal nematode commonly referred to as the pinworm or threadworm. This parasite has co-evolved with human hosts since the evolution of human hominids [100]. *Enterobius gregorii*, documented in Europe, Africa, and Asia, is now considered an immature form of *E. vermicularis* based on morphological and molecular evidence [101]. Humans are the only known host for this parasite, with an estimated 200 million infections worldwide and some reports suggesting an infection rate of over a billion people [102–104]. Pinworm infections are endemic globally, with the highest prevalence among school-aged children between 5 and 14 years with males being twice as likely to be infected as females [105].

The transmission of *E. vermicularis* is associated with inadequate hygiene, overcrowding, and low socioeconomic status, often exacerbated by poor living conditions. Despite its widespread prevalence, pinworm infection is considered the least harmful among gastrointestinal nematode helminths [106]. Since no vaccine is available, maintaining adequate hygiene remains the best preventive measure [100].

3.1.1 Morphology of Enterobius vermicularis

Enterobius vermicularis exhibits a simple life cycle within a single human host. The female parasite, characterized by a long, pointed tail, typically measures 8 to 13 mm long, while the male measures 2 to 5 mm. The organism is whitish-beige, round, and moves with a vigorous crawling motion [100, 101]. The head features three lips and a pair of wing-like cephalic alae [107]. The eggs, measuring 50 by 30 microns, are utilized in diagnostic examinations [105].

After ingestion, the eggs hatch into larvae in the small intestines and develop into adults within 1–2 months [19, 108]. The adults settle in the colon, where gravid females migrate nocturnally to the perianal region to lay eggs. The larvae inside the eggs become infective within 4–6 hours. Transmission occurs primarily through the fecal-oral route, with self-inoculation being common after individuals scratch the affected area, typically the perianal region [101]. Transmission can also occur through contact with contaminated bedding, clothing, personal care products, and furniture [105, 109]. The eggs are resilient, remaining viable in the environment for 2–3 weeks, thus increasing the risk of reinfection [109]. In rare cases, transmission can occur via inhalation followed by ingestion [110].

3.1.2 Pathogenesis of Enterobius vermicularis

Research on the pathogenesis of Enterobius vermicularis and host defense remains limited [111]. Following ingestion, it takes approximately 1–2 months for the eggs of *E. vermicularis* to develop into adults in the small intestines, typically without causing symptoms [105]. However, minor ulcerations at the mucosal attachment site may occur [112]. Exposure to nerve endings at the feeding site can lead to symptoms such as insomnia, convulsions, and nervousness [107].

Adult females migrate to the anal region at night to deposit eggs, causing pruritus [113]. Persistent scratching due to pruritus may result in bacterial superinfection. In some cases, the parasites may migrate to the vaginal area, causing vulvovaginitis and peritoneal granulomas [114]. Although rare, complications such as appendicitis may occur if the parasites obstruct the appendiceal lumen, a subject of ongoing controversy [115, 116]. The host immune response involves a type-2 immune reaction with increased eosinophil levels, although studies have reported no significant elevation in IgE levels in infected individuals [117–120].

3.1.3 Clinical manifestations of Enterobius vermicularis

E. vermicularis infection is generally considered the least harmful among gastrointestinal nematode helminths [106]. Approximately 40% of those affected are asymptomatic [121]. Symptoms, when present, may include perianal pruritus, restlessness, loss of appetite, malnutrition, anemia, insomnia, and irritability [122]. Rarely, extraintestinal enterobiasis can lead to severe health disorders such as kidney and fallopian tube penetration and, in some cases, death [123, 124]. The association between *E. vermicularis* and appendicitis remains under debate, with a meta-analysis suggesting that approximately 2% of appendicitis cases in the Americas and 8% in Africa were positive for *E. vermicularis* infection [125].

3.1.4 Diagnosis and treatment strategies for Enterobius vermicularis

Unlike most enteric nematodes, pinworm infection is not diagnosed by examining feces [111]. The gold standard for diagnosing pinworm infection is the "scotch tape" test [126]. This test involves applying clear cellulose tape to the perianal region, preferably in the morning before bathing, and then placing the tape on a glass slide for microscopic examination of eggs [127]. This process is recommended on three consecutive mornings to increase sensitivity, although it may still be low with very few eggs [100]. Recent scientific advancements include the use of mitochondrial DNA gene encoding cytochrome c oxidase subunit 1 (cox1) for genetic identification, which can be utilized with eggs collected from perianal tape or stool samples containing adult worms [128].

Treatment for *E. vermicularis* includes pyrantel pamoate, albendazole, or mebendazole, administered as a single initial dose followed by a second dose two weeks later. In cases of household infection or recurrence, it is advisable to treat all household members simultaneously [110].

3.2 Trichuris trichiura

Trichuris trichiura, commonly known as whipworm, is a parasitic nematode responsible for one of the major soil-transmitted helminth infections affecting humans. It is estimated to infect approximately 465 million people worldwide [129]. The parasite is predominantly found in tropical and subtropical regions, including parts of Asia, Africa, and Latin America, where poor sanitation practices are prevalent [130]. Transmission of *Trichuris trichiura* occurs primarily through the ingestion of embryonated eggs present in contaminated soil, food, or water [131]. The prevalence of whipworm infection can exceed 90% in impoverished conditions [132]. The species is widespread in human populations, particularly in regions where human excrement (nightsoil) is used to fertilize vegetable gardens [133]. In the United States, it is the second most common nematode, and it is more frequently observed in the rural Southeast regions [134] where conditions may favor its transmission. Whipworm infection is particularly common among children and can cause significant morbidity in heavily infected individuals.

3.2.1 Morphology of Trichuris trichiura

Whipworm is so named because of its distinctive morphology: a broad, short posterior end and a very long, narrow, whip-like anterior end. The anterior end, which contains a stichosome pharynx, is embedded in the mucosa of the lower intestines of humans, while the posterior end lies freely in the intestinal lumen [135].

During its life cycle, *T. trichiura* exhibits two forms: the adult worm and the egg. The eggs of *T. trichiura* are also distinctively barrel-shaped, bile-stained, and have a thick shell with mucus plugs at both ends [136]. They measure approximately 50–55 μm in length and 20–25 μm in width. When passed in the stool, the eggs are un-embryonated and require a period of development in the soil to become infectious [131, 137].

Juvenile worms develop in the glands of the cecal and colonic mucosa, where they molt and grow while the mature adults have their anterior ends embedded in the mucosa [138, 139].

Adult males measure 30–45 mm in length, with a coiled posterior end, whereas adult females measure 35–50 mm and have a straight posterior end [137]. The adult parasitic worms reside in the cecum, appendix, and large intestine of the human host [111].

3.2.2 Pathogenesis of Trichuris trichiura

T. trichiura infections are transmitted via the fecal-oral route, involving the ingestion of eggs with contaminated food, water, or soil. Approximately 2–3 months after encountering the parasite, the female begins laying un-embryonated eggs, with each female shedding between 3000 and 20,000 eggs daily in the cecum [19, 137]. These un-embryonated eggs, excreted in the feces, are noninfectious and take around 2–4 weeks to transition into the infectious, embryonated form [140, 141].

Upon ingestion, the eggs hatch in the small intestine, releasing larvae that migrate to the colon, where they mature and embed their anterior ends into the gastrointestinal mucosa. This results in significant cellular damage and disruption of the epithelial barrier [142]. This process triggers an immune response in the host, characterized by the recruitment of eosinophils, lymphocytes, and plasma cells to the site of infection [131]. The inflammatory response can cause a range of gastrointestinal symptoms, including rectal bleeding, abdominal pain, diarrhea, and, in severe cases, prolapse of the rectum [111, 143]. Chronic infection with *Trichuris trichiura* can lead to persistent Th2-driven immune activation and chronic intestinal inflammation, particularly in pediatric populations. Infected children often exhibit growth stunting, which is believed to be due to chronic inflammation and altered metabolic responses [144]. Chronic infection with *T. trichiura* is associated with a decrease in plasma insulin-like growth factor 1 (IGF-1) and an increase in tumor necrosis factor-alpha (TNF-α) in the colonic mucosa [144]. The chronic inflammatory response can divert nutritional resources and alter endocrine functions, further exacerbating the observed growth deficits.

3.2.3 Clinical manifestations of Trichuris trichiura

Mild infections of Trichuriasis typically manifest without observable signs or symptoms. However, more severe infections, particularly in children, can lead to gastrointestinal issues such as abdominal pain, distension, diarrhea, fecal blood, nocturnal stooling, and rectal prolapse [145, 146]. Additionally, children may experience anemia due to blood loss, growth deficiencies, and potential impairment in cognitive

- *Ascaris lumbricoides (Ascariasis)*

Host: Primary – Humans.
Transmission: Feco-oral ingestion of embryonated eggs in contaminated food (often fresh vegetables).
Pathogenesis: Eggs transform into larvae, invade intestinal mucosa, migrate to lungs, are coughed up, swallowed, and mature into adult worms in the small intestines. Eggs are excreted in stool.
Clinical Manifestations: Often asymptomatic; high burden may cause abdominal pain, obstruction, biliary blockage, appendicitis, nasopharyngeal expulsion, allergic reactions, and Loeffler's syndrome.
Diagnosis: Microscopic stool examination for oval and knobby-coated Ascaris eggs.
Drug of Choice: Mebendazole, pyrantel pamoate, or albendazole

- *Necator americanus (New World Intestinal Hookworm Disease)*

Host: Primary – Hrmrans.
Transmission: Skin penetration by filariform larvae, often through feet/ankles from walking barefoot.
Pathogenesis: Larvae migrate to lungs via bloodstream, travel to pharynx, are swallowed, and mature into adults in tire small intestines.
Clinical Manifestations: Serpiginous tunnel and severe pruritus at penetration site (Ground Itch), cough, abdominal pain, nausea, anorexia. Anemia due to blood loss at the site of attachment in the intestinal wall (Intestinal Hookworm Disease).
Diagnosis: Microscopic stool examination for thin-shelled, oval eggs with a clear, smooth outer layer.
Drug of Choice: Albendazole or pyrantel pamoate

- *Ancylostoma duodenale (Old World Intestinal Hookworm Disease)*

Host: Primary – Humans.
Transmission: Skin penetration by filariform larvae, often through feet/ankles from walking barefoot (Intestinal Hookworm Disease, Ancylostomiasis). Pathogenesis: Larvae migrate to lungs via bloodstream, travel to pharynx, are swallowed, and mature into adults in the small intestines.
Clinical Manifestations: Abdominal pain, diarrhea, exertional dyspnea, fatigue, palpitations, dizziness. Anemia may be more severe than in *N. americanus.* Oral infection (Wakana Disease).
Diagnosis: Microscopic stool examination for oval, thin-shelled eggs with a clear outer layer and segmented embryos.
Drug of Choice: Albendazole or pyrantel pamoate

- *Strongyloides stercoralis (Strongyloidiasis)*

Host: Primary – Humans, dogs and cats.
Transmission: Filariform larvae penetrate intact human skin or are ingested.
Pathogenesis: Larvae penetrate skin, enter bloodstream, migrate to lungs, are coughed up, swallowed, and mature into adult females in the duodenum and jejunum, producing rhabditiform larvae.
Clinical Manifestations: Often asymptomatic, localized pruritic rash at skin penetration site, cough, diarrhea, abdominal pain, Chronic infection may cause peripheral eosinophilia, Loeffler's syndrome.
Diagnosis: Microscopic stool examination for of rhabditiform larvae.
Drug of Choice: Ivermectin.

Box 2.
Additional Clinically Relevant Intestinal Parasitic Infections: Helminths (Nematodes) [155–162].

development. These latter effects are believed to stem from iron deficiency and nutritional inadequacies resulting from the parasitic burden rather than a direct consequence of the infestation [131].

3.2.4 Diagnosis and treatment strategies for Trichuris trichiura

Due to the substantial volume of deposited eggs, approximately 200 eggs per gram of feces per nematode pair, microscopic analysis of a single fecal smear is often sufficient for diagnosis [22]. However, egg detection may be more challenging in cases of light infections. Consequently, a concentration procedure, such as the formalin-ether concentration technique, is recommended, as it enhances egg detection by separating parasitic forms from fecal debris and then sedimenting them by centrifugation [147, 148]. Additionally, given that symptom severity correlates with parasitic burden, quantification using the Kato-Katz technique is beneficial. The Kato-Katz technique involves preparing a standardized thick smear of feces on a slide and staining it to facilitate egg counting [149]. Visualization of adult parasites may also be achieved by examining the rectal mucosa via proctoscopy or directly in cases of rectal prolapse [137, 150, 151].

Trichuris trichiura infections is treated with anthelminthic medications such as albendazole, mebendazole, or ivermectin. The standard treatment regimen for *T. trichiura* infections typically spans three days [152]. These anthelminthic agents primarily act by inhibiting the parasite's microtubule formation and inducing paralysis of the worms, facilitating their expulsion from the host; however, they do not affect the eggs [153]. Iron supplementation may be incorporated into the treatment protocol when the infected individual exhibits anemia [154]. A 2023 study highlights the superior effectiveness of Emodepside, a veterinary drug, in treating *T. trichiura* infections compared to albendazole and placebo, even at a low dose of 5 mg. This finding suggests that Emodepside could become a promising therapeutic option for soil-transmitted helminth infections, offering improved efficacy over existing treatments (**Box 2**) [163].

4. Clinically significant intestinal helminthic parasites - Cestodes

4.1 Hymenolepis nana

Hymenolepis nana, commonly known as the dwarf tapeworm, is the smallest cestode capable of infecting humans and is considered the most prevalent tapeworm worldwide. It is estimated that up to 75 million people are carriers of this parasite [22]. The endemic regions for H. nana include Asia, southern and eastern Europe, Africa, Central, and South America [164]. In the United States and other temperate regions, the incidence of H. nana is notably higher among children and institutionalized groups due to factors such as close living quarters, poor hygiene practices, and increased opportunities for fecal-oral transmission [165].

4.1.1 Morphology of Hymenolepis nana

Hymenolepis nana is a species that exhibits a direct life cycle in which humans and rodents can serve as definitive hosts. Unlike other tapeworms, H. nana does not require an intermediate host to complete its life cycle, making it unique among cestodes [166]. Humans can acquire infection by ingesting food or water contaminated with Hymenolepis nana eggs or by accidentally ingesting insects containing the cysticercoid larva [22, 167]. When the eggs are ingested, the oncospheres contained within the eggs are released and penetrate the intestinal villi, where they develop into cysticercoid larvae [168]. The villi eventually rupture, and the cysticercoids develop into adult worms within a few weeks [169, 170]. Once maturation is complete, eggs are released and passed in the stool. The adult worm, measuring approximately 15 to 40 mm in length, resides in the human small intestine [165]. It is composed of a head, neck, and strobila. The head features four suckers and a rostellum with numerous hooklets used for penetrating the intestinal mucosa. The neck is the region where segments, known as proglottids, proliferate, and the strobila is a chain of proglottids that contain both male and female reproductive organs [22].

4.1.2 Pathogenesis of Hymenolepis nana

The eggs of *Hymenolepis nana* are both the infective and diagnostic forms of the parasite, typically ranging from 30 to 50 μm in size. These eggs have two membranes: an outer eggshell, an inner embryophore, and an oncosphere with six hooklets [165]. The outer eggshell provides protection to the developing embryo, ensuring its survival in the external environment until ingestion by a host. The inner embryophore offers an additional protective layer around the oncosphere, enhancing its stability and ensuring its readiness for infection. The oncosphere, equipped with six hooklets, is crucial for penetrating the host's intestinal wall, allowing the parasite to reach the site where it can develop into a larva [171].

The adult worm has a relatively short lifespan of about 4 to 6 weeks; however, the infection persists due to internal autoinfection [172]. Although there is limited information regarding the pathogenicity of *H. nana*, species within the genus *Hymenolepis* are well-established models in cestode research using mouse models. The lack of studies specifically analyzing the immune response to *H. nana* in humans highlights the inattention given to some neglected tropical diseases [173].

4.1.3 Clinical manifestations of Hymenolepis nana

The clinical presentation of Hymenolepis nana infection is often asymptomatic. However, symptomatic cases can present with abdominal pain, headache, diarrhea, loss of appetite, and anal pruritus [174]. Symptoms are more likely to occur when the worm burden exceeds 1000 to 2000 [175]. Approximately one-third of infected individuals develop peripheral eosinophilia greater than 5% on a white blood cell differential, which can be a useful diagnostic indicator [176].

4.1.4 Diagnosis and treatment strategies for Hymenolepis nana

The established diagnostic protocol for *hymenolepiasis* involves stool examination to identify non-bile-stained eggs characterized by polar filaments between the shell membranes [177]. Additionally, some patients may exhibit eosinophilia, with levels reaching 5% or higher [22]. Although infections with *H. nana* are generally non-severe and effectively treated, there is a potential for misdiagnosis, particularly for pinworm infections [165].

Praziquantel is the treatment of choice for *H. nana* infections in adults and children. This single-dose therapy effectively targets both adult worms and cysticercoid larvae. Alternatives, such as Niclosamide and Nitazoxanide, are available but not in the United States [178]. Recent studies have explored alternative treatments for *H. nana*. Compounds from *Leucaena leucocephala (wild tamarind)* and *Artemisia absinthium* (wormwood) have shown promising results, demonstrating efficacy comparable to praziquantel [179, 180]. These findings underscore the importance of developing new treatments to prevent potential drug resistance [181].

4.2 *Diphyllobothrium latum*

Diphyllobothrium latum, also known as the broad fish tapeworm, represents the largest cestode known to infect humans, attaining lengths over 30 feet [182, 183] . This parasitic infection is of significant global health concern, primarily due to the widespread consumption of raw or undercooked fish that may contain Diphyllobothrium larvae. With an estimated global prevalence of approximately 20 million individuals, the infection is particularly common in regions within the North Temperate and sub-Arctic zones, where the consumption of freshwater fish is prevalent [184, 185]. The surge in case reports from nonendemic regions, along with improved molecular understanding of the pathogen, has recently enhanced the focus on diphyllobothriasis.

4.2.1 Morphology of Diphyllobothrium latum

Diphyllobothrium latum, an intestinal cestode parasite, manifests in three distinct forms: the adult worm, eggs, and larvae. Morphologically, the adult worm can attain lengths of 2 to 15 meters and comprises approximately 3000 proglottids [186]. The worm is anatomically divided into a head (scolex), neck, and body (strobila). The scolex is equipped with two grooves (bothria) that facilitate attachment to the small intestines [171]. The neck, representing the proliferative end, gives rise to proglottids. The strobila comprises over 3000 segments in various immaturity, maturity, or gravidity stages. A notable characteristic of the adult D. latus worm is its distinctive rosette-shaped ovaries [187].

The eggs exhibit an oval shape with dimensions ranging from 55 to 75 μm by 40 to 50 μm. One end is marked by an operculum, while the opposite end features a small knob [186]. When freshly excreted in feces, these eggs are in an unembryonated state. In a freshwater environment, the eggs develop and hatch into the first larval stage, coracidium. Small aquatic crustaceans, such as copepods, ingest the coracidium, where it transforms into the second stage, the procercoid larva. When a fish eats the infected crustacean, the procercoid larva moves into the fish's muscles and develops into the third stage, the plerocercoid larva [188]. This plerocercoid stage is recognized as the infective form for humans [189].

4.2.2 Pathogenesis of Diphyllobothrium latum

Diphyllobothrium latum has a complex life cycle involving multiple hosts, with humans serving as the definitive hosts. Infection begins when humans consume raw or undercooked fish contaminated with plerocercoid larvae [190]. Upon ingestion, these larvae attach to the intestinal mucosa using their bothria [191]. Within the intestines, the larvae mature into adult tapeworms over several weeks, growing up to 30 feet in length and producing proglottids, which contain both male and female reproductive organs. These proglottids release eggs into the host's intestines, which are subsequently excreted with feces [192]. The tapeworm lacks a digestive system and relies on direct absorption of nutrients through its tegument, a specialized surface layer [193, 194]. This tegument is highly efficient in absorbing host nutrients, particularly vitamin B12, leading to nutrient deficiencies in the host. The parasite mediates the dissociation of the vitamin B12-intrinsic factor complex in the gut, rendering vitamin B12 unavailable to the host [195]. It has been reported that the adult cestode absorbs approximately 80% of the dietary B12 intake [184]. The tegument also plays a critical role in immune evasion by secreting substance that modulate the host's immune response, allowing the parasite to persist for years without being expelled or destroyed by the host's immune system. Furthermore, the ability of *Diphyllobothrium latum* to produce large numbers of eggs (up to 1 million per day) ensures the continued propagation of the species [170, 186].

4.2.3 Clinical manifestations of Diphyllobothrium latum

Diphyllobothriasis often presents asymptomatically; however, common symptoms include gastrointestinal discomfort, diarrhea, and vomiting. In severe cases, complications such as intestinal obstruction, cholangitis, or cholecystitis may occur [184, 196]. These infections can persist for up to 20 years [197]. The tapeworms primarily inhabit the small intestines and compete with the host for dietary vitamin B12, leading to a deficiency that result in megaloblastic anemia and neuropathy in some patients [198].

4.2.4 Diagnosis and treatment strategies for Diphyllobothrium latum

The diagnostic approach for identifying *Diphyllobothrium latum* at the family level involves microscopic examination of stool samples for eggs, typically detectable around 5 to 6 weeks post-infection [186, 199]. Further confirmation can be achieved by identifying the characteristic rosette-shaped uterus in gravid proglottids [187]. However, relying solely on morphological identification poses risks of misidentification with other flukes exhibiting similar operculate eggs.

Molecular techniques are crucial for differentiating diphyllobothriideans, particularly when morphological traits and epidemiological data overlap. Species-level identification necessitates molecular diagnostics on DNA extracted from concentrated eggs or proglottids, although this method is predominantly used for research [170]. Recent advancements, such as the pyrosequencing technique, provide a more efficient diagnostic tool with a rapid completion time of 4 hours and minimal cost [200]. This technique effectively identifies larvae, eggs, and adult stages across various taxa.

The primary treatment for *D. latum* infection is a single-dose therapy with Praziquantel, which increases the permeability of the parasite's cell membranes to calcium ions. This leads to muscle contraction and paralysis of the parasite, followed by its dislodgement and expulsion from the host's body [201]. Praziquantel is generally associated with mild side effects [202, 203]. An alternative antihelminthic treatment, Niclosamide, presents fewer side effects due to its non-absorption by the gastrointestinal tract (**Box 3**) [184].

- *Taenia solium (Pork tapeworm; Taeniasis, Cysticercosis)*

Host: Primary – Humans; Secondary – Pigs.
Transmission: Ingestion of the parasite's larval cysts (cysticerci) in undercooked and infected pork
Pathogenesis: In the human intestine, tapeworm eggs hatch into microscopic larvae (oncospheres) that burrow into the bloodstream. These larvae lodge in tissues like muscles, eyes, and the central nervous system, forming fluid-filled sacs that can cause inflammation and damage.
Clinical Manifestations: Abdominal pain, anorexia, weight loss, seizures. Pruritus, appendicitis, cholangitis from proglottid migration. Risk of neurocysticercosis.
Diagnosis: Microscopy identification of eggs and proglottids in stool; Antibody detection.
Drug of Choice: Praziquantel

- *Taenia saginata (Beef Tapeworm; Taeniasis)*

Host: Primary – Humans; Secondary – Cattle.
Transmission: Ingestion of raw/undercooked beef containing parasitic cysticerci.
Pathogenesis: Ingested cysticerci mature in the small intestine, competing for nutrients and potentially causing inflammation.
Clinical Manifestations: Mostly asymptomatic, mild abdominal discomfort, nausea, diarrhea, possible weight loss.
Diagnosis Microscopy to identify eggs or proglottids in feces; antibody detection for early stages. Species-level identification requires microscopic examination of gravid (mature) proglottids.
Drug of Choice: Praziquantel.

Box 3.
Additional Clinically Relevant Intestinal Parasitic Infections: Helminths (Cestodes) [22, 203–207].

5. Clinically significant intestinal helminthic parasites – Trematodes

5.1 Fasciolopsis buski

Fasciolopsis buski, the causative agent of fasciolopsiasis, is an intestinal trematode (fluke) that inhabits the small intestines of both humans and pigs. It is commonly referred to as the "giant intestinal fluke" as it is considered the largest intestinal fluke to infect humans. Endemic to Asia and the Indian subcontinent, individuals at heightened risk include those involved in pig farming, consumers of freshwater plants, and residents in economically challenged regions with less-than-optimal socio-cultural practices [208, 209].

Despite the lack of current global prevalence data, it has been identified as one of the most common human intestinal fluke infection [210, 211]. According to extrapolated statistics from a 1999 national survey, *F. buski* infected approximately 2 million individuals across China alone [212]. Furthermore, prior data from the CDC from 2009 indicated a frequency of up to 60% in India and mainland China [213]. Further research is needed to determine the current global frequency and epidemiology of *F. buski*.

5.1.1 Morphology of Fasciolopsis buski

Fasciolopsis buski is an intestinal trematode characterized by three distinct forms: adult worm, egg, and larva. Morphologically, the adult worm is a hermaphroditic organism, measuring between 20 and 75 mm in length, and possesses both a ventral and an oral sucker. The eggs of F. buski are unembryonated, large, and ellipsoidal, with dimensions approximately 130–150 μm in length and 60–90 μm in width [209].

The life cycle of *Fasciolopsis buski* is complex, involving three hosts: a definitive host (human or pig) and two intermediate hosts (a freshwater snail and aquatic plants). Human infection typically occurs through the ingestion of contaminated water or the consumption of plants, such as bamboo shoots, watercress, or water chestnuts, bearing infectious metacercariae [214].

In the definitive host, larvae undergo excystation within the duodenum, adhering to the intestinal wall and maturing into adult flukes over approximately three months. Adult flukes have a lifespan of about one year, during which they lay unembryonated eggs. These eggs are excreted in feces and may enter freshwater environments, where they mature and hatch, releasing miracidia that infect freshwater snails. Within the snail, larvae progress through several developmental stages to the cercariae stage, which are released and encyst as metacercariae on the surfaces of aquatic plants [209, 215].

5.1.2 *Pathogenesis of* Fasciolopsis buski

Fasciolopsis buski attaches to and ulcerates the mucosa of the proximal small bowel. Adult trematodes, which grow to approximately 20 to 75 mm in length, have a lifespan of about one year. This attachment and ulceration can induce low-grade eosinophilia [216, 217]. The clinical manifestations of infection are contingent on the parasitic load, local pathological changes, and the absorption of toxic metabolites [210].

In mild cases, infection may result in lower hematocrit and serum vitamin B12 levels [218]. This is potentially due to the organism's competitive utilization of vitamin B12 or impaired absorption from the host's damaged mucosa. More severe symptoms occur in heavy infections, where worms interfere with the normal secretion of intestinal juices, cause excessive mucus secretion, and obstruct the passage of food [214].

5.1.3 *Clinical manifestations of* Fasciolopsis buski

Fasciolopsiasis is generally asymptomatic. However, in cases of heavy infection, symptoms typically manifest 30 to 60 days post-exposure and may include anorexia, vomiting, diarrhea, abdominal pain, and signs of malabsorption. Peripheral eosinophilia can also be present [209, 210]. Severe infections can lead to significant complications such as edema and ascites due to protein loss, as well as vitamin B12 deficiency and anemia [219]. There have also been reports of acute kidney injury resulting from sub-acute intestinal obstructions caused by *Fasciolopsis buski* [220].

5.1.4 *Diagnosis and treatment strategies for* Fasciolopsis buski

The standard diagnostic method for fasciolopsiasis involves microscopic examination of stool to identify operculated eggs [221]. However, a significant limitation is that these eggs are indistinguishable from those of Fasciola hepatica, Echinostoma, and Gastrodiscoides species [222]. Diagnosis can also be confirmed by the presence of the adult fluke in stool or vomitus, although this occurrence is rare [209, 223].

Praziquantel is the preferred drug for treating *Fasciolopsis buski*, administered in three divided doses over a single day. To date, no cases of drug resistance to Praziquantel have been documented [224]. Despite this, the limited number of

- *Fasciola hepatica (Fascioliasis)*

Host: Primary – Humans and wild ruminants; Secondary – Snails.
Transmission: Ingestion of freshwater plants contaminated with metacercariae.
Pathogenesis: Metacercariae excyst in the duodenum, penetrate the intestinal wall, migrate to the liver, and mature in the biliary ducts, causing inflammation, tissue damage, and obstruction in the liver and bile ducts
Clinical Manifestations: The acute phase includes abdominal pain, nausea, vomiting, hepatomegaly, RUQ pain, malaise, fever, and cough. The chronic phase involves inflammation or blockage of bile ducts.
Diagnosis: Microscopic examination of eggs in stool, duodenal, or biliary drainage. Antibody detection.
Drug of Choice: Triclabendazole

- *Schistosoma mansoni (Intestinal Schistosomiasis)*

Hosts: Primary – Humans; Secondary – Snails.
Transmission: Skin penetration by cercariae in freshwater lakes/streams.
Pathogenesis: Cercariae penetrate human skin, transform into schistosomulae, and migrate to the lungs, heart, and liver to mature. Adult worms reside in mesenteric veins, where females deposit eggs in the portal venous system. Eggs are excreted in feces and hatch in freshwater to form miracidia, which infect snails. Snails release cercariae that penetrate human skin.
Clinical Manifestations: Cercarial dermatitis presents as a maculopapular rash within 2–3 days post-invasion. Acute schistosomiasis (Katayama Fever) occurs 4–8 weeks post-infection and includes fever, rash, cough, lymphadenopathy, hepatosplenomegaly, and eosinophilia. Chronic schistosomiasis results from eggs in the intestinal wall causing inflammation and granuloma formation.
Diagnosis: Microscopic identification of eggs in stool or urine; antibody/antigen detection.
Drug of Choice: Praziquantel

- *Paragonimus westermani (Paragonimiasis)*

Hosts: Primary – Humans/Mammals; Secondary – Snails/Crustaceans.
Transmission: Ingestion of undercooked crustaceans carrying metacercariae.
Pathogenesis: Metacercariae enter the duodenum, form cysts, and transform into larvae. Larvae penetrate the intestines, migrate to the lungs, and mature into adult worms. Adults lay eggs in the lungs, which can be swallowed and passed in stool or coughed up in sputum.
Clinical Manifestations: In the acute phase, symptoms include diarrhea, abdominal pain, fever, cough, urticaria, hepatosplenomegaly, pulmonary abnormalities, and eosinophilia. In the chronic phase, pulmonary symptoms such as cough, discolored sputum, and hemoptysis occur. Severe extrapulmonary symptoms can develop if adult worms migrate, especially to the brain.
Diagnosis: Microscopic examination of sputum or feces for eggs, antibody/antigen detection, peripheral blood eosinophilia test.
Drug of Choice: Praziquantel.

- *Opisthorchis viverrini (Opisthorchiasis)*

Hosts: Primary – Humans; Secondary – Snails.
Transmission: Ingestion of raw or undercooked freshwater fish.
Pathogenesis: Metacercariae excyst in the duodenum and ascend through hepatopancreatic ampulla into the biliary ducts, where they develop into adults. Adults reside in the biliary and pancreatic ducts, and lay eggs. Eggs are excreted in stool and contaminate freshwater, where they are ingested by snails.
Clinical Manifestations: Often asymptomatic; possible symptoms include abdominal pain, fever, diarrhea, jaundice, and hepatomegaly.
Diagnosis: Microscopic identification of eggs in stool samples.
Drug of Choice: Praziquantel.

Box 4.
Additional Clinically Relevant Intestinal Parasitic infections: Helminths (Trematodes) [22, 222, 227–238].

available drugs for this infection raises concerns about potential future drug resistance. Alternative treatments, including triclabendazole, oxyclozanide, and rafoxanide, have shown favorable responses in treating infected pigs [225].

Recent research has successfully mapped the overall transcriptome and draft genome of *Fasciolopsis buski*, representing a significant advancement in understanding the parasite [226]. This genomic information could facilitate the development of improved diagnostic tools and more effective antiparasitic agents (**Box 4**).

Author details

Jyotsna Chawla*†, Joshua Bernard† and Cyril Blavo
Dr. Kiran C. Patel College of Osteopathic Medicine, Nova Southeastern University, Clearwater, USA

*Address all correspondence to: jchawla@nova.edu

† These authors contributed equally.

References

[1] Alum A, Rubino JR, Ijaz MK. The global war against intestinal parasites—Should we use a holistic approach? International Journal of Infectious Diseases. 2010;**14**(9):e732-e738

[2] Wakid MH, Azhar EI, Zafar TA. Intestinal parasitic infection among food handlers in the Holy City of Makkah during hajj season 1428 hegira. JKAU Medical Sciences. 2009;**16**:39-52

[3] Cleaveland S, Laurenson MK, Taylor LH. Diseases of humans and their domestic mammals: Pathogen characteristics, host range and the risk of emergence. Philosophical Transactions of the Royal Society of London. Series B: Biological Sciences. 2001;**356**(1411): 991-999

[4] Feleke DG et al. Intestinal parasitic infections and associated factors among street dwellers and prison inmates: A systematic review and meta-analysis. PLoS One. 2021;**16**(8):e0255641

[5] Wharton B. Diseases of children in the subtropics and tropics. Archives of Disease in Childhood. 1991;**66**(11): 1367-1367

[6] Egwunyenga OA, Ataikiru DP. Soil-transmitted helminthiasis among school age children in Ethiope east local government area, Delta state, Nigeria. African Journal of Biotechnology. 2005; **4**:938-941

[7] Obiukwu MO, Umeanaeto PU, Eneanya CI, Nworgu GO. Prevalence of gastro-intestinal helminth in school children in Mbaukwu, Anambra state, Nigeria. Annals of Tropical Medicine and Parasitology. 2008;**29**(1):705-713

[8] Eyayu T et al. Prevalence of intestinal parasitic infections and associated factors among patients attending at Sanja primary hospital, Northwest Ethiopia: An institutional-based cross-sectional study. PLoS One. 2021;**16**(2):e0247075

[9] Dunn N, Juergens A. Giardiasis. In: StatPearls. Treasure Island: StatPearls Publishing; 2019

[10] Buret AG et al. Giardia duodenalis: New research developments in pathophysiology, pathogenesis, and virulence factors. Current Tropical Medicine Reports. 2015;**2**(3):110-118

[11] Takaoka K et al. Incidence rate and risk factors for giardiasis and strongyloidiasis in returning UK travellers. Journal of Travel Medicine. 2016;**23**(5):taw050

[12] España-Cueto S et al. Epidemiological and clinical profile of adult patients with diarrhoea after international travel attended in an international health referral center. Travel Medicine and Infectious Disease. 2022;**45**:102216

[13] Adam RD. Giardia duodenalis: Biology and pathogenesis. Clinical Microbiology Reviews. 2021;**34**(4): e00024-19

[14] Nosala C, Dawson SC. The critical role of the cytoskeleton in the pathogenesis of giardia. Current Clinical Microbiology Reports. 2015;**2**(4):155-162

[15] Ortega YR, Adam RD. Giardia: Overview and update. Clinical Infectious Diseases. 1997;**25**(3):545-549

[16] Rajurkar MN. A simple method for demonstrating the giardia Lamblia Trophozoite. Journal of Clinical and Diagnostic Research. 2012;**6**(9): 1492-1494

[17] Biswal D, Mirdha B. Falling-leaf motility of Giardia lamblia. New England Journal of Medicine. 2023;**388**(22):e73

[18] Maa'Ayeh S, Svärd S. Giardia and Giardiasis. Amsterdam, Netherlands: Elsevier; 2024. pp. 3107-3119

[19] Ahmed M. Intestinal parasitic infections in 2023. Gastroenterology Research. 2023;**16**(3):127-140

[20] Tejan N et al. Trends and clinico-epidemiological profile of patients with giardiasis: Five-year experience from a university hospital of northern India. Journal of Family Medicine and Primary Care. 2023;**12**(10):2451-2455

[21] Di Genova BM, Tonelli RR. Infection strategies of intestinal parasite pathogens and host cell responses. Frontiers in Microbiology. 2016;**7**. Article 245

[22] Sastry AS, Bhat S. Essentials of Medical Parasitology. New Delhi: Jaypee Brothers Medical Publishers LTD (JP Medical Ltd); 2014. p. 51, 129, 127,131, 27, 226, 184, 185, 186, 167-175, 204-206, 198-201, 216-219, 208-210

[23] Faubert G. Immune response to Giardia duodenalis. 2000;**13**(1):35-54

[24] Escobedo AA et al. Sexual transmission of giardiasis: A neglected route of spread? Acta Tropica. 2014;**132**: 106-111

[25] Katz DE et al. Prolonged outbreak of giardiasis with two modes of transmission. Epidemiology and Infection. 2006;**134**(5):935-941

[26] Vivancos V et al. Giardiasis: Characteristics, pathogenesis and new insights about treatment. Current Topics in Medicinal Chemistry. 2018;**18**(15): 1287-1303

[27] Amin N. Giardiasis. Postgraduate Medicine. 1979;**66**(5):151-158

[28] Einarsson E, Maa'Ayeh S, Svärd SG. An up-date on giardia and giardiasis. Current Opinion in Microbiology. 2016; **34**:47-52

[29] Leder K. Patient education: Giardia (beyond the basics). In: UpToDate. Waltham, MA: UpToDate; 2023 [Accessed: January 2, 2024]

[30] Farthing MJG. GIARDIASIS. Gastroenterology Clinics of North America. 1996;**25**(3):493-515

[31] Fekete E et al. Giardia duodenalis cysteine proteases cleave proteinase-activated receptor-2 to regulate intestinal goblet cell mucin gene expression. International Journal for Parasitology. 2022;**52**(5):285-292

[32] Heresi GP, Murphy JR, Cleary TG. Giardiasis. Seminars in Pediatric Infectious Diseases. 2000;**11**(3):189-195

[33] Gardner TB, Hill DR. Treatment of giardiasis. Clinical Microbiology Reviews. 2001;**14**(1):114-128

[34] Fantinatti M, Gonçalves-Pinto M, Da-Cruz AM. Can Giardia lamblia assemblages drive the clinical outcome of giardiasis? Current Tropical Medicine Reports. 2022;**9**(4):101-106

[35] Dixon BR. Giardia duodenalis in humans and animals – Transmission and disease. Research in Veterinary Science. 2021;**135**:283-289

[36] Prevention, C.f.D.C.a. Clinical Testing and Diagnosis for Giardia Infection. 2024. Available from: https://www.cdc.gov/giardia/hcp/diagnosis-testing/

[37] Groudan K et al. Giardia lamblia diagnosed incidentally by duodenal biopsy. Journal of Investigative Medicine

High Impact Case Reports. 2021;**9**: 232470962110016

[38] Meningher T et al. Giardia lamblia miRNAs as a new diagnostic tool for human giardiasis. PLoS Neglected Tropical Diseases. 2019;**13**(6):e0007398

[39] Argüello-García R et al. Drug resistance in giardia: mechanisms and alternative treatments for giardiasis. In: Advances in Parasitology. Amsterdam, Netherlands: Elsevier; 2020. pp. 201-282

[40] Abraham RJ et al. Aminoguanidines: New leads for treatment of giardia duodenalis infection. International Journal for Parasitology: Drugs and Drug Resistance. 2019;**10**:38-44

[41] Painter JE et al. Evolving epidemiology of reported cryptosporidiosis cases in the United States, 1995–2012. Epidemiology and Infection. 2016;**144**(8):1792-1802

[42] Yang X et al. Molecular epidemiology of human cryptosporidiosis in low- and middle-income countries. Clinical Microbiology Reviews. 2021;**34**(2):e00087-19

[43] Centers for Disease Control and Prevention, Michele Hlavsa, Dawn Roellig. Cryptosporidiosis CDC Yellow Book 2024. 2024. Available from: https://wwwnc.cdc.gov/travel/yellowbook/2024/infections-diseases/cryptosporidiosis

[44] Rossle NF, Latif B. Cryptosporidiosis as threatening health problem: A review. Asian Pacific Journal of Tropical Biomedicine. 2013;**3**(11):916-924

[45] Bouzid M et al. Cryptosporidium pathogenicity and virulence. Clinical Microbiology Reviews. 2013;**26**(1): 115-134

[46] O'Hara SP, Chen X-M. The cell biology of cryptosporidium infection. Microbes and Infection. 2011;**13**(8–9): 721-730

[47] Tzipori S, Ward H. Cryptosporidiosis: Biology, pathogenesis and disease. Microbes and Infection. 2002;**4**(10):1047-1058

[48] Shirley D-AT, Moonah SN, Kotloff KL. Burden of disease from cryptosporidiosis. Current Opinion in Infectious Diseases. 2012;**25**(5):555-563

[49] Mead JR. Early immune and host cell responses to cryptosporidium infection. Frontiers in Parasitology. 2023;**2**

[50] Korich DG et al. Effects of ozone, chlorine dioxide, chlorine, and monochloramine on Cryptosporidium parvum oocyst viability. Applied and Environmental Microbiology. 1990;**56**(5):1423-1428

[51] Chalmers RM. Cryptosporidium. Amsterdam, Netherlands: Elsevier; 2014. pp. 533-545

[52] O'Connor RM et al. Expression of the highly polymorphic Cryptosporidium parvum Cpgp40/15 gene in genotype I and II isolates. Molecular and Biochemical Parasitology. 2002;**119**(2): 203-215

[53] Dhal AK et al. An update on cryptosporidium biology and therapeutic avenues. Journal of Parasitic Diseases. 2022;**46**(3):923-939

[54] Laurent F et al. Pathogenesis of infection. Microbes and Infection. 1999;**1**(2):141-148

[55] Kumar H et al. Pulmonary cryptosporidiosis in an immunocompetent host treated

successfully with nitazoxanide. Lung India. 2016;**33**(1):69

[56] Fayer R, Ungar B. Cryptosporidium spp. and cryptosporidiosis. Microbiological Reviews. 1986;**50**(4): 458-483

[57] Fahey T. Cryptosporidiosis. Primary Care Update for OB/GYNS. 2003;**10**(2): 75-80

[58] Gerace E, Presti VDML, Biondo C. Cryptosporidium infection: Epidemiology, pathogenesis, and differential diagnosis. European Journal of Microbiology and Immunology. 2019; **9**(4):119-123

[59] Khurana S, Chaudhary P. Laboratory diagnosis of cryptosporidiosis. Tropical. Parasitology. 2018;**8**(1):2

[60] Ahmed SA, Karanis P. Comparison of current methods used to detect cryptosporidium oocysts in stools. International Journal of Hygiene and Environmental Health. 2018;**221**(5): 743-763

[61] Prevention, C.f.D.C.a. Stool Specimens – Staining Procedures. 2016. Available from: https://www.cdc.gov/dpdx/diagnosticprocedures/stool/staining.html

[62] Checkley W et al. A review of the global burden, novel diagnostics, therapeutics, and vaccine targets for cryptosporidium. The Lancet Infectious Diseases. 2015;**15**(1):85-94

[63] Amadi B et al. High dose prolonged treatment with nitazoxanide is not effective for cryptosporidiosis in HIV positive Zambian children: A randomised controlled trial. BMC Infectious Diseases. 2009;**9**(1):195

[64] Maggi P et al. Effect of antiretroviral therapy on cryptosporidiosis and Microsporidiosis in patients infected with human immunodeficiency virus type 1. European Journal of Clinical Microbiology Infectious Diseases. 2000; **19**(3):213-217

[65] O'Leary JK, Sleator RD, Lucey B. Cryptosporidium spp. diagnosis and research in the 21st century. Food and waterborne. Parasitology. 2021;**24**: e00131

[66] Vinayak S et al. Genetic modification of the diarrhoeal pathogen Cryptosporidium parvum. Nature. 2015; **523**(7561):477-480

[67] Solaymani-Mohammadi S, Petri WA. Intestinal Invasion by Entamoeba histolytica. New York: Springer; 2008. pp. 221-232

[68] Ximénez C et al. Human Amebiasis: Breaking the paradigm? International Journal of Environmental Research and Public Health. 2010;7(3):1105-1120

[69] El-Dib NA. Entamoeba histolytica: An overview. Current Tropical Medicine Reports. 2017;**4**(1):11-20

[70] Kawashima A et al. Amebiasis as a sexually transmitted infection: A re-emerging health problem in developed countries. Global Health Medicine. 2023; **5**(6):319-327

[71] Kantor M et al. Entamoeba Histolytica: Updates in clinical manifestation, pathogenesis, and vaccine development. Canadian Journal of Gastroenterology and Hepatology. 2018; **2018**:1-6

[72] Prevention, C.f.D.C.a. Laboratory Diagnosis of Amebiasis *Entamoeba histolytica* and Entamoeba Dispar. Available from: https://www.cdc.gov/

dpdx/resources/pdf/benchaids/entamoeba_benchaid.pdf

[73] Tanyuksel M, Petri WA. Laboratory diagnosis of Amebiasis. Clinical Microbiology Reviews. 2003;**16**(4):713-729

[74] Fotedar R et al. Laboratory diagnostic techniques for Entamoeba species. Clinical Microbiology Reviews. 2007;**20**(3):511-532

[75] Barron Gonzalez M et al. Entamoeba histolytica: Trophozoite, Precyst and Cyst Studied by Atomic Force Microscopy. Badajoz, Spain: Formatex; 2014. pp. 153-160

[76] Que X, Reed SL. Cysteine proteinases and the pathogenesis of amebiasis. Clinical Microbiology Reviews. 2000;**13**(2):196-206

[77] Nakada-Tsukui K, Nozaki T. Immune response of Amebiasis and immune evasion by Entamoeba histolytica. Frontiers in Immunology. 2016;**7**. Article 175

[78] Hecht O et al. Solution structure of the pore-forming protein of Entamoeba histolytica. Journal of Biological Chemistry. 2004;**279**(17):17834-17841

[79] Berninghausen O, Leippe M. Necrosis versus apoptosis as the mechanism of target cell death induced by Entamoeba histolytica. Infection and Immunity. 1997;**65**(9):3615-3621

[80] Bercu TE, Petri WA, Behm BW. Amebic colitis: New insights into pathogenesis and treatment. Current Gastroenterology Reports. 2007;**9**(5):429-433

[81] Cornick S, Chadee K. Entamoeba histolytic: Host parasite interactions at the colonic epithelium. Tissue Barriers. 2017;**5**(1):e1283386

[82] Arthur Chou RLA. Entamoeba histolytica infection. In: StatPearls. Treasure Island (FL): StatPearls Publishing; 2023

[83] Espinosa-Cantellano M, Martinez-Palomo A. Pathogenesis of intestinal amebiasis: From molecules to disease. Clinical Microbiology Reviews. 2000;**13**(2):318-331

[84] Anesi JA, Gluckman S. Amebic liver abscess. Clinical Liver Disease. 2015;**6**(2):41-43

[85] Shamsuzzaman SM, Hashiguchi Y. Thoracic amebiasis. Clinics in Chest Medicine. 2002;**23**(2):479-492

[86] Stanley SL. Amoebiasis. The Lancet. 2003;**361**(9362):1025-1034

[87] Saensiriphan S et al. First report of genitourinary amoebiasis in Thailand. Tropical Biomedicine. 2015;**32**(3):551-553

[88] Prieto-Granada CN, Lobo AZC, Mihm MC. Skin Infections. Amsterdam, Netherlands: Elsevier; 2010. pp. 519-616

[89] Reyes-López M et al. Hemoglobin uptake and utilization by human protozoan parasites: A review. Frontiers in Cellular and Infection Microbiology. 2023;**13**

[90] Prevention, C.f.D.C.a. Amebiasis. 2019. Available from: https://www.cdc.gov/dpdx/amebiasis/index.html

[91] Diamond LS, Clark CG. A Redescription of Entamoeba Histolytica Schaudinn, 1903 (emended Walker, 1911) separating it from Entamoeba Dispar Brumpt, 19251. Journal of Eukaryotic Microbiology. 1993;**40**(3):340-344

[92] Gonzales MLM, Dans LF, Sio-Aguilar J. Antiamoebic drugs for treating

amoebic colitis. Cochrane Database of Systematic Reviews. 2019;**1**(1). Article number: CD006085

[93] Centers for Disease Control and Prevention, Jennifer Cope, Ibne Ali. Amebiasis CDC Yellow Book 2024. 2023. Available from: https://wwwnc.cdc.gov/travel/yellowbook/2024/infections-diseases/amebiasis

[94] Schuster FL, Ramirez-Avila L. Current world status of *Balantidium coli*. Clinical Microbiology Reviews. 2008;**21**(4):626-638

[95] Ortega YR, Cama VA. *Cystoisospora Belli* and *Sarcocystis Spp*. Cham, Switzerland: Springer International Publishing; 2018. pp. 57-72

[96] Prevention, C.f.D.C.a. Cystoisosporiasis. 2024. Available from: https://www.cdc.gov/dpdx/cystoisosporiasis/

[97] Dubey JP, Khan A, Rosenthal BM. Life cycle and transmission of Cyclospora cayetanensis: Knowns and unknowns. Microorganisms. 2022;**10**(1):118

[98] Almeria S, Cinar HN, Dubey JP. Cyclospora cayetanensis and Cyclosporiasis: An update. Microorganisms. 2019;**7**(9):317

[99] Centers for Disease Control and Prevention, Shannon M. Casillas, Carolyne Bennett, Anne Straily. Notes from the Field: Multiple Cyclosporiasis Outbreaks — United States, 2018. 2018. Available from: https://www.cdc.gov/mmwr/volumes/67/wr/mm6739a6.htm.

[100] Wendt S et al. The Diagnosis and Treatment of Pinworm Infection. Deutsches Ärzteblatt international. Cologne, Germany: Deutscher Ärzte-Verlag GmbH; 2019

[101] Prevention, C.f.D.C.a. Enterobiasis. 2019. Available from: https://www.cdc.gov/dpdx/enterobiasis/index.html

[102] Ali WAM. Enterobius Vermicularis infection: Prevalence and risk factors among primary school children in Al-mudhafar Directorate, Taiz, Republic of Yemen. Enhanced Knowledge in Sciences and Technology. 2022;**2**(1). Article number: CD006085

[103] Norhayati M et al. Intestinal parasitic infections in man: A review. Medical Journal of Malaysia. 2003;**58**(2):296-305

[104] Lohiya GS. Epidemiology and control of enterobiasis in a developmental center. Western Journal of Medicine. 2000;**172**(5):305-308

[105] Rawla P, Sharma S. Enterobius Vermicularis. In: StatPearls. Treasure Island (FL): StatPearls Publishing; 2024

[106] Khayyat R et al. Prevalence of and risk factors for Enterobius vermicularis infestation in preschool children, West Bank, Palestine, 2015. Eastern Mediterranean Health Journal. 2021;**27**(11):1052-1060

[107] MacGowan J. The Human Pinworm *Enterobius vermicularis* (Linnaeus, 1758) Leach 1853. Gainesville, Florida: Florida Department of Agriculture and Consumer Services, Division of Plant Industry; 1976

[108] Croonen B et al. Peritoneal lesions caused by Enterobius vermicularis suspected to be metastases of ovarian malignancy. BMJ Case Reports. 2021;**14**(7):e238618

[109] Burkhart CN, Burkhart CG. Assessment of frequency, transmission, and genitourinary complications of enterobiasis (pinworms). International

Journal of Dermatology. 2005;**44**(10): 837-840

[110] Centers for Disease Control and Prevention, Rebecca Chancey, Mary Kamb. Enterobiasis/Pinworm CDC Yellow Book 2024. 2023. Available from: https://wwwnc.cdc.gov/travel/yellowbook/2024/infections-diseases/enterobiasis-pinworm

[111] Cross JH. Enteric nematodes of humans. In: Baron S, editor. Medical Microbiology. Galveston (TX): University of Texas Medical Branch at Galveston; 1996

[112] Cook GC. Enterobius vermicularis infection. Gut. 1994;**35**(9):1159-1162

[113] Khubchandani IT, Bub DS. Parasitic infections. Clinics in Colon and Rectal Surgery. 2019;**32**(5):364-371

[114] Eder TIB, Wendt S, Lipek T. Extraintestinal Oxyuriasis. Deutsches Ärzteblatt International. 2018;**115**(18):326

[115] Akhigbe T et al. Pinworm and appendicitis in children. International Journal of Surgery. 2013;**30**(3):1-4

[116] Vleeschouwers W et al. Appendicitis-like clinical image elicited by Enterobius vermicularis: Case report and review of the literature. Acta Chirurgica Belgica. 2013;**113**(2):139-142

[117] Patsantara GG et al. Immune responses in children infected with the pinwormEnterobius vermicularisin Central Greece. Journal of Helminthology. 2016;**90**(3):337-341

[118] Al-Daoody AAK, Al-Bazzaz ENH. Impact of Enterobius vermicularis infection on biochemical parameters in the blood of children in Erbil Province, Iraq. BMC Infectious Diseases. 2020;**20** (1):1-6

[119] Essawy MA et al. IgE level in parasitic diseases before and after specific therapy. Journal of the Egyptian Society of Parasitology. 1989;**19**(1): 315-326

[120] Delıalıoğlu N et al. Total serum IgE levels in children with enterobiasis. Türkiye Parazitolojii Dergisi. 2005;**29** (3):180-182

[121] Kubiak K, Dzika E, Paukszto Ł. Enterobiasis epidemiology and molecular characterization of Enterobius vermicularis in healthy children in North-Eastern Poland. Helminthologia. 2017;**54**(4):284-291

[122] Song HJ et al. Prevalence and risk factors for enterobiasis among preschool children in a metropolitan city in Korea. Parasitology Research. 2003;**91**(1):46-50

[123] Serpytis M, Seinin D. Fatal case of ectopic enterobiasis: Enterobius vermicularis in the kidneys. Scandinavian Journal of Urology and Nephrology. 2012;**46**(1):70-72

[124] Pampiglione S, Rivasi F. Enterobiasis in ectopic locations mimicking tumor-like lesions. International Journal of Microbiology. 2009;**2009**:642481

[125] Taghipour A et al. The Neglected Role of Enterobius Vermicularis in Appendicitis: A Systematic Review and Meta-Analysis. San Francisco, California: PLoS One: Public Library of Science (PLOS); 2020;**15**(4):e0232143

[126] Shoup B. Diagnosis and management of pinworm infection. Primary Care Update for OB/GYNS. 2001;**8**(6):240-243

[127] Prevention, C.f.D.C.a. Diagnosing Pinworms. 2024. Available from: https://

www.cdc.gov/pinworm/diagnosing/index.html

[128] Kaneva E et al. Development and application of a method for genetic detection of enterobius vermicularis in samples of patients with enterobiasis. Journal of IMAB - Annual Proceeding (Scientific Papers). 2024;**30**(1): 4295-5300

[129] Shears RK et al. Vaccination against whipworm: Identification of potential immunogenic proteins in Trichuris muris excretory/secretory material. Scientific Reports. 2018;**8**(1). Article number: 4508

[130] Azira NM, Zeehaida M. Severe chronic iron deficiency anaemia secondary to Trichuris dysentery syndrome - a case report. Tropical Biomedicine. 2012;**29**(4):626-631

[131] Viswanath A, Yarrarapu SNS, Williams M. Trichuris Trichiura Infection, in StatPearls. Treasure Island (FL): StatPearls Publishing; 2024

[132] Else KJ et al. Whipworm and roundworm infections. Nature Reviews Disease Primers. 2020;**6**(1). Article number: 44

[133] Yusof AM. Intestinal parasites infection in vegetables: A mini. SagepublisherCom. 2020;**16**(01):49-55

[134] Bogitsh BJ, Carter CE, Oeltmann TN. Intestinal Nematodes. Amsterdam, Netherlands: Elsevier; 2019. pp. 277-311

[135] Parasitology, A.S.f. Trichuris. Classification: Taxonomic Ranks Under Review (cf. Encyclopedic Reference of Parasitology, 2001, Springer-Verlag). Available from: https://www.parasite.org.au/para-site/text/trichuris-text.html

[136] Rivero J, Cutillas C, Callejón R. Trichuris trichiura (Linnaeus, 1771) from human and non-human primates: Morphology, biometry, host specificity, molecular characterization, and phylogeny. Frontiers in Veterinary Science. 2021;**7**. Article number: 626120

[137] Prevention, C.f.D.C.a. Trichuriasis. 2024. Available from: https://www.cdc.gov/dpdx/trichuriasis/index.html

[138] Joo JH et al. Colonoscopic diagnosis of whipworm infection. Hepato-Gastroenterology. 1998;**45**(24):2105-2109

[139] Yamamoto S, Kalepouris A. Trichuris trichiura in the colon. Clinical Gastroenterology and Hepatology. 2020; **18**(10):e116

[140] Brooker SJ, Bundy DAP. Soil-Transmitted Helminths (Geohelminths). Amsterdam, Netherlands: Elsevier; 2014. pp. 766-794.e4

[141] Beer RJS. The relationship between Trichuris trichiura (Linnaeus 1758) of man and Trichuris suis (Schrank 1788) of the pig. Research in Veterinary Science. 1976;**20**(1):47-54

[142] Schachter J et al. Whipworm infection promotes bacterial invasion, intestinal microbiota imbalance, and cellular immunomodulation. Infection and Immunity. 2020;**88**(3):1-24

[143] Diniz-Santos DR et al. Massive Trichuris trichiura infection as a cause of chronic bloody Diarrhea in a child. Journal of Tropical Pediatrics. 2006;**52** (1):66-68

[144] Stephenson LS, Holland CV, Cooper ES. The public health significance of Trichuris trichiura. Parasitology. 2000;**121**(S1):S73-S95

[145] Hechenbleikner E, McQuade J. Parasitic colitis. Clinics in Colon and Rectal Surgery. 2015;**28**(02):079-086

[146] Ok K-S et al. Trichuris trichiura infection diagnosed by colonoscopy: Case reports and review of literature. The Korean Journal of Parasitology. 2009;**47**(3):275

[147] Brummaier T et al. Improved detection of intestinal helminth infections with a formalin ethyl-acetate-based concentration technique compared to a crude formalin concentration technique. Tropical Medicine and Infectious Disease. 2021;**6**(2):51

[148] Prevention, C.f.D.C.a. Stool Specimens – Specimen Processing. 2016. Available from: https://www.cdc.gov/dpdx/diagnosticprocedures/stool/specimenproc.html

[149] Bosch F et al. Diagnosis of soil-transmitted helminths using the Kato-Katz technique: What is the influence of stirring, storage time and storage temperature on stool sample egg counts? PLoS Neglected Tropical Diseases. 2021;**15**(1):e0009032

[150] Whittier L. TRICHURIASIS IN children. American Journal of Diseases of Children. 1945;**70**(5):289

[151] Manz KM. New advances in the treatment of Trichuriasis. Current Treatment Options in Infectious Diseases. 2018;**10**(3):362-372

[152] Prevention, C.f.D.C.a. Clinical Care of Soil-transmitted Helminths. 2024. Available from: https://www.cdc.gov/sth/hcp/clinical-care/index.html

[153] Albendazole. LiverTox: Clinical and Research Information on Drug-Induced Liver Injury. Bethesda (MD): National Institute of Diabetes and Digestive and Kidney Diseases; 2012

[154] Jourdan PM et al. Soil-transmitted helminth infections. The Lancet. 2018;**391**(10117):252-265

[155] de Lima Corvino DF, Horrall S. Ascariasis. In: StatPearls. Treasure Island (FL): StatPearls Publishing Copyright © 2024, StatPearls Publishing LLC; 2024

[156] Shah J, Shahidullah A. Ascaris lumbricoides: A startling discovery during screening colonoscopy. Case Reports in Gastroenterology. 2018;**12**(2):224-229

[157] Ghodeif AO, Jain H. Hookworm. In: StatPearls. Treasure Island (FL): StatPearls Publishing; 2024

[158] Prevention, C.f.D.C.a. Hookworm (Intestinal). 2019. Available from: https://www.cdc.gov/dpdx/hookworm/index.html

[159] Prevention, C.f.D.C.a. Strongyloidiasis. 2019. Available from: https://www.cdc.gov/dpdx/strongyloidiasis/index.html

[160] Jonker FAM et al. Real-time PCR demonstrates Ancylostoma duodenale is a key factor in the Etiology of severe Anemia and iron deficiency in Malawian pre-school children. PLoS Neglected Tropical Diseases. 2012;**6**(3):e1555

[161] Loukas A et al. Hookworm infection. Nature Reviews Disease Primers. 2016;**2**(1):16088

[162] Aziz MH, Ramphul K. Ancylostoma. In: StatPearls. Treasure Island (FL): StatPearls Publishing; 2024

[163] Mrimi EC et al. Emodepside for Trichuris trichiura and hookworm infection. New England Journal of Medicine. 2023;**388**(20):1863-1875

[164] King CH, Fairley JK. Tapeworms (Cestodes). Amsterdam, Netherlands: Elsevier; 2015. pp. 3227-3236.e1

[165] Prevention, C.f.D.C.a. Hymenolepiasis. 2024. Available from: https://www.cdc.gov/dpdx/hymenolepiasis/index.html

[166] Muehlenbachs A et al. Malignant transformation of Hymenolepis nana in a human host. New England Journal of Medicine. 2015;**373**(19):1845-1852

[167] Coello Peralta RD et al. Hymenolepiasis caused by Hymenolepis nana in humans and natural infection in rodents in a marginal urban sector of Guayaquil, Ecuador. American Journal of Case Reports. 2023;**24**:1-6

[168] Held M, Cappello M. Cestodes. Amsterdam, Netherlands: Elsevier; 2004. pp. 289-293

[169] Spinicci M et al. Hymenolepis nana-an emerging intestinal parasite associated with Anemia in school children from the Bolivian Chaco. The American Journal of Tropical Medicine and Hygiene. 2018;**99**(6):1598-1601

[170] Mega JD, Galdos-Cardenas G, Gilman RH. Tapeworm Infections. Amsterdam, Netherlands: Elsevier; 2013. pp. 895-902

[171] Heyneman, D., Cestodes, in Medical Microbiology, S. Baron, Editor. 1996, University of Texas Medical Branch at Galveston Galveston (TX).

[172] Elliott DE. Intestinal Infections by Parasitic Worms. Amsterdam, Netherlands: Elsevier; 2010. pp. 1921-1939.e5

[173] Hench J, Cathomas G, Dettmer MS. Hymenolepis nana: A case report of a perfect IBD camouflage warrior. Medicine (Baltimore). 2017;**96**(50): e9146

[174] Goudarzi F et al. A systematic review and meta-analysis of Hymenolepis nana in human and rodent hosts in Iran: A remaining public health concern. Comparative Immunology, Microbiology and Infectious Diseases. 2021;**74**:101580

[175] Kim BJ et al. Heavy Hymenolepis nana infection possibly through organic foods: Report of a case. The Korean Journal of Parasitology. 2014;**52**(1):85-87

[176] Feldman SH, Easton DN. Occupational Health and Safety. Amsterdam, Netherlands: Elsevier; 2006. pp. 565-586

[177] Nkouawa A et al. Cryptic diversity in hymenolepidid tapeworms infecting humans. Parasitology International. 2016;**65**(2):83-86

[178] Prevention, C.f.D.C.a. Clinical Care of Hymenolepiasis (Dwarf Tapeworm). 2024. Available from: https://www.cdc.gov/hymenolepis/hcp/clinical-care/index.html.

[179] Ma Y-H et al. Therapeutic effect and immune changes after treatment of Hymenolepis nana-infected BALB/c mice with compounds isolated from Leucaena leucocephala. Veterinary Sciences. 2022;**9**(7):368

[180] Beshay EVN. Therapeutic efficacy of Artemisia absinthium against Hymenolepis nana: in vitro and in vivo studies in comparison with the anthelmintic praziquantel. Journal of Helminthology. 2018;**92**(3):298-308

[181] Li JWH, Vederas JC. Drug discovery and natural products: End of an era or an endless frontier? Science. 2009;**325**(5937):161-165

[182] Diemert DJ. Cestode and Trematode Infections. Amsterdam, Netherlands: Elsevier; 2017. pp. 1032-1037.e1

[183] Prevention, C.f.D.C.a. About Diphyllobothrium. 2024. Available from: https://www.cdc.gov/diphyllobothrium/about/index.html.

[184] Scholz T et al. Update on the human broad tapeworm (genus Diphyllobothrium), including clinical relevance. Clinical Microbiology Reviews. 2009;**22**(1):146-160

[185] Wittner M, Tanowitz HB. Taenia and Other Tapeworms. Amsterdam, Netherlands: Elsevier; 1996. pp. 1327-1340

[186] Prevention, C.f.D.C.a. Diphyllobothriasis. 2019. Available from: https://www.cdc.gov/dpdx/diphyllobothriasis/index.html

[187] Choi H-J, Lee J, Yang H-J. Four human cases of Diphyllobothrium latum infection. The Korean Journal of Parasitology. 2012;**50**(2):143-146

[188] Durrani MI, Basit H, Blazar E. Diphyllobothriasis (fish tapeworm infection). In: StatPearls. Treasure Island (FL): StatPearls Publishing; 2024

[189] Murrell KD. Helminths and Nematodes. Amsterdam, Netherlands: Elsevier; 1999. pp. 1052-1058

[190] Jackson Y et al. Diphyllobothrium latum outbreak from marinated raw perch, Lake Geneva, Switzerland. Emerging Infectious Diseases. 2007;**13**(12):1957-1958

[191] Ivan G, Horak AAM, Colwell DD. Platyhelminthes. Amsterdam, Netherlands: Elsevier; 2019. pp. 1-133

[192] Bowman N, Donroe J, Gilman R. Cestodes. US: Springer; 2006. pp. 197-229

[193] Caira JN, Jensen K. Electron microscopy reveals novel external specialized organs housing bacteria in eagle ray tapeworms. PLoS One. 2021;**16**(1):e0244586

[194] Ríos-Valencia DG et al. What about the cytoskeletal and related proteins of tapeworms in the Host's immune response? An integrative overview. Pathogens. 2023;**12**(6). Article number: 840

[195] Maithel S et al. An unusual cause of vitamin B12 and iron deficiency. Cleveland Clinic Journal of Medicine. 2015;**82**(7):406-408

[196] Sharma K, Wijarnpreecha K, Merrell N. Diphyllobothrium latum mimicking subacute appendicitis. Gastroenterology Research. 2018;**11**(3):235-237

[197] Raether W, Hanel H. Epidemiology, clinical manifestations and diagnosis of zoonotic cestode infections: An update. Parasitology Research. 2003;**91**(5):412-438

[198] Leder K, Weller PF. Parasitic Diseases, Nervous System Effects. Amsterdam, Netherlands: Elsevier; 2017

[199] Cong W, Elsheikha HM. Biology, epidemiology, clinical features, diagnosis, and treatment of selected fish-borne parasitic Zoonoses. The Yale Journal of Biology and Medicine. 2021;**94**(2):297-309

[200] Thanchomnang T et al. Rapid identification of nine species of diphyllobothriidean tapeworms by pyrosequencing. Scientific Reports. 2016;**6**(1):37228

[201] Esmat G, Zayed N, Elbaz TM. Parasitic Liver Disease. Amsterdam, Netherlands: Elsevier; 2018. pp. 568-578.e4

[202] Erko B et al. Efficacy and side effects of praziquantel in the treatment of schistosomiasis mansoni in schoolchildren in Shesha Kekele elementary school, Wondo genet, southern Ethiopia. Asian Pacific Journal of Tropical Biomedicine. 2012;**2**(3): 235-239

[203] Cioli D, Pica-Mattoccia L. Praziquantel. Parasitology Research. 2003;**90**(S1):S3-S9

[204] Prevention, C.f.D.C.a. Cysticercosis. 2019. Available from: https://www.cdc.gov/dpdx/cysticercosis/index.html

[205] Prevention, C.f.D.C.a. Taeniasis. 2024. Available from: https://www.cdc.gov/dpdx/taeniasis/index.html

[206] Prevention, C.f.D.C.a. Clinical Treatment of Taeniasis. 2024. Available from: https://www.cdc.gov/taeniasis/hcp/clinical-care/index.html

[207] Mathison BA, Pritt BS. Parasites of the Gastrointestinal Tract. Amsterdam, Netherlands: Elsevier; 2022. pp. 136-203

[208] Saikia D et al. Fasciolopsis buski detected in humans in Bihar and pigs in Assam, India. Emerging Infectious Diseases. 2022;**28**(6):1265-1268

[209] Prevention, C.F.D.C.a. Fasciolopsiasis. 2024. Available from: https://www.cdc.gov/dpdx/fasciolopsiasis/index.html

[210] Wu X et al. Case report: Surgical intervention for Fasciolopsis buski infection: A literature review. The American Journal of Tropical Medicine and Hygiene. 2020;**103**(6):2282-2287

[211] UpToDate; Karin Leder, Peter F. Weller. Intestinal Flukes. 2023. Available from: https://www.uptodate.com/contents/intestinal-flukes/print

[212] Lv S et al. Water-related parasitic diseases in China. International Journal of Environmental Research and Public Health. 2013;**10**(5):1977-2016

[213] Biswal DK et al. An integrated pipeline for next generation sequencing and annotation of the complete mitochondrial genome of the giant intestinal fluke, Fasciolopsis buski (Lankester, 1857) Looss, 1899. PeerJ. 2013;**1**:e207

[214] Mas-Coma S, Bargues MD, Valero MA. Human fascioliasis infection sources, their diversity, incidence factors, analytical methods and prevention measures. Parasitology. 2018; **145**(13):1665-1699

[215] Jones BF, Cappello M. Trematodes. Amsterdam, Netherlands: Elsevier; 2004. pp. 523-526

[216] Sripa B et al. Food-Borne Trematodiases in Southeast Asia. Amsterdam, Netherlands: Elsevier; 2010. pp. 305-350

[217] Davidson, M.W. Differential Interference Contrast Image Gallery *Trematode (Fasciolopsis buski) Rediae*. 2015. Available from: https://micro.magnet.fsu.edu/primer/techniques/dic/dicgallery/fasciolopsisbuskismall.html

[218] Jaroonvesama N, Charoenlarp K, Areekul S. Intestinal absorption studies in Fasciolopsis buski infection. The Southeast Asian Journal of Tropical Medicine and Public Health. 1986;**17**(4): 582-586

[219] Layden AJ, Täse K, Finkelstein JL. Neglected tropical diseases and vitamin B12: A review of the current evidence. Transactions of the Royal Society of

Tropical Medicine and Hygiene. 2018; **112**(10):423-435

[220] Karthikeyan G et al. Intestinal infestation with Fasciolopsis buski leading to acute kidney injury. The Journal of the Association of Physicians of India. 2013;**61**(12):936-938

[221] Khurana S, Datta P. Fasciolopsiasis. Singapore: Springer Nature; 2022. pp. 235-244

[222] Prevention, C.f.D.C.a. Fascioliasis. 2019. Available from: https://www.cdc.gov/dpdx/fascioliasis/index.html

[223] Wattanagoon Y, Bunnag D. Liver Fluke Infections. Amsterdam, Netherlands: Elsevier; 2013. pp. 887-891

[224] Siles-Lucas M et al. Fascioliasis and fasciolopsiasis: Current knowledge and future trends. Research in Veterinary Science. 2021;**134**:27-35

[225] Datta, S., G. Mukherjee, and J. Ghosh, Comparative Efficacy of Triclabendazole, Oxyclozanide and Rafoxanide against Fasciolopsis buski in Naturally Infected Pigs. 2004

[226] Biswal DK et al. De novo genome and transcriptome analyses provide insights into the biology of the trematode human parasite Fasciolopsis buski. PLoS One. 2018;**13**(10):e0205570

[227] Prevention, C.f.D.C.a. Clinical Overview of Fasciola. 2024. Available from: https://www.cdc.gov/liver-flukes/hcp/clinical-overview-fasciola/index.html

[228] Good R, Scherbak D. Fascioliasis. In: StatPearls. Treasure Island (FL): StatPearls Publishing; 2024

[229] Prevention, C.f.D.C.a. Schistosomiasis. 2024. Available from: https://www.cdc.gov/dpdx/schistosomiasis/index.html

[230] McManus DP et al. Schistosomiasis. Nature Reviews Disease Primers. 2018;**4**:1

[231] Prevention, C.f.D.C.a. Paragonimiasis. 2024. Available from: https://www.cdc.gov/dpdx/paragonimiasis/index.html

[232] Shah P et al. Pulmonary Paragonimiasis: A case series. Journal of Nepal Medical Association. 2023;**61**(259):290-293

[233] Prevention, C.f.D.C.a. Clinical Overview of Paragonimiasis. 2024. Available from: https://www.cdc.gov/paragonimus/hcp/clinical-overview/index.html

[234] Blair D. Paragonimiasis. Cham, Switzerland: Springer International Publishing; 2019. pp. 105-138

[235] Prevention, C.f.D.C.a. About Opisthorchis. 2024. Available from: https://www.cdc.gov/liver-flukes/opisthorchis/index.html

[236] Prevention, C.f.D.C.a. Clinical Overview of Opisthorchis. 2024. Available from: https://www.cdc.gov/liver-flukes/hcp/clinical-overview-opisthorchis/index.html

[237] Prevention, C.f.D.C.a. Opisthorchiasis. 2024. Available from: https://www.cdc.gov/dpdx/opisthorchiasis/index.html

[238] Young ND et al. The Opisthorchis viverrini genome provides insights into life in the bile duct. Nature. Communications. 2014;**5**(1). Article number: 4378

Chapter 3

Burden of Enterobiasis in Africa: Overcoming Neglect and Improving Pediatric Health

Wilfred Ofosu

Abstract

Enterobiasis is a globally prevalent, difficult-to-control, but yet neglected intestinal helminthiasis. Its asymptomatic nature in most cases leads to underestimation of its impact. However, its impact on pediatric health is significant, compromising their physical and mental well-being ultimately hampering educational development. The prevalence of enterobiasis among (pre)school-aged children in Africa varies across studies due to differences in study location characteristics and diagnostic techniques. However, higher prevalences have been reported in studies utilizing the scotch tape technique emphasizing the need for its prioritization in epidemiological studies and routine parasitological examinations due to its high diagnostic efficiency. Mebendazole (100 mg orally) is the recommended first-line treatment, and administering a second dose after 14 days is crucial to prevent reinfection. The scarcity of treatment data for enterobiasis in Africa can be attributed to various factors, including underreporting of cases, limited healthcare infrastructure, and inadequate research focus on this specific parasitic infection. Overcoming the neglect of enterobiasis requires the implementation of educational and mass treatment programs, improving diagnostic capabilities, and prioritizing research and public health initiatives. Additionally, improving hygiene practices and sanitation is essential. By addressing these challenges and introducing comprehensive interventions, the neglect of enterobiasis can be overcome, leading to improved overall African pediatric well-being.

Keywords: enterobiasis, *enterobius vermicularis*, neglected, pediatric population, intestinal helminthiasis, Africa

1. Introduction

Despite advancements in healthcare, parasitic diseases continue to pose a significant global public health challenge, particularly in developing countries where besides unmet healthcare needs, risk factors for parasite transmission remain persistent [1–5]. Caused by the nematode, *Enterobius vermicularis* (pinworm), enterobiasis is the most prevalent helminth infection, affecting an estimated 4–28% of children and more than 1 billion people globally [6]. This parasite has coexisted with humans since ancient times and continues to persist in modern populations [7]. Enterobiasis is often considered a relatively mild condition characterized symptomatically by perianal pruritus (itching). While most cases are asymptomatic, rare complications have been reported [5, 8–14].

Enterobiasis is often neglected in terms of public health recognition and research funding, leading to underestimation of its burden, particularly in Africa, where parasitic diseases are highly prevalent [1, 2]. Enterobiasis is frequently underestimated in comparison to other intestinal helminths, primarily due to the absence of apparent symptoms in most cases. Additionally, factors like the nocturnal migration of the parasites and the difficulties in detecting their eggs in routine stool examinations contribute to the underestimation of the disease burden [15]. However, untreated or under-treated enterobiasis can have long-term consequences on pediatric health, including impaired growth, nutritional deficiencies, impaired cognitive development, and compromised educational attainment [16–19].

This chapter aims to highlight the burden of enterobiasis in Africa, emphasizing the need for prioritized efforts to improve pediatric health through comprehensive control measures. By doing so, the neglect of enterobiasis can be overcome, and the well-being of African pediatric populations improved.

2. Epidemiology of enterobiasis among African children: the need for more epidemiological data

Dependent on several factors including socio-demographic and economic status, hygienic factors, and diagnostic technique, the epidemiology of enterobiasis differs across different African countries and has been poorly mapped, contributing to the underestimation of the disease's true burden in the region. However, available studies highlight the persistence of enterobiasis in African countries, with possible risk factors.

A study in rural coastal Tanzania showed higher prevalence rates of pinworm infection among preschool and school-aged children compared to infants [20]. The prevalence of pinworm infection varies in different studies, ranging from as low as 0.01% to as high as 45.3% in school-aged children [20–35]. These variations are attributed mainly to differences in diagnostic techniques, with studies using scotch tape reporting higher prevalences than those using fecal analysis.

Studies have highlighted the role of the infected hand in pinworm transmission among the pediatric population, with a high prevalence of pinworm eggs found on the hands and underneath the fingernails of school children [36–40]. These studies highlight the need for improved sanitation and proper handwashing with soap in schools to prevent parasite transmission. Overcrowded living conditions have been also associated with higher prevalence rates of pinworm infection, emphasizing the importance of addressing population density in prevention efforts [41]. Environmental factors, such as temperature, may also impact the transmission and survival of pinworm eggs [20].

Street food consumers and individuals who consume raw vegetables in Africa, particularly in sub-Saharan Africa (SSA), are identified as high-risk populations for pinworm infection. Studies conducted in Ghana and Nigeria have shown the association of pinworms with food vendors/handlers and the presence of pinworms in raw vegetables sold by market vendors [42–44]. Additionally, asymptomatic migrants from developing countries may carry pinworms, as demonstrated by screening studies on sub-Saharan African and Latin American immigrants [45].

It is important to note that the true prevalence of enterobiasis in Africa may be higher than reported due to underdiagnosis and limited surveillance systems. Other parasitic diseases such as malaria and schistosomiasis, due to their significant public health impact in Africa, may divert attention and resources away from enterobiasis surveillance and control efforts [23, 24, 34, 46, 47].

3. Impact of enterobiasis on pediatric health

The weakened immune system of children makes them vulnerable to intestinal parasitic infections (IPIs). This often leads to detrimental effects on their physical and intellectual well-being. However, the impact of IPIs on pediatric health depends on the parasite species, parasitemia and course of infection, and nutritional and immunological status of children [48].

While enterobiasis is generally asymptomatic, symptomatic cases are characterized by nocturnal perianal pruritus, which can lead to auto-infection as patients inadvertently transfer eggs under their fingernails. This itching can cause discomfort, insomnia, restlessness, and daytime drowsiness, particularly in children. Secondary lesions, such as mechanical dermatitis, can develop in the perianal or vulvar areas [49].

Although rare, complications of enterobiasis include parasites invading the reproductive organs, peritoneal cavity [8, 12], leading to hepatic enterobiasis, and acute appendicitis [10, 14]. Ectopic movements of pinworms have been associated with recurrent urinary tract infections, potentially resulting in secondary gastrointestinal infections [1]. The presence of a large number of adult worms in the bowel can cause additional symptoms like abdominal pain, tenesmus, constipation, and vaginitis [9, 13, 49].

In addition to the its impact on physical well-being, enterobiasis can also hamper a child's cognitive, emotional, and educational development. Untreated and under-treated enterobiasis may result in growth retardation and insomnia, which subsequently contributes to attention deficits, learning disabilities, increased school absenteeism, and higher dropout rates [16, 19, 50]. For instance, after a night of deprived sleep resulting from perianal pruritus, children become fatigued and less active the next day, impacting their concentration and performance at school. Others may miss school not only as a result of fatigue but also to avoid stigmatization by peers.

4. Diagnosis of enterobiasis: prioritizing the scotch tape method

Accurate diagnosis of enterobiasis is crucial for estimating the disease' burden, and disease management [51]. However, in Africa, diagnosis of intestinal helminthiasis is influenced by multiple factors including healthcare accessibility, educational status, and sociocultural beliefs.

Enterobiasis can be diagnosed by symptoms such as perianal pruritus, visual examination of adult worms, and microscopic examination of eggs and adult worms [50]. However, in Africa, most cases are asymptomatic, making diagnosis challenging and leading to an underestimation of the disease burden [52]. Diagnostic resources for pinworm infection in Africa are limited, and different methods have varying levels of effectiveness.

Stool microscopy, commonly used in clinical practice and prevalence studies in Africa, is not reliable for identifying *E. vermicularis*. It underestimates the prevalence and may miss treatable cases, especially among asymptomatic individuals with low parasitemia. Scotch tape microscopy effectively detects pinworm eggs, while stool microscopy is less reliable due to the stickiness of the eggs, causing them to adhere to the perianal skin and clothes [15, 21].

A study in Ethiopia found various intestinal helminths but no *E. vermicularis* parasites using fecal analysis [53]. Meanwhile, a study in Tanzania demonstrated reasonable prevalence of *E. vermicularis*, particularly among preschool-aged children, using scotch tape microscopy for *E. vermicularis* detection in combination with stool microscopy for other helminths [20]. Likewise, a study in South Africa showed higher pinworm prevalence using scotch tape microscopy among hospitalized children compared to stool microscopy among school-going children [21]. This highlights the underestimation of pinworm prevalence by stool microscopy and emphasizes the importance of scotch tape microscopy in diagnosing and studying pinworm infection in Africa.

Serological methods are of no relevance for diagnosing pinworm infections. However, PCR is a highly precise tool for diagnosing intestinal helminth infections [54, 55]. A study proposed a PCR-based method for *E. vermicularis* diagnosis, and its high diagnostic accuracy can address and overcome the challenges posed by other methods [56]. In resource-limited settings, however, this approach may be impractical to use particularly in smaller laboratories located at the periphery [55].

The Scotch tape method for diagnosing pinworm infection is thus crucial and should be prioritized, particularly in resource-limited settings in Africa. Although the collection method may be unpleasant and cumbersome for some individuals, the advantages of this diagnostic approach such as its ease of use, rapid results, cost effectiveness, and high sensitivity make it valuable. Furthermore, the implementation of the Scotch tape method in *E. vermicularis* epidemiological studies has the potential to estimate the true burden of the disease in Africa.

5. Treatment of enterobiasis in Africa

Enterobiasis can be effectively treated using highly effective anthelminthic drugs. Initial treatment of enterobiasis may not provide complete protection as reinfection is common [20]. It is recommended to treat enterobiasis with a single dose of albendazole (400 mg orally), mebendazole (100 mg orally), or pyrantel pamoate (11 mg/kg orally). To target newly developed adult worms and prevent reinfection, a second dose should be administered 14 days later [57]. However, mebendazole is the first-line treatment for enterobiasis [50].

The available literature and research on the specific treatment outcomes, efficacy, and prevalence of drug resistance for *E. vermicularis* in African populations are limited [58]. Anthelmintic drug resistance has been highlighted in studies worldwide [59], but resistance of *E. vermicularis* to anthelminthic drugs have been poorly explored. Given the indiscriminate use of antimicrobials and practice of self-medication in several African countries, resistance patterns are frequent [60], but it is unknown whether resistance patterns of *E. vermicularis* are significant.

The scarcity of treatment data for enterobiasis in Africa may be attributed to various factors, including underreporting of cases, limited healthcare infrastructure, and inadequate research focus on this specific parasitic infection. Limited availability and utilization of standard diagnostics in routine parasitological examinations contribute to the lack of comprehensive treatment data for enterobiasis in Africa. The scotch tape test, the most effective for diagnosing enterobiasis, is less frequently employed in clinical parasitological examinations. As a result, many cases of the infection, particularly asymptomatic ones, may go undiagnosed and unreported. This underreporting further hampers the collection of accurate treatment data, making it difficult to assess the true burden and impact of enterobiasis in Africa.

Moreover, the limited healthcare infrastructure in rural areas worsens the challenges in diagnosing and treating enterobiasis. In these resource-constrained settings, the availability of healthcare facilities, trained personnel, and access to medications is inadequate. As a result, infected children who seek medical attention for symptomatic infections may face obstacles in receiving appropriate treatment. This lack of access to treatment contributes to the scarcity of treatment data and hinders the surveillance of treatment efficacy.

Conducting large-scale clinical trials and monitoring treatment outcomes in resource-limited settings can be logistically challenging [61]. Limited funding, inadequate research infrastructure, and difficulties in follow-up and data collection pose significant barriers to conducting comprehensive studies on enterobiasis treatment in Africa. These challenges further impede the generation of robust treatment data that could inform evidence-based guidelines and interventions.

6. Overcoming neglect: strategies for improved pediatric health

To mitigate the impact of enterobiasis on pediatric health in Africa, interventions are needed at both individual and community levels. These interventions should focus on improving sanitation facilities, promoting proper hygiene practices, providing access to effective treatment, and raising awareness about the importance of prevention and control measures.

Studies reporting high prevalence have highlighted that mass treatment and educational programs should be undertaken, to reduce enterobiasis reinfection and new infections to people in endemic areas [62, 63]. Furthermore, hygienic measures should be prioritized to help reduce the transmission of the parasite [39, 44, 64].

Addressing the epidemiology of enterobiasis in Africa requires the need for continuous epidemiological research [65]. These studies should utilize sensitive diagnostic methods particularly the scotch tape method to accurately determine the prevalence and distribution of enterobiasis. Moreover, the scotch tape method should be employed in routine parasitological examinations to diagnose infections accurately.

7. Conclusion and future directions

Enterobiasis is a neglected helminth infection that primarily affects children. The lack of apparent symptoms has led to the underestimation of its disease burden. However, the high prevalence of risk factors such as poor hygiene, consumption of contaminated food, and overcrowding in African countries poses a serious threat to children, particularly those in rural areas.

Traditional diagnostic methods like stool microscopy have proven ineffective in diagnosing enterobiasis due to the stickiness of the eggs, necessitating the use of the scotch tape technique, which yields higher parasitemia. Treatment should prioritize preventing reinfection by administering the recommended dose of albendazole, mebendazole, or pyrantel pamoate, with a second dose after 14 days. To overcome the neglect of enterobiasis, two key interventions are required: mass treatment and education programs. Moreover, improving sanitation facilities, and practicing proper hygiene are important preventive and control measures.

It is crucial to allocate resources and prioritize research efforts toward studies specifically focused on *E. vermicularis* in African pediatric populations. These studies should aim to gather more epidemiological and treatment data, including prevalence, transmission dynamics, treatment outcomes, and potential drug resistance patterns. By addressing these research gaps, we can better understand and combat enterobiasis in Africa, thus improving the health and well-being of affected children.

Conflict of interest

The authors declare no conflict of interest.

Author details

Wilfred Ofosu
Department of Medical Microbiology, University of Ghana Medical School, University of Ghana, Accra, Ghana

*Address all correspondence to: wilfred.ofosu.7@gmail.com

References

[1] Bharadwaj M, Bengtson M, Golverdingen M, Waling L, Dekker C. Diagnosing point-of-care diagnostics for neglected tropical diseases. PLoS Neglected Tropical Diseases. 2021;**15**(6):1-21. DOI: 10.1371/journal.pntd.0009405

[2] Sitas F, Parkin M, Chirenje Z, Stein L, Mqoqi N, Wabinga H. In: Jamison DT, Feachem RG, Makgoba MW, Bos ER, Baingana FK, Hofman KJ, et al., editors. Disease and Mortality in Sub-Saharan Africa. 2nd ed. Washington, DC: The International Bank for Reconstruction and Development/The World Bank; 2006

[3] Shahnazi M, Sharifi M, Kalantari Z, Allipour Heidari M, Agamirkarimi N. The study of consumed vegetable parasitic infections in Qazvin. Journal of Inflammation Disease. 2009;**12**(4):83-89

[4] Malakotian M, Hosseini M, Bahrami H. Survey of the parasires of vegetable in Kerman province. Medical Journal of Hormozgan University. 2009;**13**(1):55-62

[5] Mahara G, Tian C, Xu X, Wang W. Revolutionising health care: Exploring the latest advances in medical sciences. Journal of Global Health. 2023;**13**:3042

[6] Efared B, Atsame-Ebang G, Soumana BM, Tahiri L, Hammas N, El Fatemi H, et al. Acute suppurative appendicitis associated with *Enterobius vermicularis*: An incidental finding or a causative agent? A case report. BMC Research Notes. 2017;**10**(1):494

[7] Fry GF, Moore JG. Enterobius vermicularis: 10,000-year-old human infection. Science. 1969;**166**(3913):1620

[8] Pigac B, Mašić S, Mašić V. *Enterobius vermicularis* in the endometrium of the uterus: A case report. Iranian journal of parasitology. 2017;**12**:638-641

[9] Mentessidou A, Theocharides C, Patoulias I, Panteli C. Enterobius Vermicularis-associated pelvic inflammatory disease in a child. Journal of Pediatric and Adolescent Gynecology. 2016;**29**(2):e25-e27

[10] Chhetri S, Al Mamari AH, Al Awfi MM, Al Khaldi NH, Abed NM, Pandak N, et al. Enterobius vermicularis related acute appendicitis: A case report and review of the literature. Infectious Disease Reports. 2023;**15**:417-424

[11] Arkoulis N, Zerbinis H, Simatos G, Nisiotis A. *Enterobius vermicularis* (pinworm) infection of the liver mimicking malignancy: Presentation of a new case and review of current literature. International Journal of Surgery Case Reports. 2012;**3**(1):6-9

[12] Saleem F, Malik F, Fatima S. *Enterobius vermicularis* in tubo-ovarian abscess: A rare and interesting incidental finding – A case report. The Journal of the Pakistan Medical Association. 2017;**67**(4):630-633

[13] Chitnis A, Yousefi Azimi D, Sabri S, Dhebri A. *Enterobius vermicularis*: A parasitic cause of appendicular colic. Cureus. 2020;**12**:e8524

[14] Dunphy L, Clark Z, Raja MH. *Enterobius vermicularis* (pinworm) infestation in a child presenting with symptoms of acute appendicitis: A wriggly tale! BML Case Reports. 2017

[15] Fan CK, Chuang TW, Huang YC, Yin AW, Chou CM, Hsu YT, et al.

Enterobius vermicularis infection: Prevalence and risk factors among preschool children in kindergarten in the capital area, Republic of the Marshall Islands. BMC Infectious Diseases. 2019;**19**(1):536. DOI: 10.1186/s12879-019-4159-0

[16] Fauziah N, Aviani JK, Agrianfanny YN, Fatimah SN. Intestinal parasitic infection and nutritional status in children under five years old: A systematic review. Tropical Medicine in Infectious Diseases. 2022;**7**(11):371

[17] Li HM, Zhou CH, Li ZS, Deng ZH, Ruan CW, Zhang QM, et al. Risk factors for Enterobius vermicularis infection in children in Gaozhou, Guangdong, China. Infectious Disease of Poverty. 2015;**4**:28

[18] Mwandawiro C, Okoyo C, Kihara J, Simiyu E, Kepha S, Campbell SJ, et al. Results of a national school-based deworming programme on soil-transmitted helminths infections and schistosomiasis in Kenya: 2012-2017. Parasites & Vectors. 2019;**12**(1):76. DOI: 10.1186/s13071-019-3322-1

[19] Tchuem Tchuenté LA. Control of soil-transmitted helminths in sub-Saharan Africa: Diagnosis, drug efficacy concerns and challenges. Acta Tropica. 2011;**120**:S4-S11. DOI: 10.1016/j.actatropica.2010.07.001

[20] Salim N, Schindler T, Abdul U, Rothen J, Genton B, Lweno O, et al. Enterobiasis and strongyloidiasis and associated co-infections and morbidity markers in infants, preschool- and school-aged children from rural coastal Tanzania: A cross-sectional study. BMC Infectious Diseases. 2014;**14**(1):644. DOI: 10.1186/s12879-014-0644-7

[21] Mosala TI, Appleton CC. True prevalence of pinworm (*Enterobius vermicularis*) infection among children in Qwa-Qwa, South Africa. South Africa Journal of Science. 2003;**99**(9-10):465-466

[22] Ghiwot Y, Degarege A, Erko B. Prevalence of intestinal parasitic infections among children under five years of age with emphasis on schistosoma mansoni in Wonji Shoa sugar estate, Ethiopia. PLoS One. 2014;**9**(10):9-13

[23] Ibikounlé M, Gbédjissi LG, Ogouyèmi-Hounto A, Batcho W, Kindé-Gazard D, Massougbodji A. Schistosomose et géohelminthoses dans le nord-est du Bénin: cas des écoliers des communes de Nikki et de Pèrèrè. Bulletin de la Societe de Pathologie Exotique. 2014;**107**(3):171-176

[24] Agbolade OM, Agu NC, Adesanya OO, Odejayi AO, Adigun AA, Adesanlu EB, et al. Intestinal helminthiases and schistosomiasis among school children in an urban center and some rural communities in Southwest Nigeria. The Korean Journal of Parasitology. 2007;**45**(3):233-238

[25] Tefera E, Mohammed J, Mitiku H. Intestinal helminthic infections among elementary students of Babile town, eastern Ethiopia. The Pan African Medical Journal. 2015;**20**:1-10

[26] Husen EA, Tafesse G, Hajare ST, Chauhan NM, Sharma RJ, Upadhye VJ. Cross-sectional study on assessment of frequency of intestinal helminth infections and its related risk factors among school children from Adola Town, Ethiopia. BioMed Research International. 2022;**2022**:1-12

[27] de Alegría MLAR, Colmenares K, Espasa M, Amor A, Lopez I, Nindia A, et al. Prevalence of Strongyloides stercoralis and other intestinal parasite infections in school children

in a rural area of Angola: A cross-sectional study. The American Journal of Tropical Medicine and Hygiene. 2017;**97**(4):1226-1231

[28] Rugaia MAE, Imhmmed LIA, Lahwal MM, Abdulla IM, Yousef S. Infection rate of *Enterobius vermicularis* (Pinworm) among school children in Sebha, Libya. Sirte Journal of Medical Science. 2023;**2**(2):16-19. Available from: https://api.semanticscholar.org/CorpusID:267960148

[29] Gizaw Z, Adane T, Azanaw J, Addisu A, Haile D. Childhood intestinal parasitic infection and sanitation predictors in rural Dembiya, Northwest Ethiopia. Environmental Health and Preventive Medicine. 2018;**23**(1):1-10

[30] Abah AE, Arene FOI. Status of intestinal parasitic infections among primary school children in Rivers State, Nigeria. Journal of Parasitology Research. 2015;**2015**:1-7

[31] Alemayehu B, Tomass Z, Wadilo F, Leja D, Liang S, Erko B. Epidemiology of intestinal helminthiasis among school children with emphasis on Schistosoma mansoni infection in Wolaita zone, Southern Ethiopia. BMC Public Health. 2017;**17**(1):1-10

[32] Mosala TI, Appleton CC, Levin JB. Intestinal parasitism in the Drakensberg mountains of Qwa-Qwa, South Africa. South African Journal of Epidemiology Infections. 2001;**16**(2/3):71-76. Available from: https://eurekamag.com/research/003/822/003822332.php

[33] Mosala TI. Epidemiology of human intestinal parasites in Qwa-Qwa, South Africa. 1995. Available from: https://api.semanticscholar.org/CorpusID:83367954

[34] Adedoja A, Tijani BD, Akanbi AA, Ojurongbe TA, Adeyeba OA, Ojurongbe O. Co-endemicity of *Plasmodium falciparum* and intestinal helminths infection in school age children in rural communities of Kwara state Nigeria. PLoS Neglected Tropical Diseases. 2015;**9**(7):1-13

[35] Akenten CW, Weinreich F, Paintsil EK, Amuasi J, Fosu D, Loderstädt U, et al. Intestinal helminth infections in Ghanaian children from the Ashanti region between 2007 and 2008—A retrospective cross-sectional real-time PCR-based assessment. Tropical Medical Infectious Disease. 2022;**7**(11):1-12

[36] Usman A, Aisha K. Survey on Helminth parasites associated with human fingernails among primary school pupils in Batagarawa Local Government Area, Katsina State, Nigeria. UMYU Journal of Microbiology Research (UJMR). 2019;**4**:34-38

[37] Yahaya A, Tyav Y, Idris A. Prevalence of intestinal parasitic helminths from fingernails of "Almajiris" in Birnin kudu local government area, Jigawa state, Nigeria. International Journal of Tropical Disease Health. 2015;**8**(2):66-74

[38] Alo M, Ugah U, Michael. Prevalence of intestinal parasites from the fingers of school children in Ohaozara, Ebonyi State, Nigeria. American Journal of Biology and Chemical Pharmaceutical Science. 2013;**1**(5):2328-6814

[39] Cranston I, Potgieter N, Mathebula S, Ensink JHJ. Transmission of Enterobius vermicularis eggs through hands of school children in rural South Africa. Acta Tropica. 2015;**150**:94-96

[40] Tadege B, Mekonnen Z, Dana D, Tiruneh A, Sharew B, Dereje E, et al. Assessment of the nail contamination with soil-transmitted helminths in schoolchildren in Jimma Town, Ethiopia. PLoS One. 2022;**17**:1-12. DOI: 10.1371/journal.pone.0268792

[41] Otu-Bassey IB, Ejezie GC, Epoke J, Useh MF. Enterobiasis and its relationship with anal itching and enuresis among school-age children in Calabar, Nigeria. Annals of Tropical Medical Parasitology. 2005;**99**(6):611-616

[42] Ayeh-Kumi P, Quarcoo S, Kwakye-Nuako G, Kretchy JP, Osafo-Kantanka A, Mortu S. Prevalence of intestinal parasitic infections among food vendors in Accra, Ghana. Journal of Tropical Medical Parasitology. 2009;**32**:1-8

[43] Amissah-Reynolds PK, Yar DD, Gyamerah I, Apenteng OY, Sakyi S. Fresh vegetables and ready-to-eat salads: Sources of parasitic zoonoses in Mampong-Ashanti, Ghana. European Journal of Nutrition and Food Safety. 2020;**12**(2):47-55

[44] Adenusi AA, Abimbola WA, Adewoga TOS. Human intestinal helminth contamination in pre-washed, fresh vegetables for sale in major markets in Ogun State, Southwest Nigeria. Food Control. 2015;**50**:843-849

[45] Monge-Maillo B, López-Vélez R, Norman FF, Ferrere-González F, Martínez-Pérez Á, Pérez-Molina JA. Screening of imported infectious diseases among asymptomatic sub-Saharan African and Latin American immigrants: A public health challenge. American Journal of Tropical Medical Hygiene. 2015;**92**(4):848-856. Available from: https://pubmed.ncbi.nlm.nih.gov/25646257

[46] Steinmann P, Keiser J, Bos R, Tanner M, Utzinger J. Schistosomiasis and water resources development: Systematic review, meta-analysis, and estimates of people at risk. The Lancet Infectious Diseases. 2006;**6**(7):411-425

[47] Egwunyenga AO, Ajayi JA, Nmorsi OPG, Duhlinska-Popova DD. Plasmoduim/intestinal Helminth Co-infections among pregnant Nigerian women. Memórias do Instituto Oswaldo Cruz. 2001;**96**(8):1055-1059

[48] El-Sayed NM, Ramadan ME. The impact of intestinal parasitic infections on the health status of children: An overview. Journal of Pediatric Infectious Diseases. 2017;**12**(04):209-213. Available from: http://www.thieme-connect.com/products/ejournals/abstract/10.1055/s-0037-1603576

[49] Kacker PP. Vulvo-vaginitis in an adult with thread-worms in the vagina. The British Journal of Venereal Diseases. 1973;**49**(3):314-315

[50] Wendt S, Trawinski H, Schubert S, Rodloff AC, Mössner J, Lübbert C. The diagnosis and treatment of pinworm infection. Deutsches Ärzteblatt International. 2019;**116**(13):213-219. Available from: https://pubmed.ncbi.nlm.nih.gov/31064642

[51] Riaz M, Aslam N, Zainab R, Aziz-Ur-Rehman RG, Ullah MI, et al. Prevalence, risk factors, challenges, and the currently available diagnostic tools for the determination of helminths infections in human. European Journal of Inflammation. 2020;**18**:205873922095991. DOI: 10.1177/2058739220959915

[52] Khayyat R, Belkebir S, Abuseir S, Barahmeh M, Alsadder L, Basha W. Prevalence of and risk factors for *Enterobius vermicularis* infestation in preschool children, West Bank, Palestine, 2015. East Mediterr Heal J = La Rev sante la Mediterr Orient = al-Majallah al-sihhiyah li-sharq al-mutawassit. 2021;**27**(11):1052-1060

[53] Lanker KC, Muhummed AM, Cissé G, Zinsstag J, Hattendorf J, Yusuf RB, et al. Prevalence and associated risk factors of intestinal

parasitic infections among children in pastoralist and agro-pastoralist communities in the Adadle woreda of the Somali Regional State of Ethiopia. PLoS Neglected Tropical Diseases. 2023;**17**(7):e0011448

[54] Manuel M, Ramanujam K, Ajjampur SSR. Molecular tools for diagnosis and surveillance of soil-transmitted Helminths in endemic areas. Parasitologia. 2021;**1**:105-118

[55] Meurs L, Polderman AM, Vinkeles Melchers NVS, Brienen EAT, Verweij JJ, Groosjohan B, et al. Diagnosing polyparasitism in a high-prevalence setting in Beira, Mozambique: Detection of intestinal parasites in Fecal samples by microscopy and real-time PCR. PLoS Neglected Tropical Diseases. 2017;**11**(1):e0005310-e0005310. Available from: https://pubmed.ncbi.nlm.nih.gov/28114314

[56] Ummarino A, Caputo M, Tucci FA, Pezzicoli G, Piepoli A, Gentile A, et al. A PCR-based method for the diagnosis of Enterobius vermicularis in stool samples, specifically designed for clinical application. Frontiers in Microbiology. 2022;**13**:1028988. Available from: https://pubmed.ncbi.nlm.nih.gov/36466657

[57] Jones BF, Cappello M. In: Johnson LRBTE, editor. Nematodes. New York: Elsevier; 2004. pp. 692-695. Available from: https://www.sciencedirect.com/science/article/pii/B0123868602007796

[58] Temsah KA, Ahmad DA, El Kholy AA, Elsamanoudy MI. Efficacy of Albendazole mass treatment alone compared to combined Albendazole – Flubendazole regimen for treatment of resistant *Entrobius vermicularis* infection in children. Egyptian Journal of Hospital Medicine. 2021;**84**(1):2071-2077. DOI: 10.21608/ejhm.2021.180356

[59] Geerts S, Gryseels B. Anthelmintic resistance in human helminths: A review. Tropical Medicine in International Health. 2001;**6**(11):915-921. DOI: 10.1046/j.1365-3156.2001.00774.x

[60] Kimanga AN. A situational analysis of antimicrobial drug resistance in Africa: Are we losing the battle? Ethiopian Journal of Health Sciences. 2012;**22**(2):135-143

[61] Toto N, Douglas E, Gmeiner M, Barrett LK, Lindblad R, Makhaza L, et al. Conducting clinical trials in sub-Saharan Africa: Challenges and lessons learned from the Malawi Cryptosporidium study. Trials. 2020;**21**(1):680

[62] Kim BJ, Yeon JW, Ock MS. Infection rates of Enterobius vermicularis and Clonorchis sinensis of primary school children in Hamyang-gun, Gyeongsangnam-do (province), Korea. Korean Journal of Parasitology. 2001;**39**(4):323-325

[63] Bunchu N, Vitta A, Thongwat D, Lamlertthon S, Pimolsri U, Waree P, et al. Enterobius vermicularis infection among children in lower northern Thailand. Journal of Tropical Medicine and Parasitology. 2011;**34**(1):36-40

[64] Idowu OA, Rowland SA. Oral fecal parasites and personal hygiene of food handlers in Abeokuta, Nigeria. Africa in Health Science. 2006;**6**(3):160-164

[65] Amiri SAN, Rahimi MT, Mahdavi SA, Moosazadeh M, Ramzani O, Koshk AF, et al. Prevalence of Enterobius vermicularis infection among preschool children, Babol, North of Iran. Journal of Parasitic Diseases. 2016;**40**(4):1558-1562. DOI: 10.1007/s12639-015-0727-4

Chapter 4

Comprehensive Control of Toxocariasis in Communities

Dumar A. Jaramillo-Hernández

Abstract

With the purpose of understanding the complexity of actions aimed at controlling the main zoonotic soil-transmitted helminthiasis in the world, this book chapter is proposed around the comprehensive control of toxocariasis in urban communities. From the understanding of the epidemiological cycle implicit in the vertical transmission of parasites of the genus *Toxocara* in their main urban definitive hosts (canines and felines), an action that allows a "perpetuity" of the parasite in urban areas, passing through the inextricable relationships of synanthropic hosts until reaching their paratenic or accidental hosts, humans. At the same time, control strategies will be discussed in the various links of its transmission/infection chain, demonstrating that preventive medicine supported by selective strategic deworming in canines and felines within their various age ranges is the fundamental pillar in the fight against this parasitosis. Likewise, exploring the substantial advances in the development of vaccinology to integrate new strategies in the comprehensive control of toxocariasis in communities.

Keywords: preventive medicine, public health, soil-transmitted helminthiasis, *Toxocara*, zoonoses

1. Introduction

Toxocariasis is the disease caused by parasites, type roundworms (nematodes, order Ascaridida) of the genus *Toxocara*; the etymology of the scientific name is Toxo = arrow + cara = head. The species *Toxocara canis* (Werner, 1782) and *Toxocara cati* (Schrank, 1788) [1], and possibly *Toxocara vitulorum*, *Toxocara pteropodis*, *Toxocara malayasiensis*, and *Toxocara lyncus*. These last four have a category of low level zoonosis to unresolved zoonotic potential [2–4].

The definitive hosts of *T. canis* and *T. cati* are canines and felines, particularly within urban communities' domestic dogs and cats, respectively [5]. An adult female roundworm of dogs (*T. canis*) can lay 200,000 eggs a day, which are expelled in the feces of parasitized dogs. Over a period of 2–4 weeks, they embryonate in the environment, subsequently emerging as an infective larva (third-stage larvae, L3), which could accidentally parasitize humans (paratenic or accidental host); due to these characteristics, toxocariasis is the main zoonotic soil-transmitted helminthiasis in the world [6].

Humans are not the definitive host of *Toxocara*; therefore, the life cycle of this parasite is not fulfilled. What does occur is the development of various larva migrans syndromes, where L3 migrates from the intestine to various tissues, including the central nervous system (neurotoxocariasis), abdominal viscera (visceral larva migrans), and eye (ocular larva migrans) [7]. Also, a clinical presentation where patients in whom positive toxocara serology is associated with a number of systemic and localized symptoms and signs (notably abdominal pain) but not visceral or ocular larva migrans, called covert/common toxocariasis (CT) [8].

Remembering "*The Iceberg Model*" within the diagnosis of a problematic situation in public health, where only the tip of the iceberg (the observable cases of direct correspondence to the infectious agent) correspond to 10% of the true magnitude of the problem [9], we can understand the real importance of toxocariasis. *Toxocara* is associated with alterations in the immune system's response to vaccines for various preventable infectious and contagious pathologies (e.g., rabies), in addition to a series of autoimmune diseases [10–14]. Additional studies indicate that CT may represent a major cause of lung dysfunction, cognitive disturbances, and intellectual deficits in children living in poverty [15]. Thus, toxocariasis is one of the causes of the cycle of poverty in the world [16].

Added to this highly worrying panorama regarding toxocariasis, *Toxocara* spp. is considered, by the year 2050, the greatest global threat of zoonotic soil-transmitted helminthiases [17]; furthermore, one of the five most important neglected diseases in the world [18]. Due to the little investment in research in the most affected countries, economic resources must be allocated to fill the great gap in the effective control of this parasite in dog and cat populations: effective vaccines [19]. Especially in pregnant bitches, which are capable of transmitting L3 to their offspring *via* transplacental or lacteal (vertical transmission), a situation that perpetuates environmental contamination with eggs of this parasite and the risk of infection in communities [20].

The aim of this book chapter is to provide complementary information to the existing classic information regarding the understanding of the importance of toxocariasis in public health and possible comprehensive control mechanisms of this parasite within urban communities.

2. *Toxocara* and its perpetuity in urban communities

It is estimated that in the future toxocariasis will be considered the main zoonosis associated with soil-transmitted helminths, as well as the most neglected emerging parasitic zoonotic disease in the world [17, 21]. According to the World Health Organization (WHO) in its book entitled "*Ending the Neglect to Achieve the Sustainable Development Goals a roadmap for neglected tropical diseases 2021-2030*" [18], one of its main objectives is to control helminthiases transmitted by soil. Especially toxocariasis, given its important impact on public health, especially among poor people in many countries around the world.

Today, even though there are indicators of approximately 1.4 billion people exposed or infected by *Toxocara* spp., toxocariasis remains an underdiagnosed parasitic disease [22], with underestimated epidemiological rates, as well as the real impact of this pathology on global public health [12, 14, 23]. Because the diagnosis of this parasitic infection in humans is subject to serological examination that detects antibodies against *Toxocara* excretory-secretory (TES) antigens. This test, however, has low specificity (cross-reactions with other helminths) and is not capable of discriminating the asymptomatic form from those that lead to other syndromes, or historical chronic or acute infections [24, 25].

Added to these epidemiological conditions, the life cycle and transmission processes of *Toxocara* spp. between its different hosts is highly complex and has multiple variables immersed in its understanding (**Figure 1**). Although there are highly defined and understood variables: 1. The presence of dogs and cats, especially puppies, is significantly associated with the risk of exposure to L3 or embryonated eggs of *Toxocara* spp. to its different hosts, among them humans [26]. 2. The vertical transmission of *T. canis* allows early superinfection in puppies, which are a fundamental pillar in the dissemination of eggs in the environment [20]. 3. The eggs of *Toxocara* spp. are resistant to different environmental conditions, managing to reach their hosts

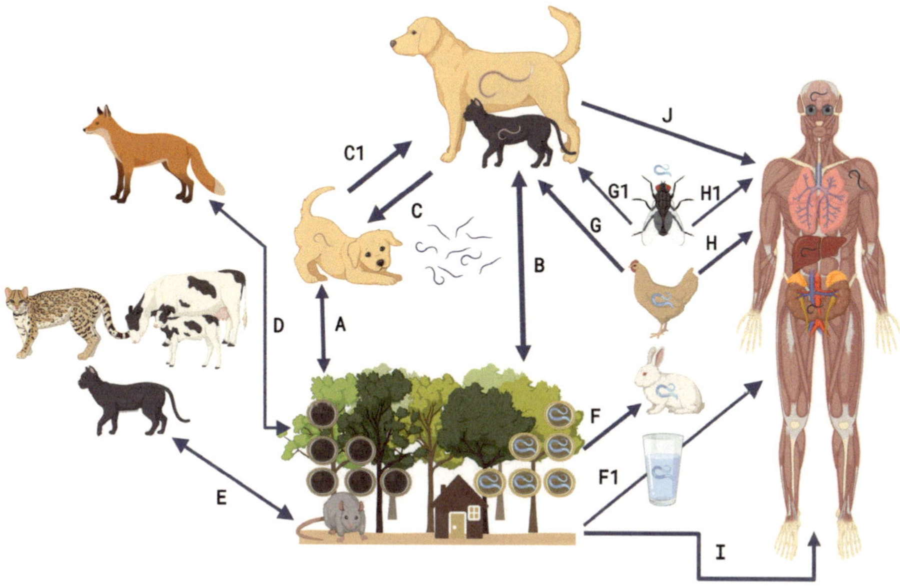

Figure 1.
Complexity of the biological cycle of Toxocara. A and B. In the intestine of dogs and cats (definitive hosts), the sexually mature forms of Toxocara are present; their unembryonated eggs come out through the feces. Under favorable environmental conditions (temperature between 25 and 30°C and relative humidity 85–95%), in 9–15 days, there is complete embryogenesis, achieving the infectious larval stage (L3). These embryonated eggs enter their definitive hosts through the oral route, hatch in the intestine, and begin migration. In puppies and kittens under 3 months of age, after migrating through the liver, kidneys, lungs, and trachea, they return to the intestinal lumen to differentiate sexually and lay eggs (prepatent period 4–5 weeks). In puppies and kittens older than 3 months, L3 migrates and encysts in various tissues, training in a state of quiescence/hypobiosis. C. Hormones associated with pregnancy in dogs, such as prolactin and progesterone, generate "awakening" from the quiescent state of L3, establishing vertical transmission (transplacental and transmammary). In queens, if Toxocara cati infection occurs during lactation, there is a probability of establishing transmammary transmission to the kittens. C1. Through the L3-contaminated emetic content of super-infected puppies or kittens, the bitches or queens can become infected. D. Wild or synanthropic (feral) canine or feline species can also spread eggs in the environment. E. Although there is no certainty about the participation of definitive atypical hosts for T. canis or T. cati (e.g., adult forms of T. canis have been found in the intestine of cats), these should be in the epidemiological research processes of this parasite. F and F1. Toxocara is considered a parasite associated with food- and waterborne diseases, especially in the consumption of paratenic hosts (e.g., poultry) without adequate cooking. G. Small mammals are suspected of contributing to the spread of Toxocara and aiding the survival of the parasite during periods when there is a temporary absence of suitable definitive hosts; if a cat preys on a paratenic host (e.g., parasitized mouse), the prepatent period could be shortened to 3 weeks. G1 and H1. Flies can be passive vectors of Toxocara. H and I. In humans, there are various routes of oral contamination with Toxocara eggs, from consumption of paratenic hosts to exposure to geophagy. After L3 infection in humans, several larva migrans syndromes can develop. J. Cats and dogs through their coat can also carry embryonated eggs or L3 of Toxocara, probably acquired in common public areas.

through various means of contamination, including water [27]. 4. The presence of the parasite is cosmopolitan, with its transmission/infection processes estimated in more than 100 countries [28], being highly related to disabling diseases that reduce the productivity of a community by up to 35% [29].

Due to the magnitude of contamination of public places with dog and cat feces, these family recreation places become important sources of exposure to infection by *Toxocara* spp. [30]. Fakhri et al. [31] published that the global prevalence of *Toxocara* eggs in public places was 21% (95%CI, 16–27%). They also estimated 13–35% of prevalence rates in different WHO regions, where a high prevalence was significantly associated with high geographical longitude, low latitude, and high relative environmental humidity. Thus, the highest prevalence was in the Western Pacific (35%; 95%CI, 15–58%) and the lowest in North and Central America (13%; 95%CI, 8–23%).

On the other hand, Rostami et al. [32] have recently published that the global *Toxocara* spp. seroprevalence rate in people was 19% (95%CI, 16.6–21.4%). A significantly higher seroprevalence was associated with a lower income level, human development index, and latitude but higher humidity, temperature, and precipitation. According to seroprevalence by WHO regions, the highest was 37.7% in the African region (95%CI, 25.7–50.6%) and lowest in the 8.2% in the Eastern Mediterranean region (95%CI, 5.1–12.0%).

This same type of study, regarding estimated global prevalences for *Toxocara*, has been carried out for dogs and cats. In dogs, it was 11.1% (95%CI, 10.6–11.7%), where a highly significant prevalence was associated with puppies (≤12 months of age), stray and rural animals, and bitches. As for the prevalence by WHO regions, Eastern Mediterranean (95%CI, 13.7–25.5%) has the highest with 19.2%, and the lowest was 6.4% for Western Pacific (95%CI, 3.3–10.2%) [33]. China draws attention, given that in that country, dogs are consumed as a source of animal protein in the diet of communities, so it is the only epidemiological indicator of direct presence of adult stages of *Toxocara* spp. in 45.2% of dogs that were slaughtered for consumption [34].

In the case of cats, the estimated *Toxocara* infection in the world was 17.0% (16.1–17.8%). The highest was associated with low-income tropical countries and stray with 28.6% (95%CI, 25.1–32.1%) and kittens (≤12 months of age) with 27.7% (95%CI, 23.4–32.0%). In turn, being the infection by *Toxocara* spp. in cats, highest in African countries 43.3% (95% CI, 28.3–58.4%) and lowest in South American countries 12.6% (95% CI, 8.2–17,0%) [35]. **Figure 2** shows the prevalence of patent *Toxocara* spp. infection (eggs in feces, coprodiagnosis) in dogs and cats in several countries around the world, allowing us to understand the cosmopolitan capacity of the parasite.

The perpetuity of *Toxocara* spp. in urban communities, even in developed countries [36], is strengthened, due to the apparent broad geographic distribution of *Toxocara* and multiple transmission routes indicating that toxocariasis is a common helminth infection in humans [21]. Likewise, based on the epidemiological principle that *T. canis* infection has a high prevalence in the entire dog population that is not treated with anthelmintics on a regular basis, and also, its infection capacity in synanthropic and wild species, which escape of the usual anthelmintic controls, makes its elimination almost impossible [37]. Additionally, *Toxocara* has characteristics of extreme hypobiosis in its paratenic hosts. Viable larvae have been found even after 9 years of residence in non-human primate tissues [38]. This information can be extrapolated to the role that small mammals play in maintaining L3 in hypobiosis in their tissues, which when preyed on by dogs or cats would help maintain the parasite cycle within urban communities [39]. For these reasons, cats are underestimated in

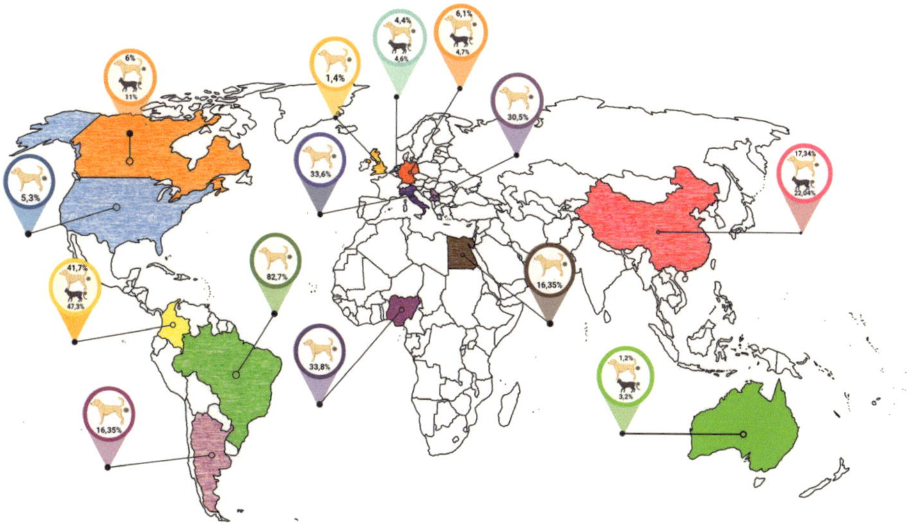

Figure 2.
Several prevalence of coprodiagnosis of Toxocara spp. infection in dogs and cats in some countries of the world.

their role in human toxocariasis, even though their offspring can become infected transmammarily, thus allowing superinfected kittens [40].

Likewise, this situation is aggravated through the cycle of uncontrolled populations of dogs and cats, especially stray animals, as well as dogs and cats from low-income families that do not have the economic requirements to access quality commercial dewormers [41]. This situation, in the case of dogs, is serious, due to the 100% risk of being born with *T. canis* infections. These puppies, which are anthropogenic beings (they arouse people's affection), access different areas of the home and public areas, managing to excrete thousands of *Toxocara* unembryonated eggs. Eggs are resistant to various environmental conditions, where they embryon and become infective [42], thus providing favorable environments to infect various hosts, among which are people. To "close" (strengthen) this cycle of perpetuity, toxocariasis is a neglected disease, a situation where governments do not specifically invest in its study and control [21, 43].

3. Approach to comprehensive control of *Toxocara*

The definition of comprehensive control refers to the holistic management of a situation, in this case knowing the multiple variables implicit in the presence and risk of infection by *Toxocara* spp. in urban communities and building a path of action possibilities (**Figure 3**). Without a doubt, dogs and cats play a predominant role in being the definitive hosts of *Toxocara* spp. [37]. Still, understanding that toxocariasis is a neglected disease and of a non-reportable nature for the world's health systems is vital [44]. For this reason, the role played by raising awareness among all members of the community regarding the health problems associated with toxocariasis should be the initial step in the integrated control work [45].

The education of communities, from their state, governmental, and social leaders to family core, must be sensitized. Topics on zoonotic soil-transmitted helminthiasis,

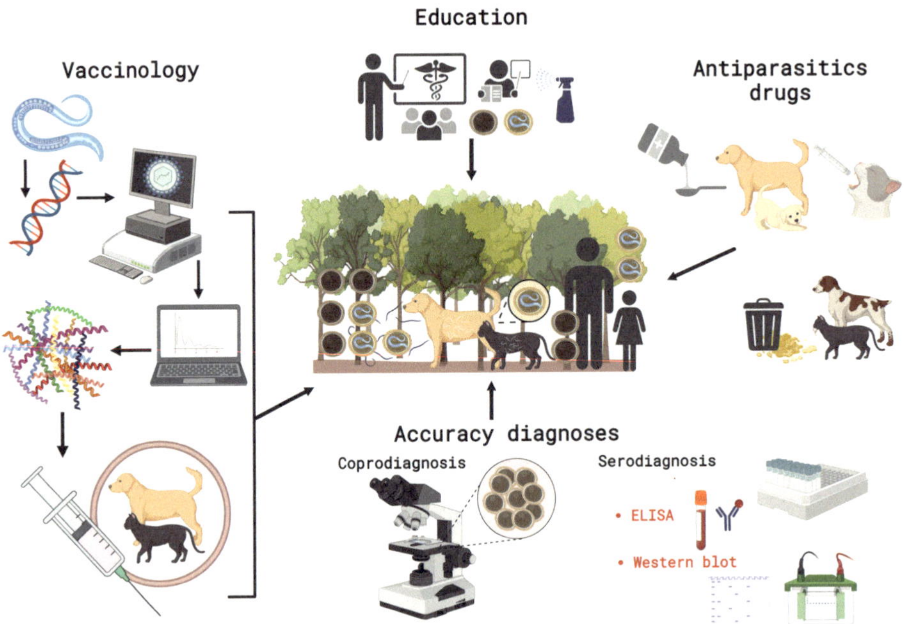

Figure 3.
Possible variables to develop in the constitution of an integrated control of Toxocara in urban communities.

responsible ownership of dogs and cats, collection of feces and its correct disposal, selective strategic deworming for *Toxocara* in dogs and cats according to their age. Also, other topics such as personal hygiene habits and good food-handling habits, among many other topics, are necessary to build knowledge, risk perception, and mitigation measures for toxocariasis in children, people with altered immune response, and nursing homes, among others [46].

The approaches of all levels of education in society are important to understand the silent scourge of toxocariasis. The use of Web-based educational resources, NEMBASE http://www.nematodes.org/nembase4, Nematode.net http://nematode.net, WormBase ParaSite http://parasite.wormbase.org/, Centers for Disease Control and Prevention (CDC, http://www.cdc.gov), and the American Association of Veterinary Parasitologists (AAVP, http://www.aavp.org/)could help in this activity. Likewise, the economic investment of States in macro research projects that allow precise epidemiological data by ecosystem regions in different countries and their communities, as well as technological developments for the control of *Toxocara* in dogs and cats (e.g. vaccines) [7, 47–49].

Within this process of educating community members, the responsible management of antiparasitic drugs is a fundamental pillar. The current guidelines of associations, the European Scientific Counsel of Companion Animal Parasites (ESCCAP; www.esccap.org), the Tropical Council for Companion Animal Parasites (TroCCAP; www.troccap.com), and the Companion Animal Parasite Council (CAPC; www.capcvet.org), recommend serial anthelmintic treatment. Every 15 days, from 2 weeks of age, puppies and kitties (under 12 weeks of age), using nematocidal antiparasitics specific to each animal species. For dogs and cats older than 12 weeks of age, selective strategic deworming should be performed every 2 to 3 months, depending on whether or not they are exposed to environments at risk of infection (e.g., visiting new parks contaminated with *Toxocara* eggs).

These deworming times are subject to: 1. Transplacentally parasitized puppies from 14 days of age begin to eliminate eggs through their feces. 2. Under most conditions, the prepatent period of *Toxocara* spp. is defined between 33 and 58 days; this being understood as the time elapsed between exposures to L3 by the host, until the moment of reaching the possibility of oviposition by the adult female [50].

Although it is not common to find effective disinfectants in the control of *Toxocara* eggs spread throughout the environment [51], in homes where there are puppies or/and kittens, there must be hygiene protocols for common family areas to which these animals have access. Recently, Zhang et al. [52] have published that the chlorocresol-based disinfectant product "Neopredisan®135–1" against to embryogenesis and viability of *T. canis* eggs. Such killing activity increases in a concentration- and time-dependent manner, with a maximum killing efficacy of 95.81% at 4% concentration and 120 min exposure time.

In turn, urban communities must group together and use antiparasitic baits for stray dogs and cats that cohabit public recreation spaces. There are examples of control of other gastrointestinal parasites in dogs and cats with this action [53–55]. This initial activity is vital to stop high loads of embryonated eggs in the environment of the urban community, in addition to reducing risks of contamination of spaces within homes where puppies and kittens are present. Nowadays, the use of parasiticide fungi, such as *Mucor circinelloides* (ovicide) and *Duddingtonia flagrans* (larvicide), has an important role in the ability to reduce the environmental load of gasrointestinal parasites, even in places with a high density of dogs and cats [56].

The biggest problem to control within the life cycle of *Toxocara* (**Figure 1**) refers to avoiding vertical transmission of the parasite, especially in bitches, which can transmit L3 to their offspring in utero and through the milk. On the other hand, the cats only transmit L3 to their offspring through milk when they suffer from *Toxocara cati* infection while they are lactating [57]. This is where homes that let their cats outside or stray can be exposed. The bitches' deworming schemes must be very precise regarding their gestation times. A macrocyclic lactone, Moxidectin, should be used on days 40 and 55 of gestation [58]. Deworming scheme based on the activation of L3 in tissues of pregnant bitches, these L3 come out of the hypostatic state at 42 days of gestation by prolactin peaks [59].

Being clear regarding the existing antiparasitic drugs protocols for the control of *Toxocara* spp. in dogs and cats, which must be socialized with responsible owners of cats and dogs [60]. The step to follow in integrated control is active epidemiological surveillance. Serial coproparasitological tests in dogs and cats are indicated to evaluate the effectiveness of antiparasitic agents and their frequency of use. The Kato-Katz technique is particularly easy to standardize in veterinary clinics or laboratories, in addition to being highly sensitive for *Toxocara* [61]. Monitoring the effectiveness of deworming through preventive coproparasitology carried out two to four times a year for puppies or kittens (<1 year old) and once or twice per year for dogs and cats (older than 1 year). Likewise, the measurement of soil contamination in common public areas (e.g., parks).

In the same way, indirect ELISA techniques use TES antigens to screen human, dog, and cat populations. Given that ELISA can generate cross-reactions with other helmint gastrointestinal infections, the results obtained from possible positives must be confirmed with the Wester blotting technique. This will provide specific epidemiological data on mitigation measures within the communities [62].

Without a doubt, the staging of a vaccine for the prevention and control of *Toxocara* spp. will be the fundamental pillar of a complete comprehensive plan for toxocariasis

[19, 63]. Vaccines are a product that stimulates the immune system to produce immunity against a specific disease, protecting the host of that disease from the infecting agent, whether bacteria, viruses, or parasites, including neoplastic cells [64]. Vaccines can stimulate the production of antibodies and cellular immunity; and in many cases, it is strictly necessary to enhance their immunogenic effect using adjuvants [65].

Reverse vaccinology allows the development of effective vaccines based on the genomic information of the infectious agent [66, 67]. In the world, there are important examples of control of gastrointestinal parasites in domestic animals through vaccination [68]. In the case of *T. canis*, the crucial point for the development of studies associated with vaccinology was the *T. canis* genome project, where Zhu et al. [69] reported that the genome of this parasite has a size of 317 Mb and encodes at least 18,596 genes that express proteins.

Based on this information, recent studies led by Zhou et al. [70] have explored details of the molecular biological processes in this parasite. They obtained high-throughput transcriptomic sequences of male and female *T. canis* of its 18,596 genes, performing a detailed bioinformatic analysis. Metabolomics studies were also carried out, where the nonprotein components of the parasite extract were characterized for the three metabolic pathways: fatty acid, amino acid, and carbohydrate metabolism [71]. Soleymani et al. [72] through proteomic analyses identified a variety of proteins from the soluble extract of *T. cati* adults, which could have a role in the host–parasite interaction, as well as 10 somatic proteins of this parasite with the capacity to generate an immune response by the host.

These studies allowed us to establish plausible bases for the identification of proteins of immunological interest for the generation of vaccines using the reverse vaccinology methodology. Recombinant proteins like potassium channel homologous protein (rTcVcam) and cadherin homologous protein (rTcCad), demonstrated immunogenicity in the murine model of toxocariasis and conferred a reduction in larval migration [73]. These proteins were selected because they were part of the cell membranes of the parasite; in theory, they behaved as hidden antigens and probably mediated the immune response to the parasite by the host [74–76].

Within reverse vaccinology, *in-silico* analyzes are important to determine the recombinant protein to be expressed. In the case of the first clinical trial in dogs [77], programs such as BLASTX (http://blast.ncbi.nlm.nih.gov/Blast.cgi) to identify possible homologous sequences, PSORT (http://www.psort.org/) to identify the cell location, TMHMM (http://www.cbs.dtu.dk/services/TMHMM-2.0/) and SOSUI (http://bp.nuap.nagoya-u.ac.jp/sosui/) to identify signal peptides and transmembrane helices, and ScanPROSITE (http://au.expasy.org/prosite/) to identify conserved domains and regions in the sequences were used.

Jaramillo-Hernández et al. [77] tested these recombinant proteins in puppies with various adjuvants, finding that rTcVcan + QuialA® promoted reduction in the parasite eggs in feces (95%) and eggs reduction obtained from the uteri of pharmacologically expelled adult females (58.38%).

In the near future, hopefully immediate, efforts should be made to research more promising antigens for the development of effective and efficient vaccines to control the vertical transmission of *T. canis* and *T. cati*. It is imperative to expand the possibility of integrated control of this zoonotic geohelminth, due to its devastating impact on the development of stable urban communities. In addition to exploring other parasite–host interactions, where the proteome composition of TES antigens has been identified, and according to the findings of computer-based analyses at the (http://crdd.osdd.net/raghava/cancerppd/index.php) site, part of the *T. canis*-secreted protein with the 18 amino acids showed a high degree of similarity (≈93%) to other anticancer agents [78].

4. Conclusion (author's opinion regarding *Toxocara* and the cycle of poverty in low-income countries, such as Colombia)

José Saramago and his masterpiece "*Blindness*" supports the power of observation, of those who can do it, the high social responsibility and preservation of the species, when others have lost that option (or have never had it). This is the case of some of the gastrointestinal parasites that can be transmitted to humans by domestic, wild, or synanthropic animals (e.g., pigeons), parasitic diseases called zoonotic geohelminthiases.

Now, the use of the Greek prefix "geo" to name these diseases refers to the high capacity of these parasites to persist and be transmitted through the soil, for example, through the green area of a park. Now, if we combine the aforementioned considerations, we can have the following picture of perfect epidemiological transmission: first, the ownership of dogs and cats—without adequate internal deworming protocols (especially in populations with limited economic resources); second, the cultural incompetence to pick up the excrement of these pets in public areas; and third, the dispersal of millions of eggs of gastrointestinal parasites, through the excrement of these dogs and cats, in the environment where humans live. Conditions that increase the probability of accidental infection, mainly in children, of these helminths (establishing parasitic zoonosis).

From the classic clinical medical perspective, this would not seem important; the learned doctors will say, "*if you have a parasite, you deworm yourself and that's it.*" But it turns out that many of these zoonotic geohelminths take humans as a "paratenic host;" that is, they infect them but do not complete the development of their entire biological cycle and end up encysted, thus leaving them outside the therapeutic effects of the classic antiparasitic agents used in medicine, considering also that they have migrated through various tissues (e.g., central nervous system) where they cause syndromes that are very difficult to diagnose.

This parasite–human interaction triggers multiple alterations, most of them subclinical (imperceptible to conventional medical examination). Of the most important alterations in the lives of people exposed at a young age to these infections, the erratic responses to vaccines stand out (e.g., alteration in the expected response to vaccination against cholera in children). Intensify the so-called "cycle of poverty", where infants and children have serious cognitive disabilities for an adequate learning process, which eventually leads them to abandon their school studies or to the impossibility of starting and/or completing their university studies. Helminthiases are the etiology for thousands of deaths and DALY (disability-adjusted life year) annually and are responsible for a 6–35.3% loss in productivity.

As I expressed previously, the majority of low-income families own pets and do not have the opportunity to deworm them adequately (most quality systemic dewormers are expensive). Therefore, it is highly likely that in these conditions, the infants will become infected and are constantly exposed to these zoonotic geohelminths, who end up being their paratenic hosts and who silently develop serious cognitive alterations that prevent them from accessing, maintaining, and graduating from higher education studies. In conclusion, without academic training that guarantees improving their economic income, it is highly likely that they will exacerbate/perpetuate their states of poverty.

This type of epidemiological-medical situations is widely unknown by the majority of the world's health systems, especially the Colombian one, where there are hardly any lines of work in public health associated with the control of the main zoonotic geohelminthiasis: toxocariasis (gastrointestinal parasite that yes or if it is transmitted to canine puppies through the placenta or milk secretion of their mothers, where approximately 14 days after birth a puppy can expel 1,000,000 eggs into the environment through its feces). This situation of hopelessness—lack of interest in working on the knowledge, status, and control of this type of diseases that afflict multiple people—determines that they are called "neglected diseases." Where not only the historical indifference of the government condemns the endemic situation (permanent in the environment), and uncontrolled of it, but also the resources and research groups that are added to the task of studying them, we are counted on the fingers that write this book chapter.

Finally, if we see the tip of the iceberg, and we are afraid of colliding with it; imagine the magnitude of the body of this phenomenon. If we make an analogy, the tip of the iceberg would be the classic diseases that must be registered in the country's precarious health system (e.g. Dengue, HIV, and COVID-19, among others), and the body would be all those that go unnoticed and ignored. As in the "Blindness," public health researchers, biologists, parasitologists, internal medicine doctors—infectious disease specialists, immunologists, veterinary doctors, and epidemiologists, among others—are called to recommend, direct, and demand from the government to generate the optimal environment to think and execute strategies that mitigate this painful public health situation, given that we are the ones who can observe this situation. If and only then, this health disaster in Colombia and others low-income countries could turn into a true change that allows everyone to have opportunities for growth in their quality of life in a fair and equitable manner.

Acknowledgements

To "Jaboneros," my lovely family.

Conflict of interest

The author declares no conflict of interest.

Appendices and nomenclature

AAVP	American Association of Veterinary Parasitologists
CDC	Centers for Disease Control and Prevention
CT	covert/common toxocariasis
DALY	disability-adjusted life year
ELISA	enzyme-linked immunosorbent assay
L3	third-stage larvae of *Toxocara* spp.
TES	*Toxocara* excretory-secretory

DOI: http://dx.doi.org/10.5772/intechopen.1005054

Author details

Dumar A. Jaramillo-Hernández
University of the Llanos, Animal Science College, Villavicencio, Colombia

*Address all correspondence to: dumar.jaramillo@unillanos.edu.co

References

[1] Holland CV, Smith HV. Toxocara: The Enigmatic Parasite. 2st ed. Wallingford: CABI Publishing; 2006. 293 p. Available from: https://goo.gl/cUATdV

[2] Moorhouse DE. Toxocariasis: A possible cause of the Palm Island mystery disease. The Medical Journal of Australia. 1982;**145**(1):172-173. DOI: 10.5694/j.1326-5377.1986.tb113732.x

[3] Gibbons LM, Jacobs DE, Sani RA. Toxocara malaysiensis (Nematoda: Ascaridoidea) from domestic cat (*Felis catus* Linnaeus 1758). Journal of Parasitology. 2001;**87**(3):660-665. DOI: 10.1645/0022-3395(2001)087[0660: TMNSNA]2.0.CO;2

[4] Macchioni G. A new species *Toxocara lyncis*, in the caracal (*Lynx caracal*). Parasitology. 1999;**41**(4):529-532 https://goo.gl/KXUSnh

[5] Holland CV. A walk on the wild side: A review of the epidemiology of *Toxocara canis* and *Toxocara cati* in wild hosts. International Journal for Parasitology: Parasites and Wildlife. 2023;**22**:216-228. DOI: 10.1016/j.ijppaw.2023.10.008

[6] Glickman LT, Schantz PM. Epidemiology and pathogenesis of zoonotic toxocariasis. Epidemiologic Reviews. 1981;**3**:230-250. DOI: 10.1093/oxfordjournals.epirev.a036235

[7] Holland C. Knowledge gaps in the epidemiology of Toxocara: The enigma remains. Parasitology. 2017;**144**(1):81-94. DOI: 10.1017/S0031182015001407

[8] Nathwani D, Laing RB, Currie PF. Covert toxocariasis—A cause of recurrent abdominal pain in childhood. British Journal of Clinical Practice. 1992;**46**(4):271

[9] Moradi G, Gholami F, Rasouli MA, Bagheri Amiri F, Moradi Y. How is the iceberg of COVID-19? Results from a rapid literature review. Medical Journal of the Islamic Republic of Iran. 2021;**35**:77. DOI: 10.47176/mjiri.35.77

[10] Maizels RM. *Toxocara canis*: Molecular basis of immune recognition and evasion. Veterinary Parasitology. 2013;**193**(4):365-374. DOI: 10.1016/j.vetpar.2012.12.032

[11] Abou-El-Naga IF, Mogahed NMFH. Potential roles of *Toxocara canis* larval excretory secretory molecules in immunomodulation and immune evasion. Acta Tropica. 2023;**238**:106784. DOI: 10.1016/j.actatropica.2022.106784

[12] Henke K, Ntovas S, Xourgia E, Exadaktylos AK, Klukowska-Rötzler J, Ziaka M. Who let the dogs out? Unmasking the neglected: A semi-systematic review on the enduring impact of toxocariasis, a prevalent zoonotic infection. International Journal of Environmental Research and Public Health. 2023;**20**(21):6972. DOI: 10.3390/ijerph20216972

[13] Mojžišová J, Süli J, Goldová M, Bajová V, Švrcek S. The effect of endoparasitism on the immune response to antirabies vaccination in puppies. Acta Parasitologica. 2007;**52**(2):176-180. DOI: 10.2478/s11686-007-0023-2

[14] Ulloque-Badaracco JR, Hernandez-Bustamante EA, Alarcón-Braga EA, Huayta-Cortez M, Carballo-Tello XL, Seminario-Amez RA, et al. Seroprevalence of human toxocariasis in Latin America and the Caribbean: A systematic review and meta-analysis. Frontiers in Public Health. 2023;**11**:1181230. DOI: 10.3389/fpubh.2023.1181230

[15] Hotez PJ. Neglected infections of poverty in the United States and their effects on the brain. JAMA Psychiatry. 2014;**71**(10):1099-1100. DOI: 10.1001/jamapsychiatry.2014.1045

[16] McGuinness SL, Leder K. Global burden of toxocariasis: A common neglected infection of poverty. Current Tropical Medicine Reports. 2014;**1**:52-61. DOI: 10.1007/s40475-013-0012-5

[17] Hotez PJ. Human parasitology and parasitic diseases: Heading towards 2050. Advances in Parasitology. 2018;**100**:29-38. DOI: 10.1016/bs.apar.2018.03.002

[18] World Health Organization. Ending the Neglect to Attain the Sustainable Development Goals: A Rationale for Continued Investment in Tackling Neglected Tropical Diseases 2021-2030 [Internet]. 2022. Available from: https://www.who.int/publications/i/item/9789240052932 [Accessed: 2024-02-29]

[19] Jaramillo-Hernández DA, Salazar-Garcés LF, Baquero-Parra MM, da Silva-Pinheiro C, Alcántara-Neves NM. Toxocariasis and Toxocara vaccine: A review. ORINOQUIA. 2020;**24**(2):79-95. DOI: 10.22579/20112629.631

[20] Lucio-Forster A, Mizhquiri JF, Mohammed HO, Kornreich BG, Bowman DD. Comparison of the prevalence of Toxocara egg shedding by pet cats and dogs in the U.S.A., 2011-2014. Veterinary Parasitology: Regional Studies and Reports. 2016;**5**:1-13. DOI: 10.1016/j.vprsr.2016.08.002

[21] Rostami A, Ma G, Wang T, Koehler AV, Hofmann A, Chang BCH, et al. Human toxocariasis—A look at a neglected disease through an epidemiological 'prism'. Infection, Genetics and Evolution. 2019;**74**:104002. DOI: 10.1016/j.meegid.2019.104002

[22] Ma G, Rostami A, Wang T, Hofmann A, Hotez PJ, Gasser RB. Global and regional seroprevalence estimates for human toxocariasis: A call for action. Advances in Parasitology. 2020;**109**:275-290. DOI: 10.1016/bs.apar.2020.01.011

[23] Rubinsky-Elefant G, Hirata CE, Yamamoto JH, Ferreira MU. Human toxocariasis: Diagnosis, worldwide seroprevalences and clinical expression of the systemic and ocular forms. Annals of Tropical Medicine and Parasitology. 2010;**104**(1):3-23. DOI: 10.1179/136485910X12607012373957

[24] Fillaux J, Magnaval JF. Laboratory diagnosis of human toxocariasis. Veterinary Parasitology. 2013;**193**(4):327-336. DOI: 10.1016/j.vetpar.2012.12.028

[25] Thu HN, Van TD, Anh VNT, Huy TT, Trung TN, Le Van N, et al. Clinical, laboratory characteristic, and treatment of human toxocariasis in northern Vietnam. Iranian Journal of Parasitology. 2022;**17**(1):1-9. DOI: 10.18502/ijpa.v17i1.9010

[26] Deplazes P, van Knapen F, Schweiger A, Overgaauw PA. Role of pet dogs and cats in the transmission of helminthic zoonoses in Europe, with a focus on echinococcosis and toxocarosis. Veterinary Parasitology. 2011;**182**(1):41-53. DOI: 10.1016/j.vetpar.2011.07.014

[27] Bowman DD. Ascaris and Toxocara as foodborne and waterborne pathogens. Research in Veterinary Science. 2021;**135**:1-7. DOI: 10.1016/j.rvsc.2020.12.017

[28] Fan CK, Liao CW, Cheng YC. Factors affecting disease manifestation of toxocarosis in humans: Genetics and environment. Veterinary Parasitology. 2013;**193**(4):342-352. DOI: 10.1016/j.vetpar.2012.12.030

[29] Anisuzzaman H, Hatta T, Labony SS, Kwofie KD, Kawada H, Tsuji N, et al. Food- and vector-borne parasitic zoonoses: Global burden and impacts. Advances in Parasitology. 2023;**120**:87-136. DOI: 10.1016/bs.apar.2023.02.001

[30] Bonilla-Aldana DK, Morales-Garcia LV, Ulloque Badaracco JR, Mosquera-Rojas MD, Alarcón-Braga EA, Hernandez-Bustamante EA, et al. Prevalence of Toxocara eggs in Latin American parks: A systematic review and meta-analysis. Le Infezioni in Medicina. 2023;**31**(3):329-349. DOI: 10.53854/liim-3103-7

[31] Fakhri Y, Gasser RB, Rostami A, Fan CK, Ghasemi SM, Javanian M, et al. Toxocara eggs in public places worldwide - a systematic review and meta-analysis. Environmental Pollution. 2018;**242**(Pt B):1467-1475. DOI: 10.1016/j.envpol.2018.07.087

[32] Rostami A, Riahi SM, Holland CV, Taghipour A, Khalili-Fomeshi M, Fakhri Y, et al. Seroprevalence estimates for toxocariasis in people worldwide: A systematic review and meta-analysis. PLOS Neglected Tropical Diseases. 2019;**13**(12):e0007809. DOI: 10.1371/journal.pntd.0007809

[33] Rostami A, Riahi SM, Hofmann A, Ma G, Wang T, Behniafar H, et al. Global prevalence of Toxocara infection in dogs. Advances in Parasitology. 2020;**109**:561-583. DOI: 10.1016/bs.apar.2020.01.017

[34] Dai RS, Li ZY, Li F, Liu DX, Liu W, Liu GH, et al. Severe infection of adult dogs with helminths in Hunan Province, China poses significant public health concerns. Veterinary Parasitology. 2009;**160**(3-4):348-350. DOI: 10.1016/j.vetpar.2008.11.002

[35] Rostami A, Sepidarkish M, Ma G, Wang T, Ebrahimi M, Fakhri Y, et al. Global prevalence of Toxocara infection in cats. Advances in Parasitology. 2020;**109**:615-639. DOI: 10.1016/bs.apar.2020.01.025

[36] Ma G, Rostami A, Wang T, Hofmann A, Hotez PJ, Gasser RB. Global and regional seroprevalence estimates for human toxocariasis: A call for action. In: Bowman DD, editor. Advances in Parasitology. Academic Press; 2020. pp. 275-290

[37] Bowman DD, editor. Toxocara and Toxocariasis, Advances in Parasitology Series. 1st ed2020. 912 p. Available from: sciencedirect.com/bookseries/advances-in-parasitology/vol/109/suppl/C

[38] Beaver PC. Toxocariasis (visceral larva migrans) in relation to tropical eosinophilia. Bulletin de la Société de Pathologie Exotique. 1962;**55**:555-576

[39] Krupińska M, Antolová D, Tołkacz K, Szczepaniak K, Strachecka A, Goll A, et al. Grassland versus forest dwelling rodents as indicators of environmental contamination with the zoonotic nematode Toxocara spp. Scientific Reports. 2023;**13**(1):3748. DOI: 10.1038/s41598-022-23891-6

[40] Jimenez Castro PD, Sapp SG. Role of cats in human toxocarosis. Companion Animal. 2020;**26**(1):1-8. DOI: 10.12968/coan.2020.0104

[41] Regis SC, Mendonça LR, Silva Ndos S, Dattoli VC, Alcântara-Neves NM, Barrouin-Melo SM. Seroprevalence and risk factors for canine toxocariasis by detection of specific IgG as a marker of infection in dogs from Salvador, Brazil. Acta Tropica. 2011;**120**(1-2):46-51. DOI: 10.1016/j.actatropica.2011.05.011

[42] Schwartz R, Bidaisee S, Fields PJ, Macpherson MLA, Macpherson CNL. The epidemiology and control of

Toxocara canis in puppies. Parasite Epidemiology Control. 2021;**16**:e00232. DOI: 10.1016/j.parepi.2021.e00232

[43] Lee RM, Moore LB, Bottazzi ME, Hotez PJ. Toxocariasis in North America: A systematic review. PLOS Neglected Tropical Diseases. 2014;**8**(8):e3116. DOI: 10.1371/journal.pntd.0003116

[44] Auer H, Walochnik J. Toxocariasis and the clinical spectrum. Advances in Parasitology. 2020;**109**:111-130. DOI: 10.1016/bs.apar.2020.01.005

[45] Quattrocchi G, Nicoletti A, Marin B, Bruno E, Druet-Cabanac M, Preux PM. Toxocariasis and epilepsy: Systematic review and meta-analysis. PLOS Neglected Tropical Diseases. 2012;**6**(8):e1775. DOI: 10.1371/journal.pntd.0001775

[46] Santarém VA, Doline FR, Ferreira IB, Farinhas JH, Biondo LM, de Souza Filho RT, et al. One health approach to toxocariasis in Brazilian indigenous populations, their dogs, and soil contamination. Frontiers in Public Health. 2023;**11**:1220001. DOI: 10.3389/fpubh.2023.1220001

[47] Overgaauw PA, van Knapen F. Veterinary and public health aspects of Toxocara spp. Veterinary Parasitology. 2013;**193**(4):398-403. DOI: 10.1016/j.vetpar.2012.12.035

[48] Bolivar-Mejia A, Alarcón-Olave C, Calvo-Betancourt LS, Paniz-Mondolfi A, Delgado O, Rodriguez-Morales AJ. Toxocariasis in the Americas: Burden and disease control. Current Tropical Medicine Reports. 2014;**1**:62-68. DOI: 10.1007/s40475-013-0010-7

[49] Vora NM, Hannah L, Walzer C, Vale MM, Lieberman S, Emerson A, et al. Interventions to reduce risk for pathogen spillover and early disease spread to prevent outbreaks, epidemics, and pandemics. Emerging Infectious Diseases. 2023;**29**(3):1-9. DOI: 10.3201/eid2903.221079

[50] Overgaauw PAM, Nederland V. Aspects of Toxocara epidemiology: Toxocarosis in dogs and cats. Critical Reviews in Microbiology. 1997;**23**(3):233-251. DOI: 10.3109/10408419709115138

[51] Ursache AL, Mircean V, Dumitrache M, Andrei S, Ştefănuţ L, Cozma V, et al. Is routine disinfection efficient in preventing contamination with Toxocara canis eggs? Journal of Helminthology. 2019;**94**:e60. DOI: 10.1017/S0022149X1900052X

[52] Zhang S, Angel C, Gu X, Liu Y, Li Y, Wang L, et al. Efficacy of a chlorocresol-based disinfectant product on *Toxocara canis* eggs. Parasitology Research. 2020;**119**(10):3369-3376. DOI: 10.1007/s00436-020-06769-2

[53] Matos M, Alho AM, Owen SP, Nunes T, Madeira de Carvalho L. Parasite control practices and public perception of parasitic diseases: A survey of dog and cat owners. Preventive Veterinary Medicine. 2015;**122**(1-2):174-180. DOI: 10.1016/j.prevetmed.2015.09.006

[54] Yu Q, Xiao N, Yang SJ, Han S. Deworming of stray dogs and wild canines with praziquantel-laced baits delivered by an unmanned aerial vehicle in areas highly endemic for echinococcosis in China. Infectious Diseases of Poverty. 2017;**6**(1):117. DOI: 10.1186/s40249-017-0329-8

[55] Alho AM, Lima C, Colella V, Madeira de Carvalho L, Otranto D, Cardoso L. Awareness of zoonotic diseases and parasite control practices: A survey of dog and cat owners in Qatar. Parasitic Vectors. 2018;**11**(1):133. DOI: 10.1186/s13071-018-2720-0

[56] Viña C, Salmo R, Pena MV, Palomero AM, Hernández JÁ, Cazapal-Monteiro C, et al. A new comestible formulation of parasiticide fungi to reduce the risk of soil-transmitted helminth infections in a canine shelter. Pathogens. 2022;**11**(11):1391. DOI: 10.3390/pathogens11111391

[57] Coati N, Schnieder T, Epe C. Vertical transmission of Toxocara cati Schrank 1788 (Anisakidae) in the cat. Parasitoly Research. 2004;**92**(2):142-146. DOI: 10.1007/s00436-003-1019-y

[58] Krämer F, Hammerstein R, Stoye M, Epe C. Investigations into the prevention of prenatal and lactogenic *Toxocara canis* infections in puppies by application of moxidectin to the pregnant dog. Journal of Veterinary Medicine. B, Infectious Diseases and Veterinary Public Health. 2006;**53**(5):218-223. DOI: 10.1111/j.1439-0450.2006.00948.x

[59] Webster GA. On prenatal infection and the migration of *Toxocara canis* Werner, 1782 in dogs. Canadian Journal of Zoology. 1958;**36**(3):435-440. DOI: 10.1139/z58-038

[60] Stull JW, Carr AP, Chomel BB, Berghaus RD, Hird DW. Small animal deworming protocols, client education, and veterinarian perception of zoonotic parasites in western Canada. The Canadian Veterinary Journal. 2007;**48**(3):269-276. DOI: 10.4141/cjas68-037

[61] Cárdenas J, Lesmes KI, Torres MC, Alcantara-Neves NM, Jaramillo-Hernández DA. Evaluación de técnicas coprodiagnósticas para *Toxocara canis*. Revista de Investigaciones Veterinarias del Perú. 2021;**32**(3):e18861. DOI: 10.15381/rivep.v32i3.18861

[62] Rudzińska M, Kowalewska B, Sikorska K. Clinical usefulness of Western blotting and ELISA avidity for the diagnosis of human toxocariasis. Parasite Immunology. 2017;**39**(1):e12400. DOI: 10.1111/pim.12400

[63] Ma G, Holland CV, Wang T, Hofmann A, Fan C-K, Maizels RM, et al. Human toxocariasis. The Lancet Infectious Diseases. 2018;**18**:e14-e24. DOI: 10.1016/S1473-3099(17)30331-6

[64] Centers for Disease Control and Prevention (CDC). Immunization: The Basics [Internet]. 2024. Available from: https://www.cdc.gov/vaccines/vac-gen/imz-basics.htm [Accessed: 2024-02-29]

[65] Pan American Health Organization (PAHO). Immunization [Internet]. 2024. Available from: https://www.paho.org/en/topics/immunization [Accessed: 2024-02-29]

[66] Delany I, Rappuoli R, Seib KL. Vaccines, reverse vaccinology, and bacterial pathogenesis. Cold Spring Harbor Perspectives in Medicine. 2013;**3**(5):a012476. DOI: 10.1101/cshperspect.a012476

[67] Kanampalliwar AM. Reverse vaccinology and its applications. Methods in Molecular Biology. 2020;**2131**:1-16. DOI: 10.1007/978-1-0716-0389-5_1

[68] Vargas L, Prieto L, Baquero M, Corredor W, Alcantara-Neves NM, Jaramillo-Hernández DA. Vaccines for gastrointestinal parasites, a pillar of preventive medicine in veterinary practice: Systematic review. Revista de Investigación Agraria y Ambiental. 2021;**13**:221-251. DOI: 10.22490/21456453.4544

[69] Zhu XQ, Korhonen PK, Cai H, Young ND, Nejsum P, von Samson-Himmelstjerna G, et al. Genetic blueprint of the zoonotic pathogen

Toxocara canis. Nature Communications. 2015;**6**:6145. DOI: 10.1038/ncomms7145

[70] Zhou RQ, Ma GX, Korhonen PK, Luo YL, Zhu HH, Luo YF, et al. Comparative transcriptomic analyses of male and female adult Toxocara canis. Gene. 2017;**600**:85-89. DOI: 10.1016/j.gene.2016.11.024

[71] Wangchuk P, Lavers O, Wishart DS, Loukas A. Excretory/secretory metabolome of the zoonotic roundworm parasite *Toxocara canis*. Biomolecules. 2020;**10**(8):1157. DOI: 10.3390/biom10081157

[72] Soleymani N, Grunberger RB, Abnous K, Borji H, Vahdati F. Identification and immunological characterization of somatic proteins from adults of *Toxocara cati* by proteomics technique. Iranian Journal of Parasitology. 2021;**16**(1):23-31. DOI: 10.18502/ijpa.v16i1.5508

[73] Salazar LF, Santiago LF, Santos SPO, Jaramillo-Hernández DA, da Silva MB, Alves VDS, et al. Immunogenicity and protection induced by recombinant *Toxocara canis* proteins in a murine model of toxocariasis. Vaccine. 2020;**38**(30):4762-4772. DOI: 10.1016/j.vaccine.2020.04.072

[74] Lightowlers MW, Rickard MD. Excretory–secretory products of helminth parasites: Effects on host immune responses. Parasitology. 1988;**96**:S123-S166. DOI: 10.1017/S0031182000086017

[75] Raulf MK, Lepenies B, Strube C. *Toxocara canis* and *Toxocara cati* somatic and excretory-secretory antigens are recognised by C-type lectin receptors. Pathogens. 2021;**10**(3):321. DOI: 10.3390/pathogens10030321

[76] Skulinová K, Novák J, Kolářová L, Kašný M. Antigenic proteins from the excretory-secretory products of *Toxocara canis* larvae and evaluation of their potential for immunodiagnostics of larval Toxocarosis. Acta Parasitology. 2022;**67**(2):705-713. DOI: 10.1007/s11686-021-00485-2

[77] Jaramillo-Hernández DA, Salazar Garcés LF, Pacheco LGC, Pinheiro CS, Alcantara-Neves NM. Protective response mediated by immunization with recombinant proteins in a murine model of toxocariasis and canine infection by *Toxocara canis*. Vaccine. 2022;**40**(6):912-923. DOI: 10.1016/j.vaccine.2021.12.052

[78] Bahadory S, Sadraei J, Zibaei M, Pirestani M, Dalimi A. In vitro anti-gastrointestinal cancer activity of *Toxocara canis*-derived peptide: Analyzing the expression level of factors related to cell proliferation and tumor growth. Frontiers in Pharmacology. 2022;**13**:878724. DOI: 10.3389/fphar.2022.878724

Chapter 5

Cryptosporidium spp.: Challenges in Control and Potential Therapeutic Strategies

Taiwo Akinnubi

Abstract

Cryptosporidium parasites (*Cryptosporidium hominis* and *Cryptosporidium parvum*) are prominent for playing a crucial role in the high prevalence of diarrheal infection across the globe, with immunocompromised individual at risk. The parasites' remarkable resilience in the environment due to several adaptive strategies is responsible for persistent challenge in control especially in regions with inadequate sanitation. In tackling these challenges, exploring promising potential therapeutic strategies to combat *Cryptosporidium* infections is of critical importance. This encompasses investigations into experimental drugs, immunotherapies, and vaccine development efforts, all aimed at reducing the burden these parasites impose. This review aims to present the current state of research and development to shed light on the future prospects for managing *Cryptosporidium* infections and their profound impact on public health.

Keywords: *Cryptosporidium*, challenges, control, therapeutic, strategies

1. Introduction

Cryptosporidium is a well-established obligate gastrointestinal protozoan parasite [1]. It is widely distributed both environmentally and geographically, encompassing numerous species with a broad host range. Over 40 species of *Cryptosporidium* have been documented, with at least 20 implicated in human infections [2, 3]. However, the predominant agents of human infection are *C. hominis* and *C. parvum*, with *C. hominis* being a predominantly human-related transmission and *C. parvum* both human- and animal-borne transmission [3].

Cryptosporidium infection occurs through the ingestion of oocysts, which are released by a host already infected with the parasite and are present in contaminated environments through oral-fecal exposure. Transmission primarily occurs *via* water and, to a lesser extent, through food. Upon ingestion of oocysts, sporozoites are liberated and subsequently adhere to intestinal epithelial cells, undergoing internalization. A thick, actin-rich layer known as the parasitophorous vacuole membrane forms, separating them from the host cytoplasm within the microvillus layer of the host cell membrane [4]. Following maturation, the organism undergoes a bifurcating life cycle. Asexual reproduction yields merozoites, which can subsequently invade further

IntechOpen

intestinal epithelial cells, perpetuating the infection within a single host. Conversely, sexual multiplication culminates in the release of oocysts, which are shed from the host and serve to establish infection in new hosts.

Cryptosporidium has become a major worldwide contributor to diarrheal illness, posing a significant health risk, especially for young children and individuals with weakened immune systems. Research indicates its substantial impact in developing countries, where it is recognized as a leading cause of moderate-to-severe gastrointestinal illness in children under 5 years old [5]. A recent in-depth investigation into gastrointestinal diseases has underscored the significant public health burden posed by *Cryptosporidium*. This study estimates that *Cryptosporidium* species caused over 1 million deaths, with nearly half occurring in children under 5 years of age. Furthermore, it resulted in more than 71 million disability-adjusted life years (DALYs) between 2005 and 2015 [6]. The data reveals that developing countries, particularly those in sub-Saharan Africa, suffer the highest mortality rates. While *Cryptosporidium* is endemic in most developing nations, it also has the potential to cause waterborne outbreaks on a large scale, impacting both developing and developed countries [7]. Especially worrisome are the long-term consequences observed in children, such as stunted growth and cognitive impairments that persist beyond the initial recovery from cryptosporidiosis [5].

Cryptosporidiosis is a noteworthy health concern not only in wild animals but also in domesticated ones. Within farm animal management, it has been linked to the development of a severe and frequently fatal diarrheal syndrome in newborn calves and other young ruminant animals. This parasite infestation leads to substantial economic losses, both directly and indirectly [8]. Furthermore, cryptosporidiosis can have lasting detrimental effects on infected animals. Studies have shown diminished weight gain and reduced production performance in both cattle and sheep [9, 10]. For example, research by [9] found that beef calves exposed to cryptosporidiosis as newborns can experience an average weight deficit of 34 kg at 6 months of age compared to their counterparts without signs of infection.

In recent times, research has been dedicated to identifying compounds with novel mechanisms of action that are effective against *Cryptosporidium* spp. Presently, only one drug, nitazoxanide, holds approval from the US Food and Drug Administration (FDA) for treating cryptosporidiosis in immune-competent individuals in the United States, excluding immunocompromised individuals like AIDS patients. However, nitazoxanide's efficacy is limited, and its mechanism of action remains unclear [11]. Compounding the challenge, there is a lack of FDA-approved medications to treat cryptosporidiosis in animals. Halofuginone lactate (Halocur), although approved for veterinary use in calves and lambs in some countries, demonstrates only partial effectiveness against *Cryptosporidium* and fails to entirely eliminate oocyst shedding [12].

Numerous obstacles in the discovery of drugs against cryptosporidiosis include the scarcity of parasite materials, lack of a robust and standardized *in vitro* cultivation system, lack of conventional drug targets, the need for the development of *in vitro* phenotypic screening platforms, the complexity of genetic manipulation techniques despite their availability, and the availability and constraints of animal models, among other challenges [13].

The complexity of combating *Cryptosporidium* spp. infections presents a formidable challenge to public health efforts worldwide. Despite significant advancements in understanding its biology and pathogenesis, effective control measures remain elusive. However, the exploration of potential therapeutic strategies offers a glimmer of hope in the quest to mitigate the impact of this ubiquitous pathogen. In this review, thelandscape of *Cryptosporidium* control is examined, with a focus on both the hurdles faced and the promising avenues for future intervention.

2. Cryptosporidiosis: transmission strategies, clinical manifestations, and public health impact

Cryptosporidium infection exhibits diverse transmission pathways. Humans can contract the parasite through direct contact with infected individuals (anthroponotic transmission) or animals (zoonotic transmission). Indirect transmission also occurs *via* contaminated food (foodborne transmission) or water (waterborne transmission). Person-to-person and waterborne transmission appear to be the most common routes, evidenced by the higher frequency of reported cases and outbreaks associated with these modes [14]. Outbreaks associated with contaminated recreational water, particularly swimming in polluted rivers, lakes, or pools, underscore the diverse modes of *Cryptosporidium* transmission [15]. Several other factors include migration, interaction with animals or young children experiencing diarrhea, and engaging in certain sexual practices (multiple sexual partner and anal intercourse) that carry a higher risk of transmission [13].

A worldwide study revealed a troubling number of waterborne protozoan illness outbreaks, totaling 936 between 1946 and 2016 [16]. *Cryptosporidium* was responsible for over half (58%) of these outbreaks. Even more concerning is its ability to bypass filtration systems, contaminating both filtered and unfiltered drinking water supplies in communities [16]. The resilience of these *Cryptosporidium* spp. Oocytes to conventional water treatment, environmental resilience, zoonotic strains and wide range of reservoir host complicate control. Oocysts can also seep from polluted surface water into groundwater [17, 18].

The most substantial outbreak of cryptosporidiosis linked to drinking water occurred in Milwaukee, Wisconsin, in 1993, impacting an estimated 403,000 individuals out of a population of around 800,000. It also resulted in high hospitalization (4400) and a hundred mortality rates [19]. The number of documented foodborne outbreaks is lower compared to waterborne incidents, potentially attributed to lack of standard foodborne oocyst detection tool and the less frequent occurrence of food contamination [20]. However, *Cryptosporidium* oocysts, the infectious stage of the parasite, have been found in a concerning variety of food products, including raw vegetables, meat, salads, fermented milk products, cider, raw milk, and apple [21]. This highlights the diverse points of contamination throughout the food chain, from production and harvest to processing, transportation, and even preparation in the home [21].

The clinical presentation of enteric cryptosporidiosis lacks distinct signs or symptoms, resembling various other forms of diarrheal diseases. Initial infections typically manifest with symptoms such as nausea, vomiting, abdominal cramps, watery diarrhea, and fatigue. Stool specimens rarely show the presence of blood or leukocytes. Unlike typical enteric infections, Cryptosporidiosis in developing countries often presents with a low-grade fever and cough less frequently [22]. Repeated exposure can lead to asymptomatic infections in children, and symptomatic cases tend to be shorter, lasting a median of just 2 days. However, weight reduction and dehydration remain a concern, especially for malnourished children or those with prolonged diarrhea [22]. In developed nations, immunocompetent individuals with Cryptosporidiosis experience severe symptoms. Diarrhea can last 9–11 days, with some requiring hospitalization [23]. Joint pain, fatigue, and other issues may also occur, especially with *C. hominis*. Cryptosporidiosis may even be linked to chronic bowel problems [22].

Cryptosporidiosis poses a greater risk for immunocompromised people. As their immune system weakens, asymptomatic infections can worsen, leading to the development of symptoms [24]. Furthermore, the parasite can invade the bile ducts, causing inflammation (cholangitis), and potentially impact the respiratory system, leading to mild oxygen deficiency and shortness of breath [24]. Previously thought uncommon, respiratory infections with *Cryptosporidium* have been identified in a surprising number of children with intestinal infections [25–28]. This suggests potential transmission through coughed-up sputum. For individuals with HIV/AIDS, Cryptosporidiosis can be life-threatening, significantly increasing mortality and shortening lifespan [28]. The severity varies greatly, with a particularly aggressive form causing massive fluid loss, severe pain, and rapid weight loss, leading to death within days or weeks. Variations in immune function, infection location, and parasite species all contribute to these differences in disease severity and patient outcomes [28].

Cryptosporidiosis poses a significant global public health concern, ranking as the sixth most frequent foodborne parasitic infection in humans and animals [29]. In developing countries, the parasite disproportionately impacts malnourished children, where it is a leading cause of death. The full scope of human *Cryptosporidium* epidemics, particularly in these less developed regions, remains unclear [30]. For children suffering from acute, chronic, or persistent diarrhea caused by *Cryptosporidium*, the consequences are severe, including stunted growth, reduced physical development, cognitive impairment, and even death [13].

Cryptosporidium species are prominent diarrheal pathogens worldwide, affecting a staggering 20% of children experiencing diarrhea in developing countries, compared to a much lower range of 1 to 5% in North America and Europe [26]. Landmark studies conducted in West Africa during the 1990s underscored the severity of this disparity. Children with Cryptosporidiosis displayed significantly higher mortality rates, with a nine-fold increase in death risk even after accounting for nutrition-related factors. Infection typically occurs earlier in life: before age 2 in developing regions and before age 5 in developed ones. Additionally, the prevalence is higher in rural areas and during rainy seasons. Exposure to the parasite appears to be continuous, as evidenced by increasing seropositivity with age [13]. However, malnutrition, HIV/AIDS, and other conditions that weaken the immune system dramatically elevate the risk, severity, and duration of Cryptosporidiosis. This makes it a defining opportunistic infection in AIDS patients and a frequent complication for malnourished children suffering from persistent diarrhea [31].

3. Current preventive and control measures and their constraints

Several control and preventive measures have been initiated toward curtailing the transmission of *Cryptosporidium* spp. most of which focus on environment-related factors and reservoir host. This is because reservoir characteristics and environmental factors significantly influence the epidemiology and transmissibility of *Cryptosporidium* spp. [32]. Oocysts, shed by the host, exhibit sensitivity to various unfavorable environmental conditions before finding a suitable new host [32]. Environmental factors like higher temperatures, age, and dryness significantly impact the survival and infectiousness of *Cryptosporidium* oocysts. While prolonged sunlight exposure completely inactivates them, traditional water treatment methods like coagulation and filtration often prove inadequate [33]. This highlights the resilience of the oocyst and the need for more robust treatment strategies. Advancements in UV disinfection research have shown promise, with UV light effectively killing *Cryptosporidium* oocysts. In addition, solar photocatalytic disinfection (SPCDIS) using titanium oxide has demonstrated effectiveness, even in less-than-ideal light conditions [33]. Chlorination has proven inadequate in removing *Cryptosporidium* spp., prompting ongoing efforts to develop vaccines for animals [34].

Similarly, [35] reported modern microbial reduction process designs, such as the integrated disinfection design framework (IDDF) which ensure the provision of low-risk drinking water by addressing the shortcomings of traditional treatment methods. Also, the prevention of reservoir hosts from contact with water supplies and the construction of wetlands for wastewater treatment have emerged as effective and cost-efficient strategies for removing parasite like *Cryptosporidium* spp. [36]. Practical measures, such as educational campaign, handwashing initiatives, and point-of-use water treatment (especially in developing nation) are key ways to curb *Cryptosporidium* transmission. Boiling water, using reliable bottled water, and home filtration units offer further protection [34]. However, in many developing countries, several challenges hinder efforts to prevent the transmission of diseases. These include a lack of access to clean water, open grazing and extensive rearing of animals, poor sanitation infrastructure leading to water source contamination, limited healthcare resources, porous borders, and high population density. These factors collectively serve as significant setbacks to various preventive measures aimed at curbing the spread of diseases.

From pharmaceutical perspective, anti-cryptosporidial agents, including paromomycin, nitazoxanide, and azithromycin, have shown limitations in treating *Cryptosporidium* enteritis. Nitazoxanide, the only FDA-endorsed medication, exhibits limitations, especially in Individuals with HIV/AIDS [37]. Studies have indicated that current chemotherapy has a limited role in managing cryptosporidiosis in immunocompromised individuals, emphasizing the importance of restoring immune status using antiretroviral drugs [37].

Research on alternative treatments involves traditional medicinal plants such as *Allium sativum* (garlic) and various plant extracts. Garlic possesses potential as a preventative measure (prophylactic) and treatment (therapeutic) for Cryptosporidiosis, with studies indicating its potential in reducing the shedding of oocysts. Furthermore, studies on plant extracts like *Peganum harmala* and *Artemesia herba*-alba have shown promising anti-parasitic activity, providing potential alternatives to conventional pharmaceuticals [38, 39]. Research into alternative treatments for *Cryptosporidium*, particularly utilizing traditional medicinal plants, faces several challenges. The lack of comprehensive scientific validation, standardization of effective dosage, bioavailability issues of active compounds, cultural variability, interactions with conventional medications, long-term effects, and many more are several issues linked with the utilization of traditional medicinal plant.

4. Existing diagnostic methods and limitation

Given that *Cryptosporidium* poses a significant threat to people with weakened immune systems and is associated with serious illness and death, it is important for clinical laboratories to come up with effective screening criteria and reliable testing methods. However there is still no agreed-upon international standard for diagnosing cryptosporidiosis [40]. In labs and field research, there are multiple ways to detect and study *Cryptosporidium* spp. Each method has its strengths and weaknesses, like sensitivity, cost, processing time, specificity, detection limits, difficulty, and equipment needs [41].

Microscopy-based methods are commonly used in identifying *Cryptosporidium* oocysts in various samples, such as water, food products, and stool. However, their reliability to identify different *Cryptosporidium* species based on Conventional microscopy alone is questioned due to the similarities in morphological characteristics among many species [42]. Also, these methods cannot determine oocyst infectivity [42]. While a range of staining techniques, such as the Ziehl–Neelsen stain (acid-fast stain) and dimethyl sulfoxide, have been utilized to distinguish *Cryptosporidium* oocysts from other particles on glass slides [41]. However, staining methods have limitations such as variation in stain uptake, low sensitivity, lack of specificity for samples with small oocyst numbers, and the need for a skilled microscopist. Furthermore, staining method is limited by its slow speed, time-consuming nature, and potential for subjectivity compared to other options [43].

Immunology-based methods, particularly immunofluorescence assays using monoclonal antibodies (mAbs), provide higher specificity and sensitivity compared to microscopy [43]. The direct fluorescent antibody (DFA) assay, which utilizes the fluorescein isothiocyanate-conjugated anti-*Cryptosporidium* mAb, is commonly employed for this purpose [43]. Commercially available kits have demonstrated high specificity and improved sensitivity [41]. However, indirect immunofluorescence assays involve additional steps compared to DFA and utilize a second fluorophore-conjugated antibody. The process is longer and potentially more prone to nonspecific binding [44].

Immunomagnetic separation (IMS) offers a valuable technique for isolating *Cryptosporidium* oocysts, particularly from samples containing low numbers of oocysts [44]. This method utilizes magnetic beads coated with specific antibodies to target and capture *Cryptosporidium* oocysts from environmental samples. Studies report high sensitivity and specificity for *C. parvum* oocysts, demonstrating its effectiveness in detecting this particular species [45]. However, a key limitation of IMS lies in its inability to differentiate between *Cryptosporidium* species or genotypes. Additionally, the time-consuming nature of the process and the high cost of commercially available IMS kits pose challenges for widespread implementation [46]. Immunochromatographic lateral-flow assays (ICLFAs) are popular rapid tests that use antibody strips to detect *Cryptosporidium* antigens in stool and water samples. Their advantages include rapid detection, cost-effectiveness, and no need for specialized equipment or trained personnel. However, despite high accuracy of ICLFA, cases of false positive and negative results have been reported. This has led to cautious consideration of positive results until further improvement of these tests [47].

The enzyme-linked immunosorbent assay (ELISA) is a widely employed method in detecting *Cryptosporidium parvum* in human and animal stool samples. ELISA offers high sensitivity for *Cryptosporidium*, exceeding acid-fast staining [48]. However, its effectiveness can vary depending on the kit and population [48, 49]. Longer processing times and potential false positives limit its use in water sample testing for *C. parvum* [50]. Flow cytometry excels in fast, large-scale analysis of cells with high accuracy, making it a valuable tool for *Cryptosporidium* detection. When combined with immunomagnetic separation (IMS), FC enhances oocyst recovery from water samples [51]. Although FC is more sensitive than traditional methods like DFA, its infrequent use in diagnostic laboratories is attributed to high costs and technical expertise requirements [43]. Cell culture immunofluorescence assays use lab-grown *C. parvum* oocysts to assess viability and infectivity. The challenges include low yields and difficulties in long-term propagation [52].

Nucleic acid methods excel in detecting parasites like *Cryptosporidium*, offering high sensitivity and improved accuracy. Conventional PCR, nested PCR, and quantitative PCR (qPCR) have been extensively used for *Cryptosporidium* detection in various samples [43, 45, 47, 50]. qPCR, in particular, allows real-time monitoring with high sensitivity and specificity [41]. Also, droplet digital PCR (ddPCR) improves nucleic acid quantification, but its use for *Cryptosporidium* detection is limited due to cost considerations [53, 54]. PCR-restriction fragment length polymorphism (PCR-RFLP) has been a useful tool for genotyping; its role is diminishing due to the affordability and accessibility of DNA sequencing technologies [55]. Furthermore, whole-genome sequencing using Sanger sequencing and next-generation sequencing platforms has also helped in understanding *Cryptosporidium* diversity [56].

DNA fingerprinting methods that include random amplified polymorphic DNA (RAPD) provide valuable information on genetic variation. However, Aptamer-based methods, which adopt synthesized molecular recognition probes, present a good approach for direct and sensitive *Cryptosporidium* detection. Aptamer's advantages over antibodies include cost-effectiveness and stability [57].

Aptamer-based aptasensors have demonstrated success in identifying *Cryptosporidium* oocysts in various samples, such as water, food products, and stool [41]. Despite challenges in aptamer research, recent advancements have addressed issues like rapid degradation and lack of standardized protocols. Emerging research suggests aptamers have the potential to become widely used in diagnostics, therapy, and biosensing applications [41].

5. Present therapeutic options

The primary pharmaceutical intervention for *Cryptosporidium* infection in children over 1 year of age remains nitazoxanide, a thiazole compound approved by the FDA in 2003. Placebo-controlled studies have demonstrated its increased efficacy in non-HIV-infected cryptosporidiosis patient [58]. The treatment's efficacy wanes in immunocompromised individuals, even when administered at higher doses for extended periods [59]. While nitazoxanide is currently the only FDA-approved treatment for *Cryptosporidium*, its effectiveness is reduced in children with malnutrition or weakened immune systems [60]. Studies have shown that nitazoxanide treatment only leads to a stop in diarrhea for 56% of malnourished children with chronic *Cryptosporidium* compared to 23% receiving a placebo [59]. Combining nitazoxanide with new anti-*Cryptosporidium* drugs may offer a more effective approach for treating malnourished children and immunocompromised patients with HIV/AIDS.

While paromomycin offers some promise and partial effectiveness in AIDS patients with *Cryptosporidium*, it lacks official treatment approval. Similarly, azithromycin shows minimal effectiveness and fails to outperform a placebo in AIDS patients with the infection [61].

Halofuginone shows promise as a treatment for coccidiosis in animals by targeting a specific parasite enzyme [62, 63]; its use in humans is limited. This compound is even licensed for cryptosporidiosis in calves in some countries [62, 63] However, unfavorable side effects on the gastrointestinal system and higher toxicity compared to other options prevent its use for human cryptosporidiosis treatment [63]. These limitations on effective drug treatments force many developing countries to rely on basic strategies like rehydration and electrolyte replacement for managing Cryptosporidiosis.

6. Challenges in the development of *Cryptosporidium* infections

Limited access to pure *Cryptosporidium* for research impedes progress. While *C. parvum* is commonly used, obtaining large quantities remains challenging [64]. Although *in vitro* culture techniques for *C. parvum* have advanced over decades, continuous cultivation faces persistent limitations. The parasite primarily replicates asexually, hindering the production of unlimited materials needed for drug discovery and a deeper understanding of the life cycle [65, 66].

Limited drug targets due to *Cryptosporidium*'s simple biology (minimal metabolism and nutrient synthesis) are a hurdle. However, recent sequencing of various *Cryptosporidium* genomes has opened exciting possibilities for identifying new drug targets [13]. While genetic manipulation tools like CRISPR/Cas9 have addressed issues in drug target validation, challenges persist in the adaptation of these tools for routine laboratory use. *C. tyzzeri*, a mouse-specific species, serves as a valuable genetic model, offering convenience for laboratory manipulation. Additionally, gene-silencing strategies have shown success in knockdown experiments [67, 68].

One major challenges of systemic drugs is inability to cross the epicellular delivery (ED) band. Significant knowledge gaps remain regarding the molecular makeup and function of the parasite–host interface, particularly the ED band. This results in unsatisfactory efficacy of some identified anti-cryptosporidial drugs *in vivo*. Systemic drugs must effectively cross the ED band; this emphasizes the importance of pharmacokinetic parameters in plasma for efficacy in mouse models. While animal experiments are informative, they are costly and time-consuming. This calls for better *in vitro* assays to evaluate how easily small molecule drugs can permeate the ED band [65]. The systemic drugs are also limited by severe watery diarrhea. This is because they can be easily flushed off from the gastrointestinal tract (GIT). Novel pharmacological modifications like exploration of the enterohepatic recycling pathway could improve drug absorption in individuals with severe diarrhea. Testing drug effectiveness in animals, especially mice that do not develop diarrhea, poses a challenge in evaluating drug absorption and efficacy [13].

An alternative strategy involves the development of drugs that target the parasite directly within the gut (nonsystemic drugs). Unlike systemic drugs, which can be flushed out by diarrhea, nonsystemic drugs offer a targeted approach. Nonsystemic drugs may serve as effective alternatives to systemic drugs. Further improvements could involve increasing its (nonsystemic drugs) adhesion to the gut lining (mucoadhesive properties) and potentially combining them with anti-diarrheal medications to maximize their effectiveness within the digestive tract [13].

7. Emerging therapeutic strategies

Significant progress has been achieved in identifying active compounds against *Cryptosporidium*, with aim of providing medication for childhood diarrhea in developing nations [69].

DOI: http://dx.doi.org/10.5772/intechopen.1005165

Benzoxaboroles, boron-heterocyclic compounds, have garnered attention globally. A compound called AN7973 shows promise as a treatment for cryptosporidiosis. This 6-carboxamide benzoxaborole inhibits the development of *C. parvum* within host cells and kills *C. hominis* parasites. AN7973 reduced fecal shedding of *C. parvum* by over 90% in both mouse models and neonatal dairy calves, suggesting its potential effectiveness. Furthermore, Pyrazolopyridines displayed over 60% inhibition of *C. parvum*. KDU731 (ayrazolopyridine) has shown efficacy against cryptosporidiosis in both immunocompromised mice and neonatal calves by reducing oocyst shedding [70].

Piperazine derivative MMV665917, initially identified in the Medicines for Malaria Venture "Malaria Box," exhibited high efficacy against *C. parvum* and *C. hominis in vitro*. In newborn calves and gnotobiotic piglets, it was discovered the MMV665917 reduced oocysts, diarrhea severity, and intestinal mucosal damage. Further investigations are required for dosage optimization and understanding mechanisms of action [64, 71].

Bicyclic azetidines, known for their effectiveness against *P. falciparum*, have demonstrated efficacy against *C. parvum* and *C. hominis* both *in vitro* and *in vivo*. Targeting phenylalanyl-tRNA synthetase, these compounds showed potent inhibition of *Cryptosporidium* growth and protective effects in mice. Bicyclic azetidines present a promising series for cryptosporidiosis treatment [72].

Recent advancements in genetic modification, particularly CRISPR-guided relinking, have enabled a broad comprehension of *Cryptosporidium* biology. This approach, known for its simplicity, supports efficient reverse genetics for the parasite. The introduction of transgenic reporter strains, like the Nluc reporter strain, has speed of the process of drug development against *Cryptosporidium*. This is achieved through the provision of a rapid and scalable screening method. These strains allow lead compound testing in both immunocompromised mouse models and *in vitro* setting. Genetic modification promises to identify crucial drug targets and understand their mechanisms, expediting drug development against *Cryptosporidium* [72].

Natural products emerge as a rich source for potential therapeutic agents. A recent study that screened 800 natural products has identified 16 compounds with low to submicromolar anti-*Cryptosporidium parvum* activity *in vitro* [73]. Compounds like Ginsenoside-Rh2, Curcurbitacin-B, flavonoids, and isoflavones displayed Anticryptosporidia activity in mouse models. Chicory, curcumin, chitosan, and others have shown efficacy against *C. parvum* both *in vivo* and *in vitro*. The investigation of novel bioactive compound and natural products holds promise in the development of effective Anticryptosporidia compounds and potent candidates [73].

Probiotics, recognized as a natural alternative therapeutic approach, demonstrate results against *Cryptosporidium* infections. Probiotics can reduce the number of oocysts shed in feces (oocyst excretion) and lessen the severity of infection [74]. Certain probiotic strains, particularly Lactobacilli, have shown potential by the clearance of *Cryptosporidium* oocysts in mice and humans. Understanding probiotic mechanisms is pertinent in the development of effective probiotic treatments against *Cryptosporidium* infections [74].

Advances in next-generation sequencing technologies allow for detailed characterization of the gut microbiota's role in various diseases, not exempting *Cryptosporidium* infection. Specific members of the microbiome, such as Megasphaera, may influence the severity of *Cryptosporidium*-induced diarrhea. Despite the complexity of the microbiota's impact on *Cryptosporidium* development, it represents a promising target for interventions. Future research should focus on understanding specific genera or phyla within the microbiota that can positively influence immune responses to *Cryptosporidium* [75].

The development of a *Cryptosporidium* vaccine is driven by the necessity for effective preventive measures. Memory T cells, essential components of immunological memory, enhance the body's ability to resist subsequent infections. This characteristic makes them a prime focus in vaccine development [76]. Identification of new vaccine candidates should prioritize antigens capable of eliciting T cell responses [77]. A molecule named gp40/15 polyprotein shows promise as a *Cryptosporidium* vaccine [78]. It triggers the production of IFN-γ, which activates memory T cells crucial for fighting off future infections. Also, Zoite surface proteins like Cpgp40 and Cpgp40/15 have demonstrated associations with the parasitophorous vacuole membrane, through the inhibition of *C. parvum* infection [79]. Antigens like gp40 elicit cellular immune responses in humans and animals, but their protective response against *Cryptosporidium* infection needs further examination. CpGP15 recombinant antigen eliminates *C. parvum* infection in cattle. It further addressed false-negative results on animal farms [80].

Furthermore, Peptides like CP15 and circumsporozoite-like antigen (CSL) stimulate antibody production and block parasite entry *in vitro* [81]. CpTSP8, a TRAP-like protein in *C. parvum*, is important for parasite movement and invasion or attachment to the host cell [82]. Despite the potential of TRAP proteins as vaccine candidates, further investigations are warranted.

Similarly, the discovery of Cp-P34, a sporozoite surface protein in *Cryptosporidium*, is crucial for developing a multiantigenic vaccine against cryptosporidiosis. This protein, primarily localized within the parasite, transiently appears on the surface of *Cryptosporidium* sporozoites, thereby stimulating host immune responses [83]. The mechanism by which Cp-P34 reaches the surface could be a valuable target for future vaccine development. Despite these advancements, further research is needed to fully understand the protective efficacy of these antigens and their potential as components of an effective vaccine against *Cryptosporidium*.

8. Conclusions

The review highlights the multifaceted challenges associated with *Cryptosporidium* spp. infections, focusing on the transmission strategies, clinical manifestations, public health impact, preventive measures, diagnostic methods, existing therapeutic options, and emerging strategies. The prevalence of waterborne and person-to-person transmission underscores the global significance of cryptosporidiosis, with substantial public health and environmental implications. The limitations of current preventive measures emphasize the need for innovative approaches to curb transmission. Diagnostic methods exhibit varied strengths and weaknesses. However, challenges like false positives and negatives persist, emphasizing the ongoing need for improvement and standardization in diagnostic techniques. Existing therapeutic options face limitations, particularly in immunocompromised patients, highlighting the necessity for novel anti-*Cryptosporidium* therapeutics. The challenges in drug development underscore the complexity of combating *Cryptosporidium* infections. Emerging therapeutic strategies, such as benzoxaboroles, pyrazolopyridines, and probiotics, show promise in preclinical studies, offering potential alternatives to current treatments. Genetic modification techniques, natural products, and the exploration of the gut microbiota's role present exciting avenues for future research and drug development. The pursuit of an effective *Cryptosporidium* vaccine remains a critical goal, with promising candidates like gp40/15 polyprotein, CpGP15 recombinant antigen, and sporozoite surface proteins showing potential. Future research should focus on refining preventive measures, improving diagnostic accuracy, advancing drug development, and ultimately developing an effective vaccine to mitigate the global impact of cryptosporidiosis.

Author details

Taiwo Akinnubi
Ambrose Ali University Ekpoma, Edo State, Nigeria

*Address all correspondence to: akinnubitaiwo2015@gmail.com; akinnubitaiwoaauekpoma@edu.ng

References

[1] Tzipori S, Widmer G. A hundred-year retrospective on cryptosporidiosis. Trends in Parasitology. 2008;**24**(4):184-189

[2] Xiao L, Feng Y. Molecular epidemiologic tools for waterborne pathogens *Cryptosporidium spp*. and *Giardia duodenalis*. Food and Waterborne Parasitology. 2017;**8**:14-32

[3] Feng Y, Ryan UM, Xiao L. Genetic diversity and population structure of *Cryptosporidium*. Trends in Parasitology. 2018;**34**(11):997-1011

[4] Ehrenman K, Wanyiri JW, Bhat N, Ward HD, Coppens I. *Cryptosporidium parvum* scavenges LDL-derived cholesterol and micellar cholesterol internalized into enterocytes. Cellular Microbiology. 2013;**15**(7):1182-1197

[5] Kotloff KL, Nataro JP, Blackwelder WC, Nasrin D, Farag TH, Panchalingam S, et al. Burden and aetiology of diarrhoeal disease in infants and young children in developing countries (the global enteric multicenter study, GEMS): A prospective, case-control study. The Lancet. 2013;**382**(9888):209-222

[6] Troeger C, Forouzanfar M, Rao PC, Khalil I, Brown A, Reiner RC, et al. Estimates of global, regional, and national morbidity, mortality, and aetiologies of diarrhoeal diseases: A systematic analysis for the global burden of disease study 2015. The Lancet Infectious Diseases. 2017;**17**(9):909-948

[7] Efstratiou A, Ongerth JE, Karanis P. Waterborne transmission of protozoan parasites: Review of worldwide outbreaks-an update 2011-2016. Water Research. 2017;**114**:14-22

[8] Olson ME, O'Handley RM, Ralston BJ, McAllister TA, Thompson RA. Update on *Cryptosporidium* and *Giardia* infections in cattle. Trends in Parasitology. 2004;**20**(4):185-191

[9] Jacobson C, Williams A, Yang R, Ryan U, Carmichael I, Campbell AJ, et al. Greater intensity and frequency of *Cryptosporidium* and *Giardia* oocyst shedding beyond the neonatal period is associated with reductions in growth, carcase weight and dressing efficiency in sheep. Veterinary Parasitology. 2016;**228**:42-51

[10] Shaw HJ, Innes EA, Morrison LJ, Katzer F, Wells B. Long-term production effects of clinical cryptosporidiosis in neonatal calves. International Journal for Parasitology. 2020;**50**(5):371-376

[11] Fox LM, Saravolatz LD. Nitazoxanide: A new thiazolide antiparasitic agent. Clinical Infectious Diseases. 2005;**40**(8):1173-1180

[12] Trotz-Williams LA, Jarvie BD, Peregrine AS, Duffield TF, Leslie KE. Efficacy of halofuginone lactate in the prevention of cryptosporidiosis in dairy calves. Veterinary Record. 2011;**168**(19):509

[13] Zhu G, Yin J, Cuny GD. Current status and challenges in drug discovery against the globally important zoonotic cryptosporidiosis. Animal Diseases. 2021;**1**(1):3

[14] Carmena D. Waterborne transmission of *Cryptosporidium* and Giardia: Detection, surveillance and implications for public health. Current Research, Technology and Education Topics in Applied Microbiology and Microbial Biotechnology. 2010;**20**:3-4

[15] Lemmon JM, McAnulty JM, Bawden-Smith J. Outbreak of cryptosporidiosis linked to an indoor swimming pool. Medical Journal of Australia. 1996;**165**(11-12):613-616

[16] dos Santos Toledo R, Martins FD, Freire RL. Waterborne Giardia and *Cryptosporidium*: Contamination of human drinking water by sewage and cattle feces. Semina: Ciências Agrárias. 2017;**38**(5):3395-3415

[17] Betancourt WQ, Rose JB. Drinking water treatment processes for removal of *Cryptosporidium* and Giardia. Veterinary Parasitology. 2004;**126**(1-2):219-234

[18] Smith HV, Rose JB. Waterborne cryptosporidiosis: Current status. Parasitology Today. 1998;**14**(1):14-22

[19] Mac Kenzie WR, Hoxie NJ, Proctor ME, Gradus MS, Blair KA, Peterson DE, et al. A massive outbreak in Milwaukee of *Cryptosporidium* infection transmitted through the public water supply. New England Journal of Medicine. 1994;**331**(3):161-167

[20] Dawson D. Foodborne protozoan parasites. International Journal of Food Microbiology. 2005;**103**(2):207-227

[21] Ryan U, Hijjawi N, Xiao L. Foodborne cryptosporidiosis. International Journal for Parasitology. 2018;**48**(1):1-2

[22] Chalmers RM, Davies AP. Minireview: Clinical cryptosporidiosis. Experimental Parasitology. 2010;**124**(1):138-146

[23] Goh S, Reacher M, Casemore DP, Verlander NQ, Chalmers R, Knowles M, et al. Sporadic cryptosporidiosis, North Cumbria, England, 1996-2000. Emerging Infectious Diseases. 2004;**10**(6):1007

[24] Angelis CD, Mangone M, Bianchi M, Saracco G, Repici A, Rizzetto M, et al. An update on AIDS-related cholangiopathy. Minerva Gastroenterologica e Dietologica. 2009;**55**(1):79-82

[25] Mor SM, Tumwine JK, Ndeezi G, Srinivasan MG, Kaddu-Mulindwa DH, Tzipori S, et al. Respiratory cryptosporidiosis in HIV-seronegative children in Uganda: Potential for respiratory transmission. Clinical Infectious Diseases. 2010;**50**(10):1366-1372

[26] Mor SM, Ascolillo LR, Nakato R, Ndeezi G, Tumwine JK, Okwera A, et al. Expectoration of *Cryptosporidium* parasites in sputum of human immunodeficiency virus–positive and–negative adults. The American Journal of Tropical Medicine and Hygiene. 2018;**98**(4):1086

[27] Sponseller JK, Griffiths JK, Tzipori S. The evolution of respiratory cryptosporidiosis: Evidence for transmission by inhalation. Clinical Microbiology Reviews. 2014;**27**(3):575-586

[28] Cama VA, Ross JM, Crawford S, Kawai V, Chavez-Valdez R, Vargas D, et al. Differences in clinical manifestations among *Cryptosporidium* species and subtypes in HIV-infected persons. The Journal of Infectious Diseases. 2007;**196**(5):684-691

[29] Bamaiyi PH, Redhuan NE. Prevalence and risk factors for cryptosporidiosis: A global, emerging, neglected zoonosis. Asian Biomedicine. 2016;**10**(4):309-325

[30] Wang ZD, Liu Q, Liu HH, Li S, Zhang L, Zhao YK, et al. Prevalence of *Cryptosporidium*, microsporidia and *Isospora* infection in HIV-infected people: A global systematic review and meta-analysis. Parasites & Vectors. 2018;**11**:1-9

[31] Cama VA, Bern C, Roberts J, Cabrera L, Sterling CR, Ortega Y, et al. *Cryptosporidium* species and subtypes and clinical manifestations in children, Peru. Emerging Infectious Diseases. 2008;**14**(10):1567

[32] Miller WA, Lewis DJ, Pereira MD, Lennox M, Conrad PA, Tate KW, et al. Farm factors associated with reducing *Cryptosporidium* loading in storm runoff from dairies. Journal of Environmental Quality. 2008;**37**(5):1875-1882

[33] Méndez-Hermida F, Ares-Mazás E, McGuigan KG, Boyle M, Sichel C, Fernández-Ibáñez P. Disinfection of drinking water contaminated with *Cryptosporidium parvum* oocysts under natural sunlight and using the photocatalyst TiO2. Journal of Photochemistry and Photobiology B: Biology. 2007;**88**(2-3):105-111

[34] Samie A, Al-Qahtani A, El Bakri A, Ehdaie B. Challenges and innovative strategies to interrupt *Cryptosporidium* transmission in resource-limited settings. Current Tropical Medicine Reports. 2015;**2**:161-170

[35] Finch GR, Belosevic M. Controlling Giardia spp. and *Cryptosporidium* spp. in drinking water by microbial reduction processes. Canadian Journal of Civil Engineering. 2001;**28**(S1):67-80

[36] Graczyk TK, Lucy FE, Tamang L, Mashinski Y, Broaders MA, Connolly M, et al. Propagation of human enteropathogens in constructed horizontal wetlands used for tertiary wastewater treatment. Applied and Environmental Microbiology. 2009;**75**(13):4531-4538

[37] Amadi B, Mwiya M, Sianongo S, Payne L, Watuka A, Katubulushi M, et al. High dose prolonged treatment with nitazoxanide is not effective for cryptosporidiosis in HIV positive Zambian children: A randomised controlled trial. BMC Infectious Diseases. 2009;**9**:1-7

[38] Gaafar MR. Efficacy of *Allium sativum* (garlic) against experimental cryptosporidiosis. Alexandria Journal of Medicine. 2012;**48**(1):59-66

[39] Al-Hamairy AK, Mugheer AH, Al-Dulaimi FA. Prevalence of *Cryptosporidium* sp. and treatment by using some plant extracts in Al-Hilla City, Babylon Province of Iraq. The Egyptian Journal of Experimental Biology (Zoology). 2012;**8**:287-293

[40] Taghipour A, Khazaei S, Ghodsian S, Shajarizadeh M, Olfatifar M, Foroutan M, et al. Global prevalence of *Cryptosporidium* spp. in cats: A systematic review and meta-analysis. Research in Veterinary Science. 2021;**137**:77-85

[41] Hassan EM, Örmeci B, DeRosa MC, Dixon BR, Sattar SA, Iqbal A. A review of *Cryptosporidium* spp. and their detection in water. Water Science and Technology. 2021;**83**(1):1-25

[42] Fall A, Thompson RC, Hobbs RP, Morgan-Ryan U. Morphology is not a reliable tool for delineating species within *Cryptosporidium*. Journal of Parasitology. 2003;**89**(2):399-402

[43] Jex AR, Smith HV, Monis PT, Campbell BE, Gasser RB. *Cryptosporidium*—Biotechnological advances in the detection, diagnosis and analysis of genetic variation. Biotechnology Advances. 2008;**26**(4):304-317

[44] Iacovski RB, Barardi CR, Simões CM. Detection and enumeration of *Cryptosporidium* sp. oocysts in sewage sludge samples from the city

of Florianópolis (Brazil) by using immunomagnetic separation combined with indirect immunofluorescence assay. Waste Management & Research. 2004;**22**(3):171-176

[45] Smith HV, Nichols RA. *Cryptosporidium*: Detection in water and food. Experimental Parasitology. 2010;**124**(1):61-79

[46] LeChevallier MW, Di Giovanni GD, Clancy JL, Bukhari Z, Bukhari S, Rosen JS, et al. Comparison of method 1623 and cell culture-PCR for detection of *Cryptosporidium* spp. in source waters. Applied and Environmental Microbiology. 2003;**69**(2):971-979

[47] Ahmed SA, Karanis P. Comparison of current methods used to detect *Cryptosporidium* oocysts in stools. International Journal of Hygiene and Environmental Health. 2018;**221**(5):743-763

[48] Ghoshal U, Jain V, Dey A, Ranjan P. Evaluation of enzyme linked immunosorbent assay for stool antigen detection for the diagnosis of cryptosporidiosis among HIV negative immunocompromised patients in a tertiary care hospital of northern India. Journal of Infection and Public Health. 2018;**11**(1):115-119

[49] Rossle NF, Latif B. Cryptosporidiosis as threatening health problem: A review. Asian Pacific Journal of Tropical Biomedicine. 2013;**3**(11):916-924

[50] Adeyemo FE, Singh G, Reddy P, Stenström TA. Methods for the detection of *Cryptosporidium* and *Giardia*: From microscopy to nucleic acid based tools in clinical and environmental regimes. Acta Tropica. 2018;**184**:15-28

[51] Hsu BM, Wu NM, Jang HD, Shih FC, Wan MT, Kung CM. Using the flow cytometry to quantify the Giardia cysts and *Cryptosporidium* oocysts in water samples. Environmental Monitoring and Assessment. 2005;**104**:155-162

[52] Miller CN, Jossé L, Brown I, Blakeman B, Povey J, Yiangou L, et al. A cell culture platform for *Cryptosporidium* that enables long-term cultivation and new tools for the systematic investigation of its biology. International Journal for Parasitology. 2018;**48**(3-4):197-201

[53] Yang R, Paparini A, Monis P, Ryan U. Comparison of next-generation droplet digital PCR (ddPCR) with quantitative PCR (qPCR) for enumeration of *Cryptosporidium* oocysts in faecal samples. International Journal for Parasitology. 2014;**44**(14):1105-1113

[54] Zahedi A, Monis P, Aucote S, King B, Paparini A, Jian F, et al. Zoonotic *Cryptosporidium* species in animals inhabiting Sydney water catchments. PLoS One. 2016;**11**(12):e0168169

[55] Dwivedi S, Purohit P, Misra R, Pareek P, Goel A, Khattri S, et al. Diseases and molecular diagnostics: A step closer to precision medicine. Indian Journal of Clinical Biochemistry. 2017;**32**:374-398

[56] Jex AR, Gasser RB. *Cryptosporidium*: Current state of genomics and systems biological research. In: *Cryptosporidium*: Parasite and Disease. Vienna: Springer Vienna; 2013. pp. 327-344

[57] Soldevilla MM, Meraviglia-Crivelli de Caso D, Menon AP, Pastor F. Aptamer-iRNAs as therapeutics for cancer treatment. Pharmaceuticals. 2018;**11**(4):108

[58] Rossignol JF, Kabil SM, El-Gohary Y, Younis AM. Effect of nitazoxanide in diarrhea and enteritis caused by *Cryptosporidium* species.

Clinical Gastroenterology and Hepatology. 2006;**4**(3):320-324

[59] Amadi B, Mwiya M, Musuku J, Watuka A, Sianongo S, Ayoub A, et al. Effect of nitazoxanide on morbidity and mortality in Zambian children with cryptosporidiosis: A randomised controlled trial. The Lancet. 2002;**360**(9343):1375-1380

[60] Rytter MJ, Kolte L, Briend A, Friis H, Christensen VB. The immune system in children with malnutrition—A systematic review. PLoS One. 2014;**9**(8):e105017

[61] Allam AF, Shehab AY. Efficacy of azithromycin, praziquantel and mirazid in treatment of cryptosporidiosis in school children. Journal of the Egyptian Society of Parasitology. 2002;**32**(3):969-978

[62] Brainard J, Hammer CC, Hunter PR, Katzer F, Hurle G, Tyler K. Efficacy of halofuginone products to prevent or treat cryptosporidiosis in bovine calves: A systematic review and meta-analyses. Parasitology. 2021;**148**(4):408-419

[63] Rahman SU, Mi R, Zhou S, Gong H, Ullah M, Huang Y, et al. Advances in therapeutic and vaccine targets for *Cryptosporidium*: Challenges and possible mitigation strategies. Acta Tropica. 2022;**226**:106273

[64] Lee S, Beamer G, Tzipori S. The piglet acute diarrhea model for evaluating efficacy of treatment and control of cryptosporidiosis. Human Vaccines & Immunotherapeutics. 2019;**15**(6):1445-1452

[65] Yarlett N, Morada M, Gobin M, Van Voorhis W, Arnold S. *In vitro* culture of *Cryptosporidium parvum* using hollow fiber bioreactor: Applications for simultaneous pharmacokinetic and pharmacodynamic evaluation of test compounds. In: Mead J, Arrowood M, editors. *Cryptosporidium*. New York: Methods in Molecular Biology Humana; 2020. pp. 335-350

[66] Baydoun M, Vanneste SB, Creusy C, Guyot K, Gantois N, Chabe M, et al. Three-dimensional (3D) culture of adult murine colon as an *in vitro* model of cryptosporidiosis: Proof of concept. Scientific Reports. 2017;**7**(1):17288

[67] Sateriale A, Šlapeta J, Baptista R, Engiles JB, Gullicksrud JA, Herbert GT, et al. A genetically tractable, natural mouse model of cryptosporidiosis offers insights into host protective immunity. Cell Host & Microbe. 2019;**26**(1):135-146

[68] Choudhary HH, Nava MG, Gartlan BE, Rose S, Vinayak S. A conditional protein degradation system to study essential gene function in *Cryptosporidium parvum*. MBio. 2020;**11**(4):10-128

[69] Huston CD, Spangenberg T, Burrows J, Willis P, Wells TN, van Voorhis W. A proposed target product profile and developmental cascade for new cryptosporidiosis treatments. PLoS Neglected Tropical Diseases. 2015;**9**(10):e0003987

[70] Manjunatha UH, Vinayak S, Zambriski JA, Chao AT, Sy T, Noble CG, et al. A *Cryptosporidium* PI (4) K inhibitor is a drug candidate for cryptosporidiosis. Nature. 2017;**546**(7658):376-380

[71] Stebbins E, Jumani RS, Klopfer C, Barlow J, Miller P, Campbell MA, et al. Clinical and microbiologic efficacy of the piperazine-based drug lead MMV665917 in the dairy calf cryptosporidiosis model. PLoS Neglected Tropical Diseases. 2018;**12**(1):e0006183

[72] Vinayak S, Jumani RS, Miller P, Hasan MM, McLeod BI, Tandel J, et al.

Bicyclic azetidines kill the diarrheal pathogen *Cryptosporidium* in mice by inhibiting parasite phenylalanyl-tRNA synthetase. Science Translational Medicine. 2020;**12**(563):eaba8412

[73] Jin Z, Ma J, Zhu G, Zhang H. Discovery of novel anti-cryptosporidial activities from natural products by *in vitro* high-throughput phenotypic screening. Frontiers in Microbiology. 2019;**10**:478846

[74] Sanad MM, Al-Malki JS, Al-Ghabban AG. Control of cryptosporidiosis by probiotic bacteria. In: International Conference on Agricultural, Ecological and Medical Sciences (AEMS-2015), Phuket (Thailand). Apr 2015. pp. 7-8

[75] Chappell CL, Darkoh C, Shimmin L, Farhana N, Kim DK, Okhuysen PC, et al. Fecal indole as a biomarker of susceptibility to *Cryptosporidium* infection. Infection and Immunity. 2016;**84**(8):2299-2306

[76] Rogawski McQuade ET, Liu J, Kang G, Kosek MN, Lima AA, Bessong PO, et al. Protection from natural immunity against enteric infections and etiology-specific diarrhea in a longitudinal birth cohort. The Journal of Infectious Diseases. 2020;**222**(11):1858-1868

[77] Mead JR. Challenges and prospects for a *Cryptosporidium* vaccine. Future Microbiology. 2010;**5**(3):335-337

[78] Preidis GA, Wang HC, Lewis DE, Castellanos-Gonzalez A, Rogers KA, Graviss EA, et al. Seropositive human subjects produce interferon gamma after stimulation with recombinant *Cryptosporidium hominis* gp 15. American Journal of Tropical Medicine and Hygiene. 2007;**77**(3):583-585

[79] Cui Z, Wang L, Wang Y, Li J, Wang R, Sun M, et al. *Cryptosporidium parvum* gp40/15 is associated with the parasitophorous vacuole membrane and is a potential vaccine target. Microorganisms. 2020;**8**(3):363

[80] Ichikawa-Seki M, Fereig RM, Masatani T, Kinami A, Takahashi Y, Kida K, et al. Development of CpGP15 recombinant antigen of *Cryptosporidium parvum* for detection of the specific antibodies in cattle. Parasitology International. 2019;**69**:8-12

[81] Avendaño C, Jenkins M, Méndez-Callejas G, Oviedo J, Guzmán F, Patarroyo MA, et al. CP15 and CSL protein-derived synthetic peptides' immunogenicity and *in vitro* seroneutralisation capability. Vaccine. 2018;**36**(45):6703-6710

[82] Deng M, Templeton TJ, London NR, Bauer C, Schroeder AA, Abrahamsen MS. *Cryptosporidium parvum* genes containing thrombospondin type 1 domains. Infection and Immunity. 2002;**70**(12):6987-6995

[83] Jaskiewicz JJ, Tremblay JM, Tzipori S, Shoemaker CB. Identification and characterization of a new 34 kDa MORN motif-containing sporozoite surface-exposed protein, Cp-P34, unique to *Cryptosporidium*. International Journal for Parasitology. 2021;**51**(9):761-775

Chapter 6

Frequency of Subtypes of *Blastocystis* spp. in Children from Vulnerable Populations

Janeth Oliva Guangorena-Gómez and Claudia Muñoz Yañez

Abstract

Blastocystis is a very common gastrointestinal protozoan globally distributed; it colonizes humans and non-humans, and in some communities, it reaches prevalences of up to 100%. *Blastocystis* is transmitted through the fecal-oral route, contaminated food and water, and close contact with animals. There are 34 known subtypes of *Blastocystis*, and subtypes 1 to 4 (ST1–ST4) are the most common in humans. It should be remembered that its pathogenicity is controversial since some studies have shown that *Blastocystis* is more prevalent in healthy individuals; who have greater diversity and richness of the intestinal microbiota; other studies suggest that *Blastocystis* infections occur in individuals with intestinal dysbiosis. In America and Africa, a high incidence of ST1 and ST2 is observed in rural areas. Recent data indicate that *Blastocystis* is linked with specific gut microbiota profiles and health indicators. Convincing information and tools that distinguish asymptomatic colonization from infection in children have yet to be demonstrated. Although this protozoan can cause disease under certain circumstances, but the attention of *Blastocystis* may change, as the frequency of *Blastocystis* subtypes in children may vary depending on the geographic area and local health conditions.

Keywords: *Blastocystis*, controversial pathogenicity, frequency, health, gut microbiota

1. Introduction

A complex and diverse population of microorganisms lives in the human intestine: bacteria, fungi, viruses, archaea, and protozoans [1]. *Blastocystis* spp. is a very common protozoan; it is a Stramenopile or Heterokonta Eukaryote [2], and it has different forms: vacuolar, avacuolar, granular, cystic, and amoeboid [3]. It colonizes a wide diversity of species in the world, such as humans and non-humans; approximately one billion individuals in the world are infected by this protozoan [4]. It is known that this protist is one of the most prevalent; in some communities, it reaches prevalence of up to 100% [5]. The fecal-oral route *Blastocystis*, through contaminated food and water and close contact with animals, which are the best-known transmission sources for *Blastocystis* [6, 7]. Studies have reported that it can cause diarrhea accompanied by abdominal pain, dizziness, vomiting, and weight loss, among others [8, 9].

Blastocystis infection is mainly associated with nonspecific gastrointestinal symptoms, both acute and chronic [10].

It has been identified 34 subtypes of *Blastocystis* [11–13], but only 17 are recorded, subtypes one to subtype nine are found in humans (ST1–ST9), and subtypes one to four (ST1–ST4) are the most frequent [14, 15]. It is worth noting that there are studies where *Blastocystis* is more prevalent in healthy individuals [16] who have a greater diversity and richness of the intestinal microbiota [17] and have even been postulated as a viable probiotic agent [18]. Other research suggests that *Blastocystis* infection occurs in individuals with intestinal dysbiosis and irritable bowel syndrome [19, 20]. The clinical significance of *Blastocystis* is still inconclusive [18, 21, 22]. All this dissimilarity may be due to the diversity of coexisting subtypes [15].

In America, a high incidence is observed for ST1 and ST2 [23]. In Mexico, higher prevalence was reported for ST1 (51%) [24] in 2023. A global prevalence of 44.0% was reported in school-age children in a rural area, with a prevalence of 56.5% for ST1, followed by ST2 (26.3%) and ST3 (19.7%). In Colombian children, a study carried out in 2021 reported a global prevalence of 58.2% of *Blastocystis*, and the first identification of Subtype 16 in humans was made [13]. Also, previously in Colombia, a study in 2015 found that subtype 3 is associated with urticaria in Argentine patients and that allele a134 predominated in patients with symptoms [25]. Later, in 2017, another study in the pediatric population found no statistical association between *Blastocystis* infection and subtypes with variables such as sex, age, symptoms or sociodemographic stratification [26]. Another study in Panama in apparently healthy school-age children from rural areas in 2020 found a global prevalence of *Blastocystis* of 74.2%, and the prevalence of ST1 was 42.2% [27].

Some African countries have reported a high prevalence of *Blastocystis* infection, although data on the prevalence and distribution of *Blastocystis* subtypes still needs to be available. On this continent, a multicenter study was carried out among certain villages in Senegal. An essential variation in prevalence was observed between the villages, 51.7–100% in this study; additionally, the first report of subtypes 10 and 14 in humans was made [28].

The classification of *Blastocystis* as pathogenic or non-pathogenic has been problematic since a direct causal link has not been demonstrated [22]. However, some explanations for its pathogenicity are the excretion of proteases and the presence of more than five parasites per field in the intestine, mainly causing an inflammatory process at lamina propria level. Also, the composition of the intestinal microbiota, the immune system, and the nutritional status of the host are some of the decisive factors for the presence of the parasite and its pathogenicity [29, 30]. It is known that *Blastocystis* and the intestinal microbiota cohabit in the intestinal tract of the host and can interact with each other [31–38]. Bacteria are the most abundant in the intestinal microbiota, and two main phyla are present: Firmicutes and Bacteroidetes (representing 80%). At lower levels, *Proteobacteria*, *Actinobacteria*, *Fusobacteria*, and *Verrucomicrobia* are present [39, 40]. Recent data suggest that *Blastocystis* is associated with specific gut microbiota profiles and health indices. Stensvold et al. (2022) used metabarcoding analyses to identify variations in fecal microbiota diversity between *Blastocystis*-carrying and non-carrying individuals. Alpha diversity was considerably higher in *Blastocystis* carriers. Subjects with *Blastocystis*-positive stools had gut microbiomes associated with eubiosis, while in individuals with negative feces for *Blastocystis*, the intestinal microbiome was similar to those associated with dysbiosis [41]. Importantly, clinical data were not obtained from the subjects from whom feces were obtained, so the role of *Blastocystis* as a potential modulator of the intestinal microbiota needs to be known with greater scrutiny.

More sensitive tools that differentiate asymptomatic colonization from infection in children have yet to be demonstrated. Although the parasite can cause disease under certain circumstances, the focus on *Blastocystis* may shift from a clinical to a public health perspective [42]. On the other hand, the frequency of *Blastocystis* subtypes in children may vary depending on the geographic area and local health conditions. Since in developing countries, drinking water and hygiene are scarce, in rural communities, contact with animals and children is more frequent, and it is a population that is more vulnerable to infection through the anus-oral route.

2. *Blastocystis* spp.

It was described for the first time in 1912 [43] by Alexeieff, who named it considered it a yeast and named it *Blastocystis enterocola*; Brumpt described the parasite and named it *Blastocystis hominis* [44]. Zierd et al. classified it as a parasite, and using ribosomal DNA sequences, *Blastocystis* was classified within the kingdom Chromista by Silberman. It was not until 1997 that Clark described the polymorphisms of this protozoan [45].

2.1 Taxonomy

Blastocystis belongs to the kingdom Chromista, Subkingdom Chromobiota, Subphylum Opalinata, class Blastocystea [46]. It is the main unicellular eukaryotic protozoan found in the intestine of mammals [47]. It presents characteristics of the protist kingdom with one or more nuclei, strict anaerobe, and sensitivity to O_2. It measures 5–40 μm and reproduces mainly by binary fission.

2.2 Morphology

There are many variations between sizes and the form of presentation according to subtypes, but the primary peculiarity is the appearance of a central vacuole (occupies 90% of the cytoplasm) with metabolic and storage functions, easily observable after staining [48]. In humans, different forms of *Blastocystis* have been described including vacuolar, avacuolar, granular, multi vacuolar, cystic, and amoeboid form, which is more prevalent in symptomatic individuals [3].

It presents four well-differentiated morphological stages:

2.2.1 Vacuolar form

The form most easily identified in feces, they have a size of 5–15 μm and binary fission reproduction. The diagnosis is made based on vacuolar form. They have a central corpuscle or vacuole composed of lipids and carbohydrates with reserve functions, which compress the cell nucleus and cytoplasm [49].

2.2.2 Ameboid form

This form measures 10 μm, does not have a central body, but has 1 or 2 slow-moving pseudopodia. Cellular debris has been found inside, which suggests that it has a significant role in the nutrition of the microorganism [49].

2.2.3 Granular form

It has 1 to 4 nuclei and measures between 6 and 8 μm. This form is scarce, and three types of granules are distinguished: metabolic, reproductive, and lipidic [50].

2.2.4 Cyst form

They measure 3–10 μm and are ovoid or spherical; the cells include lipid and glycogen deposits and vacuoles. Generally, the isolated nuclei are binucleate. They survive approximately 1 month at room temperature; however, they are sensitive to disinfectants and extreme temperatures [49].

2.3 Life cycle

The life cycle is similar to most protists. Two types of cycles have been described: binary fission and autogamy for the formation of cysts that can be thick or thin-walled, which help in the transmission of the parasite. The avacuolar cell is present in the intestine, passing through the intestinal tract. After the disintegration of vesicles in the cytoplasm, the multi-vacuolar form is generated, which is covered by a thick cell wall. The cystic wall forms under the cell cover disintegrates, resulting in a cyst, which is the infectious cell of *Blastocystis* spp. Ingestion by a host completes the cycle; excystment is the final route of infection caused by exposure to gastric acid and intestinal enzymes [51].

2.4 Transmission

Blastocystis is found in the feces of mammals (humans and primates), as well as amphibians, birds, livestock, and reptiles [52]; its exposure is usually incidental, and the transmission of fecal-oral has been reported as the primary form of transmission. Recent studies suggest that it is present in contaminated water, although exposure to these factors is usually insufficient for infection. Among the risk factors associated with *Blastocystis* infection are overcrowding, same-sex relationships, contaminated water, low educational level, travelers, living with infected animals, and poor hygiene (**Figure 1**) [53].

2.5 Pathogenicity

The pathophysiology of *Blastocystis* is not entirely known; it is believed to lie mainly in apoptosis, degradation of transmembrane proteins that results in exaggeration of intestinal permeability, induction of pro-inflammatory cytokines and the regulation of nitric oxide [3, 48].

2.5.1 Blastocystis *and immune system*

Blastocystis spp. can degrade immunoglobulin A (An antibody present in mucosal secretions, predominating in tears, saliva, and gastrointestinal secretions) [48]. Although it is generally accepted that *Blastocystis* is not an invasive pathogen and cannot phagocytose the host microbiota, pathogenicity depends on the subtype and the *Blastocystis* proteases [54]; for example, one study described that hydrolases alter the colonic mucus layer.

DOI: http://dx.doi.org/10.5772/intechopen.1004780

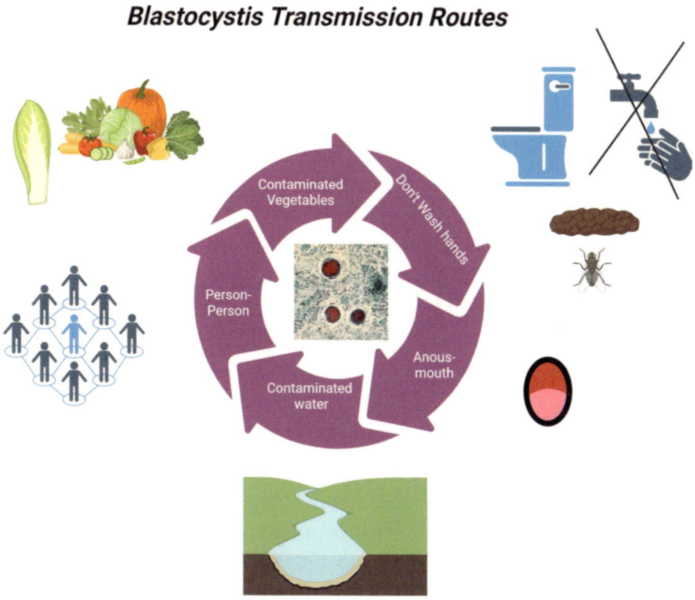

Figure 1.
Blastocystis *spp. transmission routes.* Blastocystis *can be transmitted through fecal-oral routes, such as water and food contaminated with infected feces. It can also spread from person to person through direct contact with contaminated fecal matter.*

In vivo, studies with rats have shown that the microorganism's proteases stimulate the production of Interleukin 8 (IL-8) by colon epithelial cells through mechanisms dependent on nuclear factors, which are responsible for fluid loss and intestinal inflammation in affected individuals. Therefore, it is believed that these enzymes produce hyperplasia of the goblet cells and cecal mucosa in infected rats [49]. It was also experimentally demonstrated that *Blastocystis* spp. can trigger increased cell proliferation in human colorectal cancer, causing interferon-gamma (IFN γ) and p53 expression deregulation. The subtype with the most pathogenic relationship is ST3, which increases the proliferation of cancer cells by decreasing the apoptosis of these cells and severe inflammatory reactions [55]. Regarding other classes of enzymes, the gene encoding the beta-1,3-galactosyltransferase (b1,3GalT), was acquired laterally by this protozoan and was duplicated several times in its genome; the encoding proteins are involved in molecular mimicry, which helps *Blastocystis* to camouflage [56].

Blastocystis has been reported in immunocompromised patients, and those under stress since the overproduction of oxygen and hydroxyl free radicals causes oxidation of lipids and proteins, resulting in poor functioning of the body's tissues and deficient antibody production [57]. Blasto-Ag (an antigen produced by *B. hominis*) is responsible for the downregulation of peripheral blood cells, and this inhibitory effect is more significant in asymptomatic individuals. In the infection, it is expected to find low levels of IgA with high levels of immunoglobulin G (predominant antibody in cerebrospinal fluid, peritoneal fluid, and blood, which responds to the presence of viruses and bacteria), associated with the overproduction of eosinophils (which suppress infection). In this context, there are studies of children with leukemia where immunoglobulin M (the first antibody produced to fight infections found in blood and lymph) and IgG are high compared to IgA [58].

However, it should be noted that recent studies have identified *Blastocystis* as part of the microbiota, found in more than 50% of the healthy population, with a tendency to long-term colonization, with the same microorganism found 10 years later [56].

2.6 Subtypes

As previously mentioned, 34 subtypes of *Blastocystis* spp. have been identified. STs 1–4 are the most prevalent in 90% of carriers; these subtypes are found in 95% of patients with a single infection [14].

2.6.1 Distribution of subtypes by hosts

ST1 and ST2 are also found in other animal species, including monkeys, cows, chickens, pigs, rats, dogs, and nonhuman primates. ST3 has been found in nonhuman primates, pigs, and cattle. ST4 has been described in rodents and monkeys. The rarer subtypes in humans (ST5–8) are found most frequently in other hosts: ST5 is common in cattle, apes, pigs, rats, dogs, and Old World monkeys, while ST6 and ST7 are mainly found in birds and cattle (ST6). ST8 has been recognized in marsupials, different species of captive primates and their caretakers. These rarer subtypes in humans have been suggested to be of zoonotic derivation, and there is some confirmation that ST8 has been found in zookeepers of nonhuman primates [15, 59].

Based on next-generation sequencing [60], *Blastocystis* co-infection using suitable for subtyping (STS) and polymerase chain reaction (PCR) in fecal samples has been established. The mixed subtypes most frequently found are ST1 + ST3, ST1 + ST2, and ST2 + ST3—Figure 4. A case of co-infection by three different subtypes (probably from the same strain) was recently described. This assumption is supported by the polymorphism observed among the 38 sequences belonging to subtype 3 [44].

2.6.2 Prevalence of Blastocystis *subtypes according to geographic region*

Blastocystis spp. worldwide prevalence is around 25% in humans [45], with a marked superiority in some developing countries with an approximate prevalence of 55–100% [28], while in developed countries, the prevalence reported is 10–15%; this difference has been attributed to hygiene levels and the presence or absence of contact with animals and contaminated water and food [61]. *Blastocystis* colonizes between one and two million people globally and is one of humans and animals most common intestinal parasites. Humans are primarily colonized by subtypes 1–4, but the relative prevalence of these subtypes appears to differ substantially between regions [23]. According to reports, in Europe, ST1–4 are found more frequently and specifically in the North and South America, since a higher prevalence was found subtypes (ST1–3). The countries with greater variety of these subtypes are the United States, Brazil, and Colombia, with 14, 9 and 8 subtypes, respectively [59].

2.6.3 Differences between subtypes

Currently, the *Blastocystis*'s subtype is the most accepted approach to explain its pathogenicity *Blastocystis* [62]. Also, intrasubtypic variations have been observed, thus suggesting that not all strains of a particular subtype are pathogenic and that the subtype does not predict pathogenicity [50].

Subtype 3 (ST3) is one of the most common in humans, as well as the most frequently found in fecal samples from patients with both gastrointestinal and dermatological clinical manifestations (urticaria) [62]. About the pathogenicity of ST4, in a meta-analysis that included studies from Europe, Asia, Africa, and South America this subtype has a much higher global sequence conservation than the others. Furthermore, heat shock proteins (such as 0PHA3 and KOG3047, a ubiquitously expressed prefoldin-like chaperone) and cytosolic Ca^{2+} ion-dependent cysteine proteases (such as KOG0045, which is a cysteine-like peptidase similar to calpain) were found in the ST4 genomes that were not present in other ST genomes, which may represent virulence factors unique to ST4 [63]. The activities of cysteine proteases in ST4 and ST7 isolates have shown significant variations, which may be one of the reasons for the differences in their virulence [10]. Several studies worldwide have demonstrated that ST5 is derived from animals since it has been found in people who live in rural areas and have close contact with animals. In addition, poor hygiene plays a vital role in contagion [62, 64].

About subtype 7 (ST7), in vitro assays revealed that this subtype caused alterations in the intestinal epithelial barrier by altering binding proteins such as occludin and zonula occludens-1 (ZO-1) [38], which was associated with greater adhesiveness to intestinal epithelial cells and more significant cysteine protease activity than ST4. In the same study, histopathological results showed that mice infected with ST7 had more colon damage and ulceration than control mice [32]. Also, it has shown that ST7 in isolate H (with greater adhesiveness than other isolates) binds preferentially to colonic tissue concerning the cecum and terminal ileum. ST7 has also been associated with more significant colonization of other parasites [60]. Furthermore, comparing sensitivity and resistance to certain antibiotics showed that ST7 has greater resistance to metronidazole than ST4 whereas it has greater sensitivity to emetine than ST4 [61]. In ST7, the 0IZK7 Cystatin B has a potential role in parasitic cysteine protease function and inhibition of host proteases; this protein is also present in ST2 but not in ST1, ST3 and ST4 [62].

2.6.4 Distribution of subtypes in children from different countries

With the advent of new-generation sequencing (**Figure 2**), since 2020, more *Blastocystis* subtypes have been identified; for example, in North Thailand the child population in rural areas, which is a vulnerable group to poverty and poor sanitation conditions (**Table 1**). The authors suggest that the main transmission routes of *Blastocystis* to humans are soil and water [11]. Contrary to another study in the Thai-Myanmar Border, Ratchaburi Province (Thailand) in the same year, 2023 [69], in which the prevalence of *Blastocystis* was very low (3.35%). In Thailand, *Blastocystis* infection rates are 0.7–45.2% in school-age children, and the highest rates are found in young children living in orphan homes in Pathum Thani province; this is consistent with several studies that mention that the prevalence of *Blastocystis* is higher in developing countries where the prevalence reaches 100% [28]. This is the case in children in Senegal, where open defecation of the population of these regions is attributed to the lack of latrines and water. Conversely, data on the prevalence and distribution of *Blastocystis* subtypes remain scarce in Africa; however, a multicenter study in 2020 with a total of 731 stool samples collected from healthy children living in 10 villages in the region northwest of Senegal showed significant variation of *Blastocystis* infections between villages from 51.7 to 100%, the overall prevalence was 80.4% and mixed infections 23%, the possible potential sources of transmission in this population are

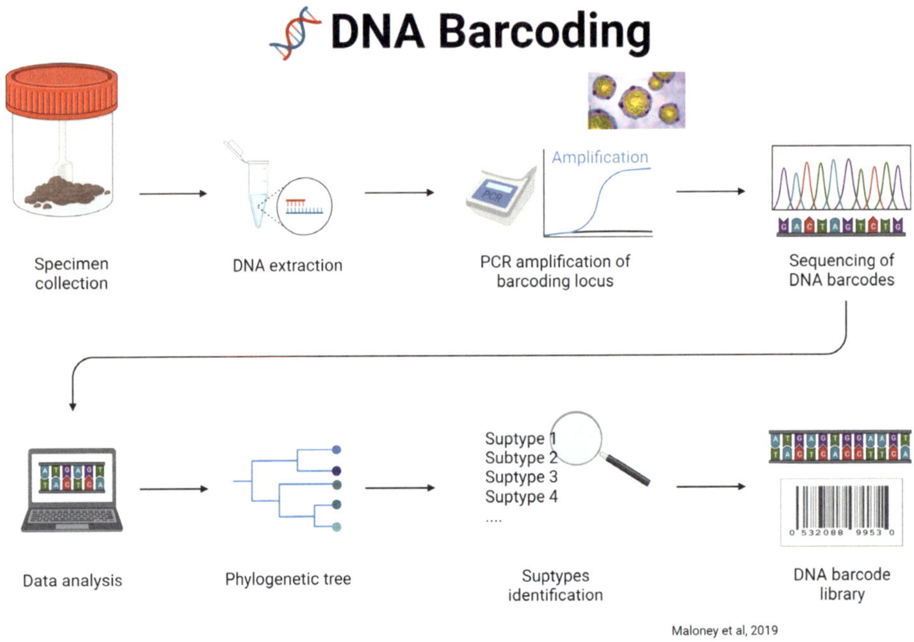

Figure 2.
Next generation sequencing method for the subtyping of Blastocystis. *Next-generation sequencing (NGS) in the context of barcoding refers to applying high-capacity DNA sequencing technologies to identify and characterize multiple species, in this case, those of Blastocystis, using genetic barcodes. This involves the massive generation of DNA sequences from multiple samples simultaneously.*

suggested to be person-person transmission, zoonotic and transmission through contaminated water, also, this is the first report of subtype 10 and 14 in humans [28].

In Latin America, in a study carried out in Colombia in a child population that attended daycare centers in Medellín, where the population was urban, the global prevalence of *Blastocystis* was 36.6% by microscopy and 58.2% by polymerase chain reaction (PCR); this is the first report of subtype 16 identification in humans [13]. In other studies in rural areas of Panama and Mexico, the prevalence of Blastocystis was of 74.2% and 44.0%, respectively. Additionally, in apparently healthy school-aged children in Panama, *Blastocystis* subtype infection was not associated with gastrointestinal symptoms except for diarrhea in these children [27]. In children from Mexico, the frequency of *Blastocystis* subtypes was related to ingesting contaminated foods such as sweets, snacks, and artisanal foods at food stalls [24]. As previously described, the child population in developing countries is the most affected by *Blastocystis* infection. The studies in the child population aim to understand the dynamics of transmission and its consequences for the health of this group. In this regard, the relationship between age and epidemiological and molecular characterization of *Blastocystis* infection is vital since the lack of information of long-term parasite stability in asymptomatic children makes it difficult to interpret the transmission and pathogenesis (**Table 1**).

2.6.5 Association of Blastocystis *and the gut microbiota*

The association of *Blastocystis* and the fecal microbiota in children has been little studied; recently a study with 57 samples of school-age children in Colombia

Country	Year	Age (years)	N of samples sequenced n	ST1	ST2	ST3	ST4	ST5	ST6	ST7	ST16	ST26	Methodology	Reference
Jakarta	2018	6–12	16	12 (67.95%)	5 (26.4%)	2 (3.8%)	1 (1.9%)	—	—	—	—	—	Sanger	[65]
Panama	2020	1–12	49	28 (57.1%)		21 (42.8%)	—	—	—	—	—	—	Sanger	[27]
Senegal	2020	6–19	588	113 (19.2%)	226 (38.4%)	107 (18.19%)	—	—	—	—	—	—	Genoscreen	[28]
Colombia	2021	0–5	59	12 (20.3%)	14 (23.7%)	18 (30.5%)	3 (5.0%)	—	1 (1.7%)	—	9 (15.3%)	—	Barcoding	[13]
Azerbaijan	2021	6.4–13.4	22	3 (14%)	5 (23%)	14 (64%)	0	—	0	—	—	—	Barcoding	[66]
Czechia	2021	8.1–12.7	8	1 (13%)	3 (38%)	3 (38%)	1 (25%)	—	0	—	—	—	Barcoding	[66]
Jordan	2021	7.9–13.4	5	1 (20%)	1 (20%)	4 (80%)	0	—	0	—	—	—	Barcoding	[66]
Nigeria	2021	13.9–16.9	14	8 (57%)	4 (29%)	5 (36%)	0	—	1 (7%)	—	—	—	Barcoding	[66]
Sudan	2021	7.4–12.9	24	14 (58%)	5 (21%)	10 (42%)	0	—	0	—	—	—	Barcoding	[66]
Tanzania	2021	11.1–14.6	8	2 (25%)	2 (25%)	4 (50%)	0	—	0	—	—	—	Barcoding	[66]
Tukey	2022	1–18	14	3 (21.4%)	6 (42.8%)	5 (35.7%)	—	—	—	—	—	—	Sanger	[67]
Thailand	2023	4–12	17	5 (29.4%)	1 (5.8%)	11 (64.7%)	—	—	—	—	—	—	Barcoding	[68]

Country	Year	Age (years)	N of samples sequenced n	ST1	ST2	ST3	ST4	ST5	ST6	ST7	ST16	ST26	Methodology	Reference
Rural Thailand	2023	6–14	93	7 (7.5%)	19 (20.4%)	42 (45.1%)	—	1 (1.07%)	—	14 (15.05%)	—	1 (1.07%)	Barcoding	[69]
Ecuador	2023	3–11	84	22 (26.2%)	22 (26.2%)	24 (28.6%)	12 (14.3%)	—	—	—	—	—	Bigdye Terminator	[70]
Mexico	2023	3–15	78	43 (56.5%)	18 (23.6%)	15 (19.7%)	—	—	—	—	—	—	Barcoding	[24]

n number of samples; % of sequenced samples.

Table 1.
Sequence types of Blastocystis *found in the populations of children studied.*

showed that the composition of the intestinal bacterial community was not different between colonized children and those not colonized by *Blastocystis*; however, a greater microbial richness was observed in the fecal microbiota of children colonized by *Blastocystis*, Firmicutes was the most predominant phylum in both groups, and a more significant proportion of Bacteroidetes was found in children not colonized [36].

A previous study in 2016 with subjects aged 9 to 70 years found a higher relative abundance of Bacteroides in *Blastocystis*-negative samples and a low abundance of *Prevotella* and a higher abundance of the Clostridial group XIVa in *Blastocystis*-negative samples. *Blastocystis* is associated with fecal microbiota characterized by low relative abundances of *Bacteroides*, Clostridial group XIVa, and high levels of *Prevotella* [71].

3. Conclusions

The studies described above aim to understand the dynamics of the transmission of *Blastocystis* according to subtypes, and implications on health mainly in children. For this reason, it is crucial to characterize *Blastocystis* infection epidemiologically and molecularly to generate conclusive epidemiological information in developing countries. However, information on stability and epidemiology in asymptomatic children complicates the interpretation of the transmission and pathogenesis of the subtypes of this protozoan. A host can harbor more than two subtypes; however, the extent of subtype diversity within the host is poorly understood. New studies have emerged in which *Blastocystis* is considered a member of the healthy intestinal microbiota. This disparity is suggested to be due to the high variability between subtypes and host immunity, so it is necessary to know and evaluate the diversity of *Blastocystis* subtypes; this is crucial to understanding the epidemiology and sources of transmission to humans and, subsequently, depending on the patient's symptoms, give appropriate treatment. It is crucial to investigate the alterations in the structure of the gut microbiota related to the presence of *Blastocystis*.

Conflict of interest

The authors declare no conflict of interest.

Author details

Janeth Oliva Guangorena-Gómez* and Claudia Muñoz Yañez
Faculty of Health Sciences, University Juarez of State of Durango,
Gómez Palacio, Durango, México

*Address all correspondence to: janethguangorenagomez@gmail.com

References

[1] Alam A, Neish A. Role of gut microbiota in intestinal wound healing and barrier function. Tissue Barriers. 2018;**6**:1-21

[2] Farré EM. The brown clock: Circadian rhythms in stramenopiles. Physiologia Plantarum. 2020;**169**:430-441

[3] Tan TC, Suresh KG. Predominance of amoeboid forms of *Blastocystis hominis* in isolates from symptomatic patients. *Parasitology Research*. 2006;**98**(3):189-193. Epub ahead of print. DOI: 10.1080/01421590500312847

[4] Scanlan PD, Stensvold CR. *Blastocystis*: Getting to grips with our guileful guest. Trends in Parasitology. 2013;**29**:523-529

[5] El Safadi D, Gaayeb L, Meloni D, et al. Children of Senegal River Basin show the highest prevalence of *Blastocystis* sp. ever observed worldwide. BMC Infectious Diseases. 2014;**14**:1-11

[6] Tan KSW. New insights on classification, identification, and clinical relevance of *Blastocystis* spp. Clinical Microbiology Reviews. 2008;**21**:639-665

[7] Zou Y, Bin YW, Zou FC, et al. Molecular detection and subtype distribution of *Blastocystis* in farmed pigs in southern China. Microbial Pathogenesis. 2021;**151**:104751

[8] Domínguez-Márquez MV, Guna R, Muñoz C, et al. High prevalence of subtype 4 among isolates of *Blastocystis hominis* from symptomatic patients of a health district of Valencia (Spain). Parasitology Research. 2009;**105**:949-955

[9] Ramírez JD, Sánchez LV, Bautista DC, et al. *Blastocystis* subtypes detected in humans and animals from Colombia. México: Infection, Genetics and Evolution. 2014;**22**:223-228

[10] Kumarasamy V. *Blastocystis* sp., parasite associated with gastrointestinal disorders: An overview of its pathogenesis, immune modulation and therapeutic strategies. Current Pharmaceutical Design. 2018;**24**:3172-3175

[11] Jinatham V, Maxamhud S, Popluechai S, et al. *Blastocystis* one health approach in a rural community of Northern Thailand: Prevalence, subtypes and novel transmission routes. Frontiers in Microbiology. 2021;**12**:746340. Epub ahead of print. DOI: 10.3389/fmicb.2021.746340

[12] Maloney JG, Molokin A, Seguí R, et al. Identification and molecular characterization of four new *Blastocystis* subtypes designated ST35-ST38. Microorganisms. 2023;**11**:46. Epub ahead of print. DOI: 10.3390/microorganisms11010046

[13] Osorio-Pulgarin MI, Higuera A, Beltran-álzate JC, et al. Epidemiological and molecular characterization of *Blastocystis* infection in children attending daycare centers in medellín, Colombia. Biology (Basel). 2021;**10**:669. Epub ahead of print. DOI: 10.3390/biology10070669

[14] Alfellani MA. Genetic diversity of *Blastocystis* in livestock and zoo animals. Protist. 2013;**164**:497-509

[15] Skotarczak B. Genetic diversity and pathogenicity of *Blastocystis*. Annals of Agricultural and Environmental Medicine. 2018;**25**:411-416

[16] Scanlan PD, Stensvold CR, Rajilić-Stojanović M, et al. The microbial eukaryote *Blastocystis* is a prevalent and diverse member of the healthy human gut microbiota. FEMS Microbiology Ecology. 2014;**90**:326-330

[17] Lukeš J, Stensvold CR, Jirků-Pomajbíková K, et al. Are human intestinal eukaryotes beneficial or commensals? PLoS Pathogens. 2015;**11**:e1005039. Epub ahead of print. DOI: 10.1371/journal.ppat.1005039

[18] Andersen LO, Stensvold CR. *Blastocystis* in health and disease: Are we moving from a clinical to a public health perspective? Journal of Clinical Microbiology. 2016;**54**:524-528

[19] Nourrisson C, Scanzi J, Pereira B, et al. *Blastocystis* is associated with decrease of fecal microbiota protective bacteria: Comparative analysis between patients with irritable bowel syndrome and control subjects. PLoS ONE. 2014;**9**:1-9

[20] Lepczyńska M, Dzika E, Kubiak K, et al. The role of *Blastocystis* sp. as an etiology of irritable bowel syndrome. Polish Annals of Medicine. 2016;**23**:57-60

[21] Yakoob J, Jafri W, Beg MA, et al. *Blastocystis hominis* and *Dientamoeba fragilis* in patients fulfilling irritable bowel syndrome criteria. Parasitology Research. 2010;**107**:679-684

[22] Audebert C, Even G, Cian A, et al. Colonization with the enteric protozoa *Blastocystis* is associated with increased diversity of human gut bacterial microbiota. Scientific Reports. 2016;**6**:1-11

[23] Seyer A, Karasartova D, Ruh E, et al. Epidemiology and prevalence of *Blastocystis* spp. in North Cyprus. The American Journal of Tropical Medicine and Hygiene. 2017;**96**:1164-1170

[24] Hidalgo-Gonzalez LA, Salgado-Lopez J, Pineda-Rodriguez SA, et al. Identification of *Blastocystis* sp. in school children from a rural Mexican village: Subtypes and risk factors analysis. Parasitology Research. 2023;**122**:1701-1707

[25] Casero RD, Mongi F, Sánchez A, et al. *Blastocystis* and urticaria: Examination of subtypes and morphotypes in an unusual clinical manifestation. Acta Tropica. 2015;**148**:156-161

[26] Ramírez JD, Flórez C, Olivera M, et al. *Blastocystis* subtyping and its association with intestinal parasites in children from different geographical regions of Colombia. PLoS ONE. 2017;**12**:1-13

[27] Perea M, Vásquez V, Pineda V, et al. Prevalence and subtype distribution of *Blastocystis* sp. infecting children from a rural community in Panama. Parasite Epidemiology and Control. 2020;**9**:1-8

[28] Khaled S, Gantois N, Ly AT, et al. Prevalence and subtype distribution of *Blastocystis* sp. in Senegalese school children. Microorganisms. 2020;**8**:1-17

[29] Lepczyńska M, Dzika E. The influence of probiotic bacteria and human gut microorganisms causing opportunistic infections on *Blastocystis* ST3. Gut Pathogens. 2019;**11**:1-11

[30] Becerril-Flores MA. Blastocystosis. In: *Parasitología Médica*. México: McGraw Hill; 2019. pp. 165-167

[31] Stensvold CR, van der Giezen M. Associations between gut microbiota and common luminal intestinal parasites. Trends in Parasitology. 2018;**34**:369-377

[32] Gentekaki E, Curtis BA, Stairs CW, et al. Extreme genome diversity in the hyper-prevalent parasitic eukaryote *Blastocystis*. PLoS Biology. 2017;**15**:1-42

[33] Forsell J, Bengtsson-Palme J, Angelin M, et al. The relation between *Blastocystis* and the intestinal microbiota in Swedish travellers. BMC Microbiology. 2017;**17**:1-9

[34] Kodio A, Coulibaly D, Koné AK, et al. *Blastocystis* colonization is associated with increased diversity and altered gut bacterial communities in healthy Malian children. Microorganisms. 2019;7:1-11

[35] Tito RY, Chaffron S, Caenepeel C, et al. Population-level analysis of *Blastocystis* subtype prevalence and variation in the human gut microbiota. Gut Microbiota. 2019;**68**:1180-1189

[36] Castañeda S, Muñoz M, Villamizar X, et al. Microbiota characterization in *Blastocystis*-colonized and *Blastocystis*-free school-age children from Colombia. Parasit Vectors. 2020;**13**:521. Epub ahead of print. DOI: 10.1186/s13071-020-04392-9

[37] Nieves-Ramírez ME, Partida-Rodríguez O, Laforest-Lapointe I, et al. Asymptomatic intestinal colonization with protist *Blastocystis* is strongly associated with distinct microbiome ecological patterns. mSystems. 2018;**3**:1-18

[38] Yason JA, Liang YR, Png CW, et al. Interactions between a pathogenic *Blastocystis* subtype and gut microbiota: In vitro and in vivo studies. Microbiome. 2019;7:1-13

[39] Foster JA, Rinaman L, Cryan JF. Stress & the gut-brain axis: Regulation by the microbiome. Neurobiology of Stress. 2017;7:124-136

[40] García Peña C, Álvarez Cisneros T, Quiroz Baez R, et al. Microbiota and aging. A review and commentary. Archives of Medical Research. 2017;**48**:681-689

[41] Stensvold CR, Sørland BA, Berg RPKD, et al. Stool microbiota diversity analysis of *Blastocystis*-positive and *Blastocystis*-negative individuals. Microorganisms. 2022;**10**:1-6

[42] Deng L, Wojciech L, Gascoigne NRJ, et al. New insights into the interactions between *Blastocystis*, the gut microbiota, and host immunity. PLoS Pathogens. 2021;**17**:1-15

[43] Yoshikawa H, Nagano I, Wu Z, et al. Genomic polymorphism among *Blastocystis hominis* strains and development of subtype-specific diagnostic primers. Molecular and Cellular Probes. 1998;**12**:153-159

[44] Poirier P, Meloni D, Nourrisson C, et al. Molecular subtyping of *Blastocystis* spp. using a new rDNA marker from the mitochondria-like organelle genome. Parasitology. 2014;**141**:670-681

[45] Zhan T, He S, Liu T, et al. A novel genotype screening and phylogenetic analysis of *Blastocystis* hominis based on EF-1α. International Journal of Clinical and Experimental Pathology. 2017;**10**:8314-8323

[46] Sierra RL, Muñoz SGD, Lora SFM, et al. Identificación de subtipos de *Blastocystis* sp. asociados a fuentes de transmisión en una zona rural del departamento del Quindío. Revista de la Asociación Colombiana de Ciencias Biológicas. 2023;**35**:113-127

[47] Stensvold CR, Traub RJ, von Samson-Himmelstjerna G, et al. *Blastocystis*: Subtyping isolates using pyrosequencing™ technology.

Experimental Parasitology. 2007;**116**:111-119

[48] Ajjampur SSR, Tan KSW. Pathogenic mechanisms in *Blastocystis* spp.—Interpreting results from in vitro and in vivo studies. Parasitology International. 2016;**65**:772-779

[49] del Coco VF, Molina NB, Basualdo JA, et al. *Blastocystis* spp.: Advances, controversies and future challenges. Revista Argentina de Microbiología. 2017;**49**:110-118

[50] Jeremiah S, Parija S. *Blastocystis*: Taxonomy, biology and virulence. Tropenmedizin und Parasitologie. 2013;**3**:17

[51] Popruk S, Adao DE V, Rivera WL. Epidemiology and subtype distribution of *Blastocystis* in humans: A review. Infection, Genetics and Evolution. 2021;**95**:1-14

[52] Mohamed RT, El-bali MA, Mohamed AA, et al. Subtyping of *Blastocystis* sp. isolated from symptomatic and asymptomatic individuals in Makkah, Saudi Arabia. Parasites & Vectors. 2017;**10**:1-7

[53] Basak S, Rajurkar MN, Mallick SK. Detection of *Blastocystis hominis*: A controversial human pathogen. Parasitology Research. 2014;**113**:261-265

[54] Andersen LOB, Bonde I, Nielsen HBHB, et al. A retrospective metagenomics approach to studying *Blastocystis*. FEMS Microbiology Ecology. 2015;**91**:1-9

[55] Kurt Ö, Doğruman Al F, Tanyüksel M. Eradication of *Blastocystis* in humans: Really necessary for all? Parasitology International. 2016;**65**:797-801

[56] Stensvold CR, Clark CG. Current status of *Blastocystis*: A personal view. Parasitology International. 2016;**65**:763-771

[57] Eme L, Gentekaki E, Curtis B, et al. Lateral gene transfer in the adaptation of the anaerobic parasite *Blastocystis* to the gut. Current Biology. 2017;**27**:807-820

[58] Chandramathi S, Suresh K, Sivanandam S, et al. Stress exacerbates infectivity and pathogenicity of *Blastocystis hominis*: In vitro and in vivo evidences. PLoS ONE. 2014;**9**:1-11

[59] Jiménez PA, Jaimes JE, Ramírez JD. A summary of *Blastocystis* subtypes in North and South America. Parasites & Vectors. 2019;**12**:1-9

[60] Maloney JG, Molokin A, Santin M. Next generation amplicon sequencing improves detection of *Blastocystis* mixed subtype infections. Infection, Genetics and Evolution. 2019;**73**:119-125

[61] Mohamed AM, Ahmed MA, Ahmed SA, et al. Predominance and association risk of *Blastocystis hominis* subtype I in colorectal cancer: A case control study. Infectious Agents and Cancer. 2017;**12**:1-8

[62] Cakir F, Cicek M, Yildirim IH. Determination the subtypes of *Blastocystis* sp. and evaluate the effect of these subtypes on pathogenicity. Acta Parasitologica. 2019;**64**:7-12

[63] Beghini F, Pasolli E, Truong TD, et al. Large-scale comparative metagenomics of *Blastocystis*, a common member of the human gut microbiome. ISME Journal. 2017;**11**:2848-2863

[64] Yañez CM, Hernández AM, Sandoval AM, et al. Prevalence of *Blastocystis* and its association with *Firmicutes/Bacteroidetes* ratio in clinically

healthy and metabolically ill subjects. BMC Microbiology. 2021;**21**:1-11

[65] Sari IP, Benung MR, Wahdini S, et al. Diagnosis and identification of *Blastocystis* subtypes in primary school children in Jakarta. Journal of Tropical Pediatrics. 2018;**64**:208-214

[66] Cinek O, Polackova K, Odeh R, et al. *Blastocystis* in the faeces of children from six distant countries: Prevalence, quantity, subtypes and the relation to the gut bacteriome. Parasites & Vectors. 2021;**14**:1-16

[67] Semra Güreser A, Comba A, Karasartova D, et al. Detection of *Blastocystis* subtypes in children with functional abdominal pain and celiac disease in Çorum, Turkey. Iranian Journal of Parasitology. 2021;**17**:296-305

[68] Abu A, Sutthikornchai C, Mahittikorn A, et al. Prevalence and subtype distribution of *Blastocystis* isolated from school-aged children in the Thai-Myanmar Border, Ratchaburi Province, Thailand. International Journal of Environmental Research and Public Health. 2022;**20**:1-9

[69] McCain A, Gruneck L, Popluechai S, et al. Circulation and colonisation of *Blastocystis* subtypes in schoolchildren of various ethnicities in rural northern Thailand. Epidemiology and Infection. 2023;**151**:e85. Epub ahead of print. DOI: 10.1017/S0950268823000596

[70] Tapia-Veloz E, Gozalbo M, Guillén M, et al. Prevalence and associated risk factors of intestinal parasites among schoolchildren in Ecuador, with emphasis on the molecular diversity of *Giardia duodenalis*, *Blastocystis* sp. and *Enterocytozoon bieneusi*. PLoS Neglected Tropical Diseases. 2023;**17**:1-21

[71] O'Brien Andersen L, Karim AB, Roager HM, et al. Associations between common intestinal parasites and bacteria in humans as revealed by qPCR. European Journal of Clinical Microbiology and Infectious Diseases. 2016;**35**:1427-1431

Chapter 7

Intestinal Tapeworm (Cestode)

Samatar Abshir Mahamed

Abstract

Adult tapeworms, known as cestodes, reside in the small intestine where they feed off the host's food. They are attached to the intestinal wall by a structure called the scolex, which is connected to a chain of segments known as proglottids that make up the strobila. Each proglottid contains both male and female reproductive systems and are categorized as immature, mature, or gravid based on their stage of development. Gravid proglottids are found at the end of the strobila and contain a fully developed uterus filled with eggs, which is often used for identification purposes. The eggs and the scolex can also be used to identify the specific species of the tapeworm. Cestodes have complex life cycles that involve intermediate and definitive hosts. In some cases, humans can be the definitive hosts with adult worms living in the intestine (*Diphyllobothrium latum, Taenia saginata, Hymenolepis diminuta,* and *Dipylidium caninum*), while in other cases humans can serve as both the definitive and intermediate hosts (*T. solium* and *H. nana*). Tapeworms have been documented as far back as 1500 BC and are among the oldest known human parasites. The prevalence of human intestinal tapeworms is not well understood, but it is estimated that millions of people are infected with various species of tapeworms. While the presence of adult tapeworms in the intestine is not typically life threatening, infection with larval tapeworms can be serious and potentially fatal.

Keywords: intestine, tapeworm, cestode, parasite, taeniasis

1. Introduction

Tapeworms are flatworms that live in the intestinal tracts of their hosts. Beyond depriving their hosts of certain micronutrients, like vitamins, adult tapeworms do little harm to their hosts. The size of adult tapeworms ranges from 0.04 inches to 50 feet long, and they are visible to the unaided eye. Cestodiasis is the name for a tapeworm infection. Tapeworms are flatworms that live in the digestive tracts of their hosts. They are classified into two orders: Pseudophyllidea and Cyclophyllidea. The heads (scolex), neck, and proglottids (strobila) are the three components that make up an adult worm. Succkers or grooves, depending on the order, can be found on the scolex, the organ that attaches to the intestinal mucosa. New proglottids form in the growth region of the neck. The proglottids are divided into three segments: premature, adult, and gravid, with the gravid segment containing eggs in the uterus. Tapeworms possess both male and female reproductive systems in every segment, making them hermaphrodites. They lack bodily cavities or alimentary canals, through which nutrients are absorbed by their outer layer. The two orders of tapeworms,

Characteristic	*Diphyllobothrium latum*	*Taenia saginata*	*Taenia saginata asiatica*	*Taenia solium*	*Hymenolepis nana*	*Hymenolepis diminuta*	*Dipylidium caninum*
Common intermediate hosts	Fish and copepods	Cattle	Pig	Pig	1: different arthropods (fleas, beetles); or none	2: Different arthropods (beetles, fleas)	1: different arthropods (fleas, dog, lice)
Source of infection	consuming plerocercoid (sparganum) from fish that has been infected	Consumption of beef contaminated with cysticercus	consumption of infected tissue, mainly liver with cysticercus	Cysticercus consumption in contaminated pork	Consumption of an egg directly or consuming a cysticercoid within an infected arthropod; autoinfection is also a possibility.	Consumption of cysticercoid in an infected arthropod	Consumption of cysticercoid within fleas, lice
The prepatent phase	3 to 5 weeks	10 to 12 weeks	10 to 12 weeks	5 to 12 weeks	2 to 3 weeks	About 3 weeks	3 to 4 weeks
The average life span	A maximum of 25 years	A maximum of 25 years	A maximum of 25 years	A maximum of 25 years	Due to autoinfection, possibly for a number of years	Usually less than a year	Usually less than a year
Size	4 to 10 meters	4 to 12 meters	4 to 8 meters	1.5–8 meters	2.5 to 4 cm	20 to 60 cm	10 to 70 cm
Scolex	With two shallow grooves (bothria) and a spatulate, 3 × 1 mm shape, it lacks rostellum and hooklets.	Four suckers, quadrate, 1–2 mm in diameter, without rostellum or hooklets	Four suckers, quadrate, 1–2 mm in diameter, without rostellum or hooklets	Four suckers, rostellum, hooklets, and a quadrate with a diameter of 1 mm.	Has four suckers, rostellum, and hooklets; knoblike but rarely seen	Has four suckers; rostellum but no hooklets; knoblike but rarely found	0.2–0.5 mm in diameter, with four suckers and a conical, retractile rostellum equipped with four to seven rows of tiny hooklets.

Table 1.
Intestinal tapeworm (Cestode) characteristics.

Cyclophyllidea and Pseudophyllidea, differ in terms of their eggs. Cyclophyllidea eggs contain hexacanth embryos equipped with hooklets, while Pseudophyllidea eggs have operculums (**Table 1**) [1].

2. *Diphyllobothrium latum*

D. latum is a member of the group of tapeworms known as pseudophyllideans. One distinguishing feature of this group is the presence of two bothria, or sucking organs, on the scolex [1]. This is in contrast to the Taenia tapeworms, which have a scolex with four suckers. The common name for *D. latum* is fish tapeworm or broad tapeworm (**Table 1**) [2].

2.1 Distribution

This disease is prevalent worldwide.

2.2 Predilection site

In the human small intestine, the ileum is where the adult worm is normally found.

2.3 Morphology

Adults can reach a length of 10 m or more and have up to 3000 proglottids inside of them [3]. This is the biggest tapeworm that lives in the human small intestine. The spoon-shaped, elongated scolex of *D. latum* measures approximately 2–3 mm in length and 1 mm in width. It features two long sucking grooves (**Figure 1a**), one on the ventral surface (bothria) and the other on the dorsal surface. The neck lacks segmentation and is thin. Strobila is made up of approximately 3000–4000 proglottids [3]. The width of a plottid is greater than its length (**Figure 1b**). Midventrally, the genital pores open. The egg has a thick, light brown shell and is roughly ovoid, measuring 65 by 45 μm (**Figure 1c**). At one end, it has an operculum. It grows fully in freshwater and is excreted in feces [5]. Humans are not infected by the egg [2].

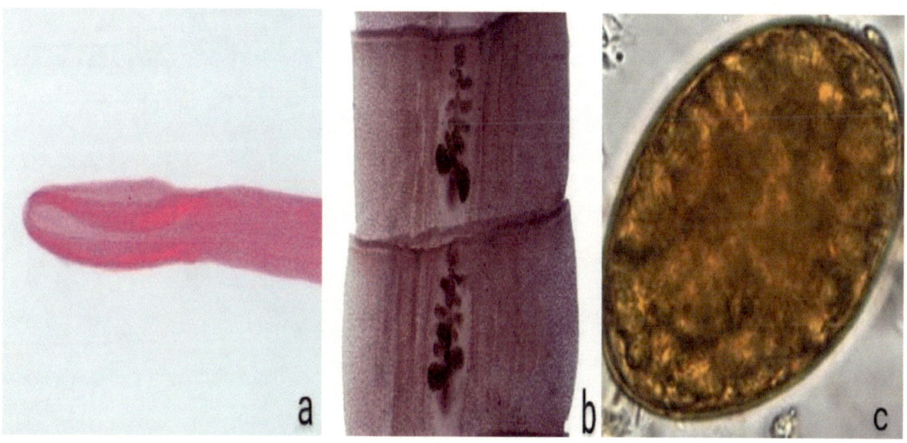

Figure 1.
Diphyllobothrium latum. (a) Scolex, (b) gravid proglottids, (c) egg [4].

2.4 Life cycle

(1) Infected humans excrete feces that contain immature eggs. Secondly, eggs develop in water. (3) Crustaceans consume the coracidia after they hatch from their eggs. (4) The body cavity of crustaceans is where procercoid larvae develop. (5) Procercoid larvae become plerocercoid larvae after being eaten by small freshwater fish that have come into contact with the contaminated crustaceans. (6) Small infected fish are eaten by predator fish. (7) Humans become infected when they consume raw or undercooked fish that is contaminated with pleurocercoid larvae. In the small intestine, adults develop. (9) Immature eggs released by proglottids are excreted in the feces. In the body cavity of crustaceans, procercoid larvae develop. (5) When an intermediate host, such as fish, reptiles, or amphibians, consumes infected crustaceans, the procercoid larvae transform into plerocercoid larvae. (6) Predators, including dogs and cats, consume the infected second intermediate host. (7) The small intestines of dogs and cats are where plerocercoid larvae mature into adults. Of procercoid larvae in crustaceans or plerocercoid larvae in second intermediate hosts, or the application of raw poultices made of second intermediate hosts containing plerocercoid larvae for medicinal purposes on open wounds, lesions, or the eyes, can result in infection in humans (**Figure 2**) [4].

2.5 Pathogenesis and clinical symptoms

In the human gut, the second intermediate host—amphibians, reptiles, and fish—releases the sparganum, or plerocercoid larvae. Infected water can also infect humans

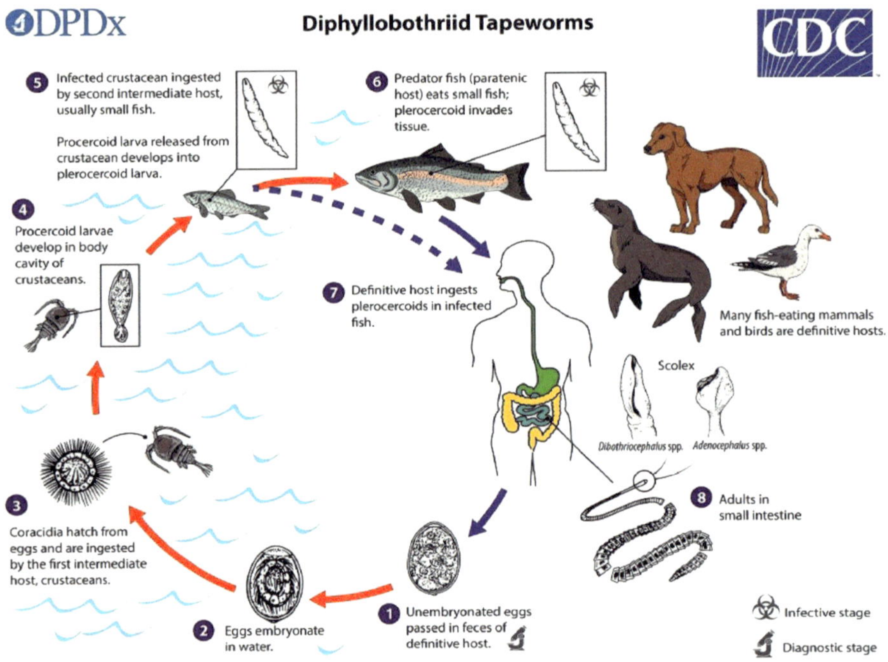

Figure 2.
Life cycle of Diphyllobothrium latum [4].

if they consume cyclops that contain procercoid larvae. The larvae of procercoid will mature into plerocercoid larvae, which will migrate to other organs and subcutaneous tissue after penetrating the intestinal wall. Early migration phases do not cause any symptoms. As it reaches its destination, it starts to spread and inflame the tissues around it, causing pain. No encyst occurs in the larvae. The organs or tissues that are affected by sparganosis determine its clinical features, which can include subcutaneous nodules, periorbital edema, seizures, parasthesias, and hemiparesis in the central nervous system [6]. While Intestinal obstruction is a possible presentation in some patients, infections can also be asymptomatic [2]. The typical symptoms include anemia, weakness, diarrhea, nausea, and abdominal pain [7, 8]. The worms reside in the ileum, which is also the site of vitamin B12 absorption. It can cause anemia by competing with the host for vitamin B12 [3].

2.6 Diagnosis

2.6.1 Microscopical examination

Typically, the diagnosis is made after the proglottids, or characteristic eggs, have been recovered and identified [3]. The operculum should be visible after closely examining the eggs. Tapping on the wet preparation's coverslip can cause it to pop open if it is difficult to see. To make the operculum easier to see, the light should be turned down a little. Proglottids are frequently passed in chains that range in length from a few inches to several feet. Furthermore, the uterine structure is visible in the center of the gravid proglotids, which are significantly wider than long (rosette).

2.6.2 Molecular diagnoses

PCR analysis of clinical specimens [9].

There is no risk of cysticercosis from handling the specimens, but all fecal specimens should be handled carefully as they may contain other organisms that could be infectious.

2.7 Treatment

Oral praziquantel (5–10 mg/kg in one dose) [10]. Anemia caused by a vitamin B12 deficiency should be treated with parenteral vitamin B12 [3].

2.8 Prevention and control

1. Cook fish properly
2. Deep freeze fish at −10°C for 24–48 hours
3. Maintain proper hygiene
4. Periodically deworm pets like cats and dogs.
5. Treat infected cases

3. *Taenia saginata* and *Taenia solium*

Beef tapeworm (*Taenia saginata*) and pork tapeworm (*Taenia solium*) are common intestinal parasites [1].

3.1 Distribution

Worldwide distribution is observed for *Taenia saginata* and *Taenia solium* [11].

3.2 Predilection site

Both *Taenia saginata* and *Taenia solium* adult worms reside in the human small intestine.

3.3 Morphology

The adult *Taenia saginata* is segmented and flattened dorsoventrally, with a length of 5–10 m. With four suckers for attachment, *T. saginata*'s scolex has a diameter of approximately 1–2 mm. There are no hooklets or rostellum on the scolex (**Figure 3A**). The shape of the neck is long and narrow. There are 1000–2000 proglottids in each strobila. They have the characteristics of a hermaphrodite. The lateral branches of each gravid segment range from 15 to 30, and each gravid segment is roughly 20 mm in length and 5 mm in width (**Figure 3a**). The segments of gravid material separate and exit separately through the anus of the host. It is possible to see the gravid segment moving actively. Both *T. solium* and *T. saginata* have identical eggs. They have a diameter of 31–43 μm, are brown, and are spherical. As shown in **Figure 3**, the shell

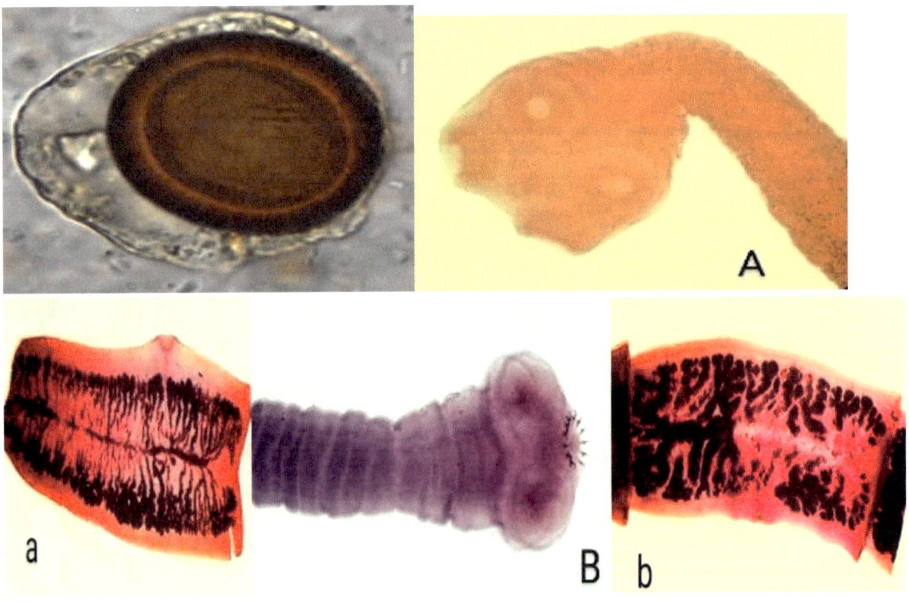

Figure 3.
Taenia sp. egg. (A) Scolex of T. saginata. Note the four large suckers and lack of rostellum and rostellar hooks. (a) Mature proglottid of T. saginata. (B) Scolex of T. solium. Note the four large suckers and rostellum containing two rows of hooks. (b) Mature proglottid of T. solium [12].

has striating radially. Six hooklets are present in the embryo (oncosphere). The larva of *Taenia saginata* is called *Cysticercus bovis*. The stage at which humans are infected is the larva. It is a single perforated scolex (bladder worm) inside a milky-white, ovoid, fluid-filled, opalescent vesicle that measures approximately 5 by 10 mm in diameter. Infected cattle's muscles contain cysticerci. In the contaminated beef (measly beef), they are obscenely visible as white dots. At 2–3 meters in length, the mature *T. solium* is segmented and flattened dorsoventrally. *T. solium* has four suckers on its scolex, which has a diameter of approximately 1 mm. A rostellum and hooklets are present on the scolex (**Figure 3B**). It has a short neck. Less than 1000 proglottids make up the strobila. Each gravid segment has seven to thirteen lateral uterine branches, and they are roughly 12 mm long and 6 mm broad (**Figure 3b**). They possess hermaphrodite properties. Through the host's anus, the gravid segments are released in chains. The human-infecting form of *T. solium* is known as *Cysticercus cellulosae*, which is also its larval form. Both in humans and in pigs, it can develop in different organs. It resembles *Cysticercus bovis* in morphology. The adult scolex of *Taenia solium* and the invaginated scolex of *Cysticercus cellulosae* share a similar morphology [1].

3.4 Life cycle

The life cycle is depicted in **Figure 4** (1). Infected humans excrete eggs or gravid proglottids. (2) Ingestion of vegetation contaminated with eggs or gravid proglottids causes infection in cattle (*Teania saginata*) and pigs (*Taenia solium*). (3) After emerging from the eggs, oncospheres pass through the intestinal wall and travel to the muscles, where they mature into cystcerci. (4) Humans become infected by consuming raw or undercooked infected meat containing larvae. The larvae. (5) In the human

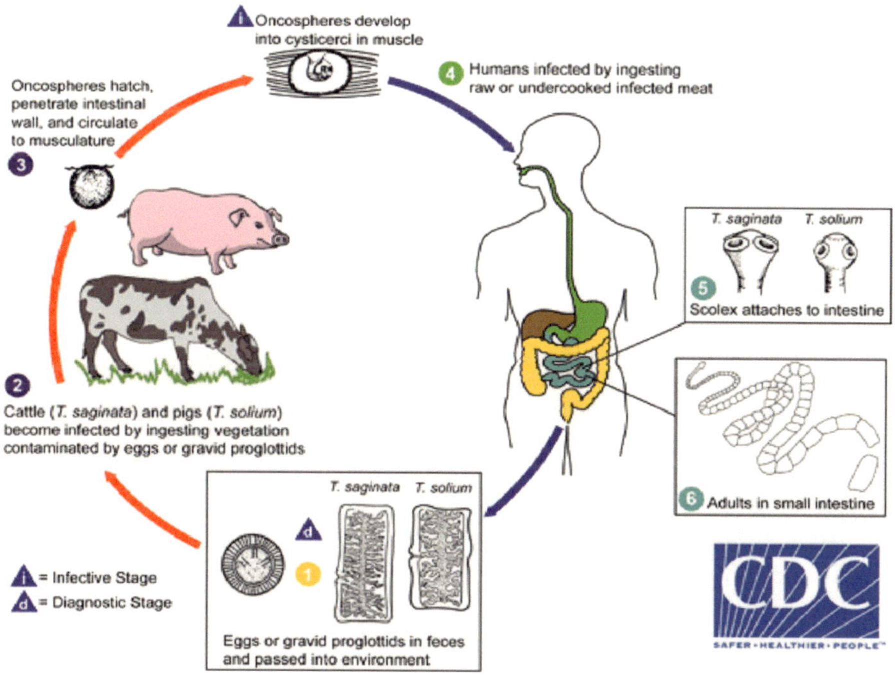

Figure 4.
Life cycle of Taenia saginata and T. solium [12].

small intestine, the larvae mature into adult tapeworms. (6) The tapeworm's head, or scolex, adheres to the small intestine mucosa [1, 13].

3.5 Pathogenesis and clinical symptoms

T. saginata and *T. solium* cause intestinal taeniasis. Symptomatic infection leads to nausea, diarrhea, indigestion, weight loss, and vague abdominal pain. The larval stages of *T. solium* (cysticercus cellulosae) cause cysticercosis [11, 14]. Humans become infected after consuming *T. solium* eggs in contaminated food or water. It can affect any organ or tissue, but the brain, eyes, and subcutaneous tissues are the most commonly affected. Except in the eye and brain ventricles, the cysticercus is encased in a fibrous capsule. The cellular response induced by degenerating larvae involves neutrophils, eosinophils, lymphocytes, and plasma cells. Calcification results from the subsequent fibrosis and larval death. The affected site influences the clinical signs. Acute myositis is the symptom of muscular cysticercosis; subcutaneous nodules are usually asymptomatic. The most prevalent and dangerous type, known as neurocysticercosis (brain cysticercosis), results in adult-onset epilepsy [15]. Another common condition is headaches. Vision loss or blurriness are common symptoms of ocular cysticercosis [16].

3.6 Diagnosis

Specimen: blood, muscle tissue, CSF, and feces.

1. *Macroscopic examination:* Specimen examined for segments or proglottids. Dark yellow feces contrast sharply with the whitish segment. Identification of distinct eggs, gravid proglottids, or scolex (*Taenia soluim* has a row of hooks, whereas *Taenia saginata* does not) in feces. Acid-fast staining can be used to diagnose the species because the eggs of *T. soluim* and *T. saginata* are similar. While *T. saginata* eggs are acid-fast, *T. soluim* eggs are not [13, 14].

2. *Antigen detection:* Employed for screening intestinal taeniasis. Polyclonal antisera is used in ELISA to capture antigens.

3. *Serodiagnosis:* Anti-cysticercus antibodies in serum or CSF are found via serological tests. ELISA and immunoelectrotransfer blot were employed [14].

4. *Histopathological diagnosis:* NCC is diagnosed by demonstrating cysticerci in brain biopsy tissue. Skeletal cysticercosis is diagnosed by histological examination of biopsy [13].

5. *Imaging:* X-rays and CT scans are used to detect dead, calcified, and multiple cysts in different body regions. MRI shows mural nodules as pathognomonic for NCC [13–15].

6. *Other tests:* Elevated CSF protein levels and lymphocytosis are commonly observed in neurocysticercosis. Glucose levels may be low. Eosinophils in CSF are common but nonspecific [17].

3.7 Treatment

Praziquantel (5–10 mg/kg orally, given as a single dose) is the recommended treatment for intestinal taeniasis. An alternative would be to take 2 g of niclosamide orally in one dose [16]. When cysts are accessible, excision is the most effective treatment for cysticercosis. For cerebral cysticercosis, two possible treatments are albendazole (15 mg/kg daily, up to 800 mg/day for 8 days) and praziquantel (50 mg/kg in three divided doses daily for 15 days). To lessen inflammatory responses brought on by dead cysticerci, corticosteroids may be given in combination with albendazole or praziquantel. It is necessary to administer antiepileptic medications. Hydrocephalus requires surgical intervention [18].

3.8 Prevention and control

1. Ensuring that beef and pork are cooked thoroughly.

2. Maintaining proper sanitation practices.

3. Practicing good personal hygiene.

4. Avoiding eating raw veggies cultivated in contaminated soil to stop cysticercosis from developing.

5. Treat individuals with *Taeniasis solium*, as they are at risk of developing cysticercosis through self-infection.

4. *Taenia saginata asiatica* (*Asian Taenia* or *Taenia asiatica*)

There is a close relationship between *Taenia saginata asiatica* and *T. saginata*. Though it is smaller in size, its morphology is similar to that of *T. saginata*. Its intermediate host is the pig, and its cysticerci are mostly found in the pig's liver. Treatment, diagnosis, and clinical characteristics are comparable to *T. saginata*.

4.1 Distribution

Taenia saginata asiatica is found mainly in Asia. Originally identified as Taiwan Taenia sp., this cestode was initially found in Taiwanese aboriginal people [19].

4.2 Predilection site

The human intestine and the liver of pigs and wild boars are the sites of *T. asiatica* infection.

4.3 Morphology

Similar to other species of taenia, the eggs of *T. asiatica* measure 30–35 micrometers in diameter and have radial striations (**Figure 3**). The oncosphere inside the eggs has six refractile hooks. The scolex of *T. asiatica* has rudimentary hooklets arranged in a wart-like formation. The proglottids of *T. asiatica* resemble those of T. saginata and have more than 12 primary uterine branches (**Figure 3A**) [12]. *T. asiatica* larvae develop in the liver of pigs, cattle, and goats, not in their muscles like *T. saginata* or *T. solium*. The mature worm in *T. asiatica* still has an armed protoscolex, but the hooklets are absent; unlike *T. saginata*, the adult *T. asiatica* worm is smaller, measuring 4 to 8 m long and having 300 to 1000 proglottids. Furthermore, the cysticerci of *T. asiatica* are significantly smaller, with dimensions of approximately 0.5 to 1.7 mm by 0.5 to 2.0 mm, compared to *T. saginata* or *T. solium*. mm by 0.5 to 2.0 mm, compared to *T. saginata* or *T. solium* [2].

4.4 Life cycle

Although *T. asiatica* cysticerci are smaller and form in the liver of pigs, cattle, and goats rather than the muscles of cattle like *T. saginata* or *T. solium*, their life cycle is similar to that of *T. saginata* (**Figure 4**) [12].

4.5 Pathogenesis and clinical symptoms

Generally, taeniasis brought on by *T. solium* or *T. saginata* is characterized by mild, nonspecific symptoms [20]. Many individuals with taeniasis asiatica also do not experience symptoms and only become aware of the infection when they pass proglottids in their feces. Even though there are no symptoms, patients infected with the tapeworm can experience emotional distress for a prolonged period while expelling the proglottids. When taeniasis asiatica is symptomatic, it exhibits similar mild and nonspecific signs. Some of the main clinical symptoms include the shedding of proglottids in the stools, abdominal pain, nausea, diarrhea, constipation, dizziness, increased appetite, headache, and itching around the anus [2].

4.6 Diagnosis

The diagnosis of *T. asiatica* and *T. saginata* is challenging due to their similar morphologies [17]. Previously, diagnosing human intestinal taeniasis relied on finding bile-stained eggs and gravid proglottids in the feces. However, recent studies suggest that microscopic examination alone is not reliable for distinguishing *T. saginata* from *T. asiatica* due to their similarities [16]. This raises the possibility that the true prevalence of *T. asiatica* may be underestimated. To address this, newer and more reliable detection methods, such as serological and molecular techniques, have been developed.

4.7 Treatment

Praziquantel or niclosamide are recommended for treating taeniasis. The adult worm is eliminated using the same treatment strategy that is employed for *T. solium* and *T. saginata*. Generally, therapy is highly effective. Retreatment is required if proglottids reappear in the stool or emerge from the anus [16].

4.8 Control and prevention

1. Ensure thorough cooking of pig liver.

2. Practice proper sanitation.

3. Maintain good personal hygiene.

4. Treat individuals with *T. asiatica* to prevent self-infection and the development of cysticercosis

5. *Hymenolepis nana*

H. Nana has been referred to as the dwarf tapeworm. The life cycle does not require an intermediate host.

5.1 Distribution

Its distribution is worldwide. Infection is most prevalent in children.

5.2 Predilection site

Adult worms live in the ileum of humans.

5.3 Morphology

Morphologically, *Hymenolepis nana* is the smallest cestode that can infect humans. The adult worm is less than 1 mm thick and ranges in length from 5 to 45 mm. It has a retractile rostellum with a single row of hooklets and a scolex with four suckers (**Figure 5A**). With a narrow neck, the worm has a strobila made up of at least 200 proglottids, which are wider than they are long. The uterus has three round testes. Gravid segments disintegrate to release eggs into the intestine. The eggs are roughly spherical or ovoid, approximately 30–40 μm in size. They have an inner embryophore that encloses the hexacanth oncosphere and a thin outer membrane (**Figure 5B**). Between the two membranes, there are 4–8 thread-like polar filaments that arise from two knobs on the embryophore. Eggs are immediately infectious when passed in feces [20].

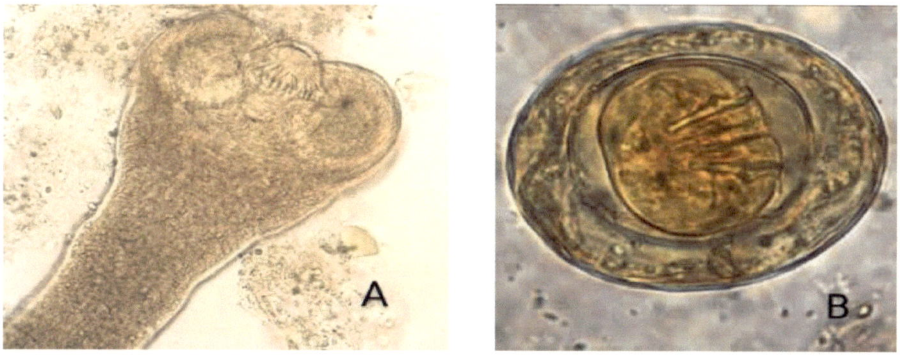

Figure 5.
(A) Scolex of H. nana. H. nana Egg in an unstained formalin ethyl acetate (FEA) wet mount is shown in (B) Four of the oncosphere hooks can be seen clearly in this image [21].

5.4 Life cycle

(1) Infected humans pass out embryonic eggs in their feces. (2) Insects (flea, beetle) ingest the eggs and develop into cysticercoid larvae. (3) When humans or rodents consume arthropods contaminated with cysticercoid mites, they become infected. (4) Consuming embryonated eggs from contaminated food, water, or hands can also expose humans to infection. (5) In the intestinal villus, the egg hatches and releases an oncosphere that matures into a cysticercoid. (6–7) The larva develops into an adult worm after emerging from the villus in the small intestine lumen. The adult worm's scolex is attached to the small intestine's ileal region. (8) The gravid proglottids release the eggs, which are then excreted in feces (**Figure 6**) [21].

5.5 Pathogenesis and clinical symptoms

In humans, adult *H. nana* worms mainly reside in the upper section of the ileum. A *H. nana* infection may be asymptomatic, even if there is a high number of worms present [22]. Symptoms that can occur include headache, Anal pruritus, dizziness, loss of appetite, abdominal pain, diarrhea, and possible irritability, particularly when there are 1000 to 2000 worms [22, 23]. Some patients may experience mild eosinophilia (5% or more). Young children with severe infections may have loose stools or diarrhea with mucus. The most common symptom reported is

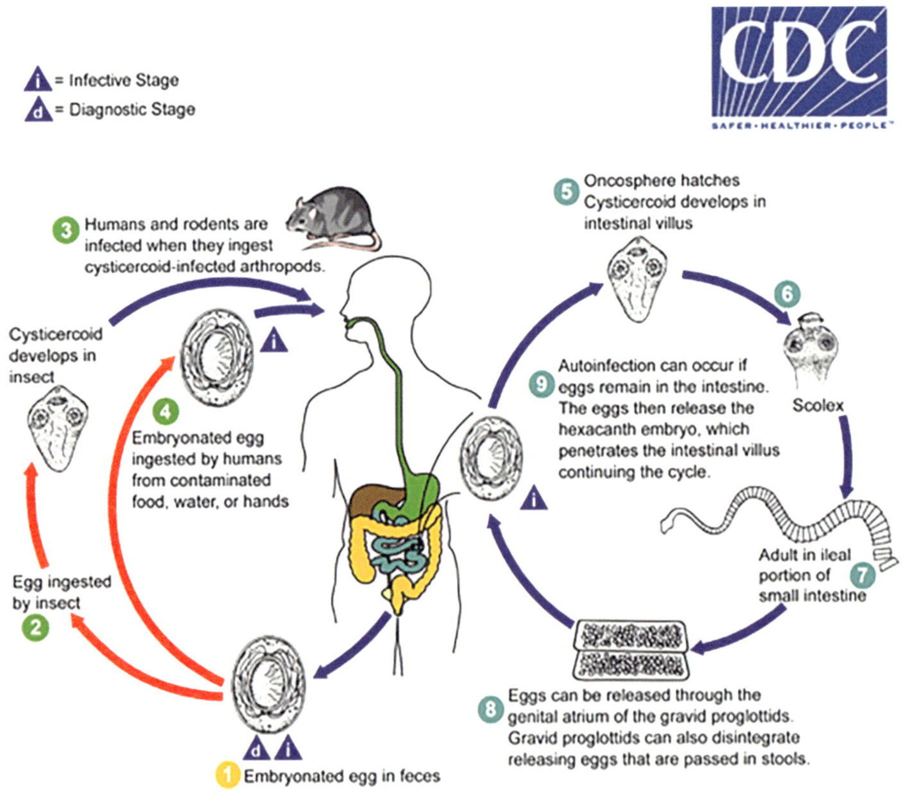

Figure 6.
Life cycle of Hymenolepis nana [21].

persistent, widespread abdominal pain [24]. Heavy infections in humans can be caused by internal autoinfection, where the eggs hatch in the intestine and complete the normal life cycle to become adult worms. This feature of the life cycle can lead to complications in individuals with weakened immune systems [25].

5.6 Diagnosis

1. Adult worms or proglottids are seldom observed in stool samples.

2. Microscopic examination: the presence of characteristic eggs with a thin shell, a six-hooked oncosphere, and polar filaments confirms the infection

3. Egg morphology is best observed in fresh specimens or those preserved in formalin-based fixatives.

4. It is important to note that works against the intestinal villi's cysticercoids as well as the adult worms. The eggs are infectious, so caution should be exercised when handling unpreserved stools.

5.7 Treatment

The preferred treatment is praziquantel (25 mg/kg in a single dose). It acts both against the adult worms and the cysticercoids in the intestinal villi. Nitazoxanide is an alternative drug [23].

5.8 Prevention and control

1. Maintain good personal hygiene.

2. Ensure proper sanitation practices.

3. Steer clear of consuming food and water that may be contaminated by fleas or beetles.

4. Implement effective rodent control methods.

6. *Hymenolepis diminuta*

H. diminuta is rarely found in humans, despite being frequently found in rats and mice.

6.1 Distributions

H. diminuta has a worldwide distribution.

6.2 Morphology

In terms of morphology, *H. diminuta* differs from *H. nana* in that the scolex of *H. diminuta* lacks hooks on the rostellum. It is common to find multiple worms, each

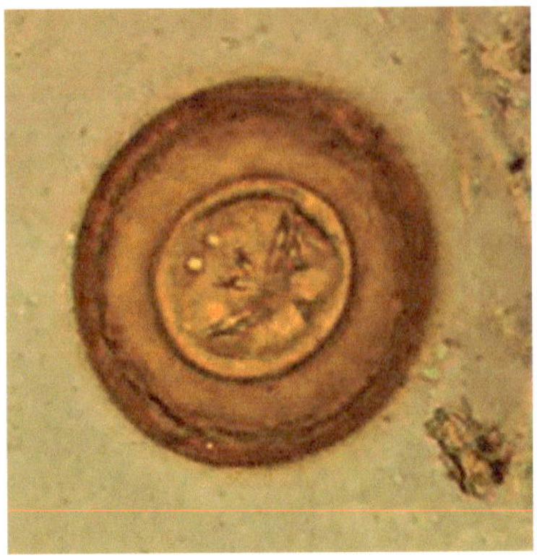

Figure 7.
Egg of H. diminuta in a wet mount stained with iodine. Four of the hooks are visible at this level of focus [21].

shorter in length than a single worm. While some adult worms (measuring 20 to 60 cm long) may occasionally be passed in the stool, eggs are usually obtained and identified. These eggs resemble those of *H. nana*, but they are larger and measure between 60 and 79 µm. They contain a six-hooked oncosphere and a clear area without polar filaments, unlike *H. nana*, which has polar filaments that arise from polar thickenings. This area in *H. diminuta* contains a gelatinous matrix (see **Figure** 7) [21, 26].

6.3 Life cycle

The eggs of *Hymenolepis diminuta*, a parasite found in rodents and humans, are passed out through feces. (1). These mature eggs are consumed by intermediate hosts like arthropods. (2). once ingested, oncospheres are released from the eggs and penetrate the host's intestinal wall (3). Then they develop into cysticercoid larvae. Tribolium species commonly serve as intermediate hosts for *H. diminuta*. Mammals become infected with *H. diminuta* by ingesting an intermediate host carrying the cysticercoid larvae (4). Humans can accidentally contract the infection by ingesting insects present in precooked cereals, other food items, or directly from the environment (especially children exploring orally). After ingestion, the arthropod tissue is digested, releasing the cysticercoid larvae in the stomach and small intestine. Shortly after being released, the larvae evaginate their scoleces. (5). Using the scolex's four suckers, the parasite attaches to the small intestine wall. Within 20 days, the parasites mature and can grow up to an average length of 30 cm. (6). Gravid proglottids in the small intestine release eggs (7), which are expelled into the environment through the mammalian host's feces (**Figure** 8) [21].

6.4 Pathogenisis and clinical symptoms

Most tapeworm infections in humans are typically well-tolerated, often without any noticeable symptoms. While the majority of infections have been observed in children under the age of 3, cases of infected adults have also been documented. In some instances, symptoms such as diarrhea, loss of appetite, nausea, headaches, and dizziness have been reported, primarily in children with severe infection [2].

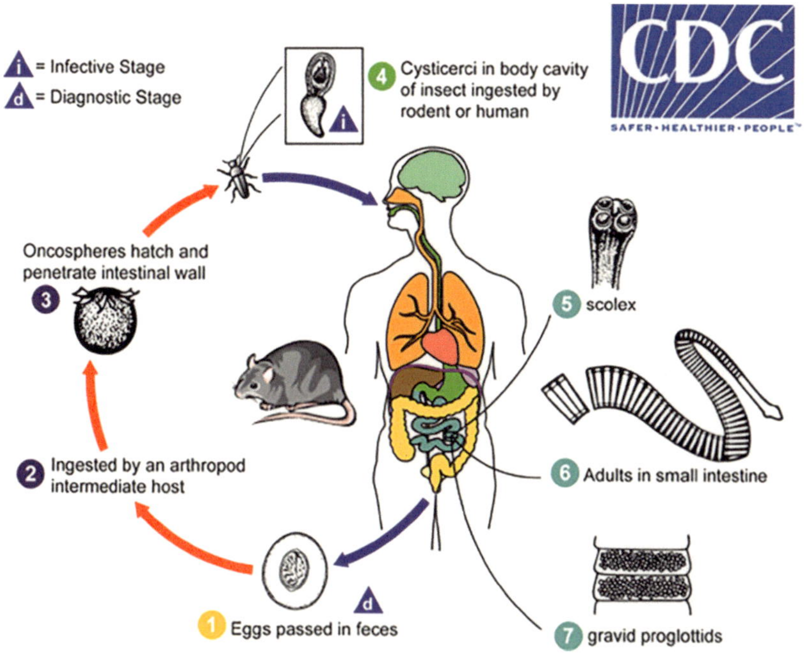

Figure 8.
Life cycle of Hymenolepis diminuta [21].

6.5 Diagnosis

1. Although human infection is uncommon, it can be diagnosed by recovering and identifying the distinctive eggs, which have a thin shell, a six-hooked oncosphere, and no polar filaments.

2. As part of proficiency testing programs, laboratories may occasionally receive these eggs for identification, and it is crucial to distinguish them from *H. nana* eggs.

3. Unlike *H. nana* eggs, the eggs of *H. diminuta* are not contagious between individuals.

6.6 Treatment

Praziquantel is recommended as a single dose of 5 to 10 mg/kg of body weight [27].

6.7 Prevention and control

To prevent the infection, it is advised to avoid accidentally ingesting intermediate arthropod hosts. Implementing rat control programs may also reduce the risk of human exposure.

7. *Dipylidium caninum*

This common double-pore tapeworm of dogs and cats may cause human infection, mainly in children.

7.1 Distribution

Dipylidium caninum is distributed globally.

7.2 Predilection site

The adult tapeworm resides in the small intestine of the host.

7.3 Morphology

The adult intestinal worm measures approximately 10–70 cm in length. Its scolex features four prominent suckers and a retractable rostellum with up to seven rows of spines (**Figure 9B**). It consists of 60–175 proglottids that resemble melon seeds. Each mature proglottid has two genital pores, one on each side. Gravid proglottids, which contain egg packets enclosed in capsules, are released through the host's anus individually or in clusters (**Figure 9B**) [2, 21, 28, 29].

7.4 Life cycle

(1–2) Eggs or proglottids from dogs and cats are consumed by larvae of dog fleas (Ctenocephalides canis) and cat fleas (*C. felis*). (3) Oncospheres hatch and enter the intestinal wall, developing into cysticercoids in the body cavity of the flea larvae. (4) Adult fleas carry the infectious cysticercoids. (5–7) Definitive hosts, including humans, become infected by ingesting fleas that contain cysticercoids. (8) The adult worm develops with its scolex attached to the small intestine (**Figure 10**) [28].

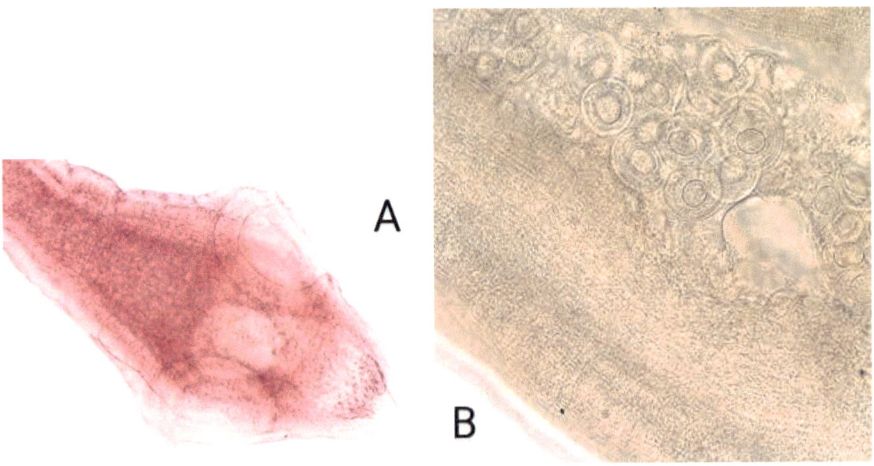

Figure 9.
(A) D. caninum scolex. (B) D. Caninum proglottid partially cleared with lactophenol, showing eggs and egg packets [28].

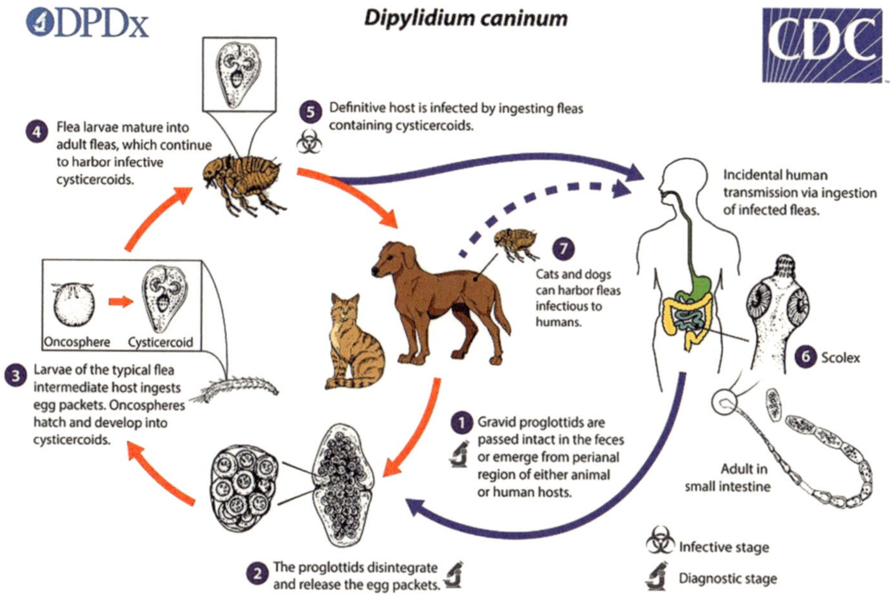

Figure 10.
The life cycle of Dipylidium caninum [28].

7.5 Pathogenesis and clinical symptoms

It is possible for gravid proglottids to actively migrate out of the anus. Human infections are usually asymptomatic. Some patients may experience abdominal pain, diarrhea, or anal pruritus.

7.6 Diagnosis

1. The diagnosis is often made using highly distinctive egg packets.

2. The shape of the proglottids (rice grains when dry, cucumber seeds when fresh) and the presence of recoverable egg packets from a ruptured proglottid are used to identify them.

7.7 Treatment

The drug of choice is praziquantel (5–10 mg/kg orally in a single-dose therapy).

7.8 Prevention and control

1. Regular deworming of infected dogs and cats

2. Prevention of flea infestation to avoid reinfection of the animals

3. Treating affected cases.

Author details

Samatar Abshir Mahamed
Jigjiga University, Ethiopia

*Address all correspondence to: samedeeq@yahoo.com

References

[1] Mahmud R, Lim YAL, Amir A. Medical Parasitology. Gewerbestrasse, Switzerland: Springer International Publishing; 2017. DOI: 10.1007/978-3-319-68795-7

[2] Garcia LS. Diagnostic medical parasitology. Santa Monica, California: ASM Press eBooks; 2016. DOI: 10.1128/9781555819002

[3] Scholz T, Garcia HH, Kuchta R, Wicht B. Update on the human broad tapeworm (genus diphyllobothrium), including clinical relevance. Clinical Microbiology Reviews. 2009;**22**(1):146-160. Table of Contents

[4] CDC - Dpdx - Diphyllobothriasis. 2019. Centers for Disease Control and Prevention. Available from: www.cdc.gov/dpdx/diphyllobothriasis/index.html

[5] Kuchta R, Radačovská A, Bazsalovicsová E, Viozzi G, Semenas L, Arbetman M, et al. Host switching of zoonotic broad fish tapeworm (*Dibothriocephalus latus*) to salmonids, patagonia. Emerging Infectious Diseases. 2019;**25**(11):2156-2158

[6] Choi HJ, Lee J, Yang HJ. Four human cases of Diphyllobothrium latum infection. The Korean Journal of Parasitology. 2012;**50**(2):143-146

[7] Tsuboi M, Hayakawa K, Yamasaki H, Katanami Y, Yamamoto K, Kutsuna S, et al. Clinical characteristics and epidemiology of intestinal tapeworm infections over the last decade in Tokyo, Japan: A retrospective review. PLoS Neglected Tropical Diseases. 2018;**12**(2):e0006297

[8] Sharma K, Wijarnpreecha K, Merrell N. *Diphyllobothrium latum* mimicking subacute appendicitis. Gastroenterology Research. 2018;**11**(3):235-237

[9] Waeschenbach A, Brabec J, Scholz T, Littlewood DTJ, Kuchta R. The catholic taste of broad tapeworms - multiple routes to human infection. International Journal for Parasitology. 2017;**47**(13):831-843

[10] Lloyd AE, Honey BL, John BM, Condren M. Treatment options and considerations for intestinal helminthic infections. The Journal of Pharmacy Technology. 2014;**30**(4):130-139

[11] Dermauw V, Dorny P, Braae UC, Devleesschauwer B, Robertson LJ, Saratsis A, et al. Epidemiology of *Taenia saginata* taeniosis/cysticercosis: A systematic review of the distribution in southern and eastern Africa. Parasites & Vectors. 2018;**11**(1):578

[12] CDC - Dpdx – Taeniasis. Available from: www.cdc.gov/dpdx/taeniasis/index.html [Accessed: March 2, 2024]

[13] Garcia HH, O'Neal SE, Noh J, Handali S. Cysticercosis working Group in Peru. Laboratory diagnosis of Neurocysticercosis (*Taenia solium*). Journal of Clinical Microbiology. 2018;**56**(9):e00424-e00418

[14] Silva CV, Costa-Cruz JM. A glance at Taenia saginata infection, diagnosis, vaccine, biological control and treatment. Infectious Disorders Drug Targets. 2010;**10**(5):313-321

[15] Reddy DS, Volkmer R. Neurocysticercosis as an infectious acquired epilepsy worldwide. Seizure. 2017;**52**:176-181

[16] Okello AL, Thomas LF. Human taeniasis: Current insights into prevention and management strategies in endemic countries. Risk Management and Healthcare Policy. 2017;**10**:107-116

[17] Yamasaki H, Allan JC, Sato MO, Nakao M, Sako Y, Nakaya K, et al. DNA differential diagnosis of *Taeniasis* and cysticercosis by multiplex PCR. Journal of Clinical Microbiology. 2004;**42**:548-553. DOI: 10.1128/JCM.42.2.548-553.2004

[18] Webb CM, White AC. Update on the diagnosis and Management of Neurocysticercosis. Current Infectious Disease Reports. 2016;**18**(12):44

[19] Ooi HK, Ho CM, Chung WC. Historical overview of *Taenia asiatica* in Taiwan. The Korean Journal of Parasitology. 2013;**51**:31-36. DOI: 10.3347/kjp.2013.51.1.31

[20] King CH, Mandell GL, Bennet JE, Dolin R. Mandel, Douglas and Bennett's Principles and Practice of Infectious Disease. 7th ed. Philadelphia: Churchill Livingstone Elsevier; 2010. Cestodes (tapeworms)

[21] CDC - Dpdx - Hymenolepiasis. Centers for Disease Control and Prevention. 2017. Available from: www.cdc.gov/dpdx/hymenolepiasis/index.html

[22] Cabada MM, Morales ML, Lopez M, Reynolds ST, Vilchez EC, Lescano AG, et al. *Hymenolepis nana* impact among children in the highlands of Cusco, Peru: An emerging neglected parasite infection. The American Journal of Tropical Medicine and Hygiene. 2016;**95**(5):1031-1036. DOI: 10.4269/ajtmh.16-0237

[23] O'Dempsey T, Finch RG, Greenwood D, Norrby SR, Whitley RJ. Helminthic infections. In: Antibiotic and Chemotherapy. 9th ed. New York: Saunders Elsevier; 2011

[24] Muehlenbachs A, Bhat Nagar J, Agudelo CA, Hidron A, Eberhard ML, Mathison BA, et al. Malignant transformation of Hymenolepis nana in a human host. The New England Journal of Medicine. 2015;**373**(19):1845-1852. DOI: 10.1056/NE-JMc1600490

[25] Thompson RC. Neglected zoonotic helminths: *Hymenolepis nana*, *Echinococcus canadensis* and *Ancylostoma ceylanicum*. Clinical Microbiology and Infection. 2015;**21**(5):426-432. DOI: 10.1016/j.cmi.2015.01.004

[26] Rozario T, Newmark PA. A confocal microscopy-based atlas of tissue architecture in the tapeworm *Hymenolepis diminuta*. Experimental Parasitology. 2015;**158**:31-41. DOI: 10.1016/j.exppara.2015.05.015

[27] Woolsey ID, Fredensborg BL, Jensen PM, Kapel CMO, Meyling NV. An insect–tapeworm model as a proxy for anthelminthic effects in the mammalian host. Parasitology Research. 2015;**114**:2777-2780. DOI: 10.1007/s00436-015-4477-0

[28] CDC - Dpdx - Dipylidium Caninum. Centers for Disease Control and Prevention. 2019. Available from: www.cdc.gov/dpdx/dipylidium/index.html#tabs-1-2

[29] Benitez-Bolivar P, Rondón S, Ortiz MI, Díaz-Díaz J, León C, Riveros J, et al. Morphological and molecular characterization of the parasite Dipylidium caninum infecting an infant in Colombia: A case report. Parasites & Vectors. 2022;**15**(1):463. DOI: 10.1186/s13071-022-05573-4

Chapter 8

Neurocysticercosis and the Central Nervous System: Advancements in Diagnosis, Treatment, and Future Prospects

Nicholas Aderinto, Gbolahan Olatunji, Emmanuel Kokori, Ismaila Ajayi Yusuf, Chimezirim Ezeano, Muili Abdulbasit and Timilehin Isarinade

Abstract

Neurocysticercosis presents a formidable global health challenge. This parasitic infection induces cystic lesions, primarily in the brain and spinal cord, leading to neurological symptoms and complications. Global prevalence varies, driven by socioeconomic conditions, cultural practices, and dietary habits, particularly in low and middle-income countries. Diagnosis remains challenging, relying on clinical, serological, and neuroimaging findings, with advanced tools like CT and MRI scans enhancing accuracy. Treatment strategies involve antiparasitic medications, anti-inflammatory drugs, and surgical interventions. Ongoing research explores innovative diagnostics and treatments, emphasising a comprehensive, individualised approach. A One Health approach, integrating human, animal, and environmental health, is crucial for effective prevention. Exploring the socioeconomic impacts, ethical considerations, and technology integration, including telemedicine, is paramount. Understanding cultural factors influencing healthcare-seeking behaviour contributes to culturally sensitive interventions. Technology integration can improve diagnostic capabilities and healthcare access, especially in regions with limited resources.

Keywords: neurocysticercosis, Taenia solium, central nervous system, diagnosis, treatment, epidemiology

1. Introduction

Neurocysticercosis is a formidable intersection of parasitology and neurology, presenting a global health challenge [1]. This condition arises from the infestation of the central nervous system by the larval form of Taenia solium, the pork tapeworm [2]. Neurocysticercosis is a parasitic infection caused by the cysticerci of Taenia solium, primarily found in pork [3]. Upon ingesting undercooked or raw infected pork, humans become inadvertent hosts to the tapeworm larvae [4]. The larvae then migrate to various tissues, with the central nervous system being a prime target [5]. The resulting neurocysticercosis manifests as cystic lesions in the brain, spinal cord, or other neural tissues, leading to neurological symptoms and complications [6].

The impact of neurocysticercosis on the central nervous system cannot be overstated. Cysticerci in neural tissues triggers inflammatory responses and immune reactions, culminating in neurological symptoms such as seizures, headaches, and cognitive impairments [7]. The significance of this parasitic infection extends beyond its immediate clinical manifestations, as it poses substantial challenges to public health systems, particularly in regions where the disease is endemic [8]. Moreover, neurocysticercosis is a leading cause of acquired epilepsy worldwide. The burden of neurological sequelae resulting from this parasitic infection emphasises the necessity for advancements in diagnosis and treatment strategies [9]. Addressing neurocysticercosis not only requires a comprehensive understanding of its pathogenesis but also necessitates a holistic approach to mitigate the socio-economic impact on affected communities [10].

The link between the tapeworm Taenia solium and neurocysticercosis underscores the importance of studying this parasitic infection's intestinal and neurological aspects [11]. The life cycle of *T. solium* involves a complex interplay between humans and pigs [12]. Understanding the dynamics of the tapeworm's transmission from the intestines to the central nervous system sheds light on potential intervention points for preventing and treating neurocysticercosis [13]. This chapter explores the intestinal relationship between Taenia solium and neurocysticercosis, exploring the pathways of transmission, risk factors, and preventive measures.

2. Epidemiology

2.1 Global prevalence and distribution

Neurocysticercosis exhibits a notable global prevalence, with specific regions experiencing a disproportionately high incidence. According to the World Health Organisation, neurocysticercosis affects around 50 million people worldwide and is a major cause of epilepsy and seizures across the globe [14]. The disease is associated with poor sanitation and is highly prevalent in Sub-Saharan Africa, Latin America and Asia [15]. Endemic hotspots include areas with poor sanitation and limited access to healthcare, particularly in low and middle-income countries. Latin America, sub-Saharan Africa, Southeast Asia, and parts of India have been identified as regions with a high prevalence of neurocysticercosis [16]. Within these areas, the transmission dynamics of Taenia solium, the causative agent, play a crucial role in shaping the epidemiological landscape [16]. Various factors contribute to the variations in neurocysticercosis prevalence across different regions. Socioeconomic conditions, inadequate sanitation infrastructure, and limited resources for public health interventions create an environment conducive to transmitting the parasite [17]. Furthermore, cultural practices, dietary habits, and local customs can influence the risk of infection, adding complexity to the epidemiological profile of neurocysticercosis [17].

2.2 High-risk populations

Neurocysticercosis often disproportionately affects individuals in lower socioeconomic strata [3]. Limited access to clean water, sanitation facilities, and healthcare services heightens the risk of infection [6]. Poverty-driven practices such as backyard pig farming and consumption of undercooked pork contribute to the prevalence of *T. solium* infestation in these vulnerable populations [9].

Cultural practices, including open defecation and insufficient hygiene practices, can facilitate the spread of *T. solium* eggs [18]. Dietary habits, especially the consumption of raw or undercooked pork in traditional dishes, contribute significantly to the transmission of neurocysticercosis. Understanding the interplay between culture, lifestyle, and disease transmission is crucial for effective public health interventions.

The ingestion of contaminated food, particularly undercooked pork containing viable cysticerci, serves as the primary mode of transmission for neurocysticercosis [12]. Improperly cooked pork acts as a vehicle for the tapeworm larvae, initiating the cycle of infection when consumed by humans. While less common, person-to-person transmission of neurocysticercosis can occur in specific circumstances. Poor hygiene practices, particularly in settings with inadequate sanitation, may lead to the faecal-oral transmission of *T. solium* eggs, perpetuating the infection cycle within communities.

Neurocysticercosis places a considerable burden on healthcare systems, particularly in regions with high incidence. The complex nature of the disease, coupled with the neurological complications it induces, demands specialised medical attention. Diagnostic challenges and the long-term management of affected individuals contribute to the strain on healthcare resources. The economic implications of neurocysticercosis extend beyond healthcare costs. The disease can lead to productivity losses due to the chronic nature of neurological symptoms, impacting affected individuals' ability to work. Additionally, public health interventions and preventive measures require substantial financial resources, emphasising the economic burden of neurocysticercosis.

3. Life cycle of Taenia solium

Taenia solium follows a complex lifecycle primarily involving humans and pigs and, less commonly, direct transmission between humans. Upon excretion of gravid proglottids or eggs from humans contaminating food and water, these proglottids or eggs find their way into the pig intermediate host [19]. When pigs ingest the tapeworm eggs, the eggs hatch, releasing oncospheres – young organisms encased in an embryonic shell [20]. These oncospheres travel through the pig's vasculature, spreading to various body parts, including viscera, skeletal muscles, subcutaneous tissues, and the cerebral parenchyma [19].

In the human host, the lifecycle continues with the consumption of raw or undercooked pork containing tapeworm larvae, known as cysticerci. These cysts adhere to the small intestine, initiating a multi-month developmental process [21]. Mature tapeworms, reaching lengths of up to 8 meters [22], are morphologically characterised by four muscular, circular suckers, an anterior scolex, and a rostellum with two rows of hooks [23]. These features enable them to adhere to the intestinal wall with minimal inflammation, often leading to mild or no symptoms.

The maturation process culminates in the release of tiny segmented proglottids, each containing thousands of eggs (up to 60,000) and exhibiting uteri with side branches resembling a "Christmas tree" [24]. These proglottids detach from the tapeworm, pass through the digestive tract, and exit the human host through excrement. Failure to observe proper hygiene during food preparation can contaminate various food sources, setting the stage for potential foodborne infections [19]. Notably, the subtle proliferation of these proglottids poses a serious threat, particularly in regions where pigs have access to human waste or lax cleanliness regulations. Alternatively, *T. solium* eggs can be ingested directly through the faecal route. Due to their sticky nature, these eggs can persist on hands and surfaces for several months under specific conditions [19, 25].

Crucial stages in the life cycle involve tissue invasion and migration, initiated when cysticerci mature within the human intestine [26]. The larvae's first stage's oncosphere hatches inside the intestine and penetrates the intestinal wall. Subsequently, these larvae enter the bloodstream, migrating across different organs and tissues. The ability of cysticerci to spread throughout the body, including the central nervous system (CNS), introduces a range of possible clinical outcomes [25]. Once in the bloodstream, these larvae have the potential to migrate to various tissues and organs, with a higher likelihood of reaching the central nervous system. This migration to the CNS is particularly significant, presenting a spectrum of clinical consequences and potential complications [25].

4. Transmission to the central nervous system

Rather than solely serving as the definitive host, humans can also act as the intermediate host for *T. solium* through feco-oral transmission [19]. Following ingestion, the eggs hatch into larvae within the human gastrointestinal tract [19]. This larval stage traverses the gastrointestinal tract walls, migrating to the tissues and causing tissue cysticercosis [19]. Host factors, including the immune system and specific genetic factors, influence the potential migration from the gastrointestinal tract to tissues [27]. Cysticercosis often exhibits a predilection for the brain, subcutaneous tissue, and the eye, although migration to other organs is possible [27]. Migration to the brain results in neurocysticercosis [27].

The encysted larva (cysticercus) gains access to the brain by disrupting the protective blood–brain barrier (BBB) and blood-cerebrospinal fluid barrier [28]. Studies in animal models of neurocysticercosis reveal increased expression of markers for BBB destruction, such as the endothelial barrier antigen and immunoglobulin G [28]. Upon entering the brain, the cysticercus may form either a parenchymal lesion within the brain substance or an extra-parenchymal lesion in the cerebrospinal fluid (CSF), subarachnoid space, ventricles, and cisterns [28].

Cysticerci exhibit remarkable longevity within the brain, often surviving for several years, achieved through modulation of the host immune system and the induction of immune tolerance [29]. This modulation involves the secretion of compounds such as prostaglandins and cytokines, including paramyosin and taenia-statin [29]. The cellular immune system is influenced by the induction of immunoregulatory cytokines like IL-10 and TGF-B [30]. Suppressed by the cysticercus, the immune system shifts to a Th2 response, facilitating the formation of a granuloma in the brain [30]. The granuloma comprises parasites, multinucleated giant cells, a surrounding fibrous collagen layer, CD68 macrophages, and various T cell subtypes [30].

While the cysticercus can inhibit the host system for extended periods, its modulatory effects eventually diminish [30]. Albendazole or Praziquantel initiates a switch to a Th1 immune response, leading to an inflammatory response and cyst degeneration [3, 30]. However, the degeneration of the cyst and the inflammatory response during treatment may exacerbate symptoms [3]. Therefore, anti-inflammatory medications such as corticosteroids are often prescribed with Praziquantel and Albendazole [31, 32]. Moreover, treating immunodeficiency states contributes to the reconstitution of the immune system against brain cysts [33]. Patients with neurocysticercosis (NCC) and human immunodeficiency virus (HIV) co-infections typically remain asymptomatic initially. However, after initiating antiretroviral therapy (ART), these patients develop robust cellular and humoral immune responses [33]. Following CNS access, the manifestations of neurocysticercosis vary, with clinical presentations determined by factors such as the number, location, size of cysts, cyst viability, and the host immune response [3].

5. Diagnosis

Neurocysticercosis (NCC) presents a diagnostic challenge due to the difficulty in histologically confirming the presence of the parasite in most cases. As a result, the diagnosis is primarily based on a combination of clinical, serological, and neuroimaging findings. Recognising the ongoing difficulty of proper diagnosis, this section delves into a review of advanced diagnostic approaches used in identifying NCC.

5.1 Imaging

5.1.1 Computed tomography (CT) scan findings in neurocysticercosis diagnosis

CT is valuable for identifying calcifications in NCC. Calcifications resembling buckshot-shaped nodules, especially in endemic areas, indicate NCC. Well-defined, round cystic lesions with smooth walls, presenting a "Swiss cheese" appearance, are characteristic. CT also reveals pericyst inflammation through enhancement, indicating the degenerative process of cysts [34–36].

5.1.2 MRI in neurocysticercosis diagnosis

MRI improves soft tissue resolution and provides enhanced details. Viable cysts appear hypointense on T1 and FLAIR MRI scans. Contrast-enhanced MRI reveals unique enhancement patterns, aiding in differentiating cysticerci phases. MRI is superior at detecting meningeal involvement, offering extensive information on the central nervous system's inflammatory response and disease severity [34, 36, 37]. Despite advances in neuroimaging, diagnosing NCC remains challenging. Developed in 1996 and subsequently reviewed, diagnostic criteria include absolute major and minor neuroimaging criteria. These criteria aid in standardising the diagnosis [38–40].

5.2 Laboratory tests

5.2.1 Serological tests

Serum Western blot with a specific proportion of *T. solium* cysts is a successful method, confirming exposure or sickness precisely. Monoclonal antibody-based antigen detection assays are useful for verifying continued infection. The enzyme-linked immunoelectrotransfer blot test (EITB) is an effective serological technique, particularly for patients with multiple brain cysts [41–45].

5.2.2 Cerebrospinal fluid analysis

Serological tests in CSF, including ELISA, remain feasible options, especially in individuals with viable neurocysticercosis infections. Antigen detection in serum and CSF is a cyst viability biomarker crucial for monitoring anthelmintic medication effectiveness [45–47].

Clinical/exposure criteria, such as identifying specific antibodies or antigens, extraneural cysticercosis, evidence of household contact, and clinical signs, provide circumstantial evidence to support the diagnosis. Symptomatic NCC patients often present with seizures, headaches, focal neurologic abnormalities, and cognitive deterioration [40]. Definitive and probable diagnoses have evolved, incorporating neuroimaging criteria, clinical/exposure criteria, and additional evaluations. Criteria for definitive and probable diagnoses involve various combinations of neuroimaging and clinical/exposure criteria [40].

5.3 Advanced diagnostic tools

The widely accepted LLGP-EITB test is the standard for antibody detection, demonstrating remarkable diagnostic performance in clinical settings. Monoclonal antibody-based techniques, such as B158/B60 Ag-ELISA and HP10 assays, have emerged as effective tools for establishing the presence of live parasites. Recent research proposes innovative techniques, including urine assays for *T. solium* DNA and portable fluorescence sensors for on-the-spot diagnostics. Continued progress in neuroimaging, exemplified by portable MRI machines, enhances accessibility, particularly in low- and middle-income countries (LMICs) [18, 48–55].

6. Treatment

The therapeutic management of neurocysticercosis aims to alleviate symptoms, treat the parasitic infection, combat the inflammatory process, and manage complications. It is best approached from an individualised, patient-specific perspective [56]. The treatment approaches vary based on factors such as the viability of cysts, age (children or adults), location, number, and size of the cysts, among others. There are two major components to managing neurocysticercosis: pharmacological and surgical approaches.

6.1 Antiparasitic treatment

Antiparasitic treatment is recommended, and its use alone is reserved for patients without complications like untreated hydrocephalus, cerebral oedema, and other causes of raised intracranial pressure. The recommended antiparasitic regimen for cases with ≤2 viable parenchymal cysticerci is a monotherapy of oral Albendazole at 15 mg/kg/day divided into 2 daily doses for 10–14 days with food, up to a maximum dose of 1200 mg/day.

In cases with >2 viable cysticerci, combination therapy of albendazole (15 mg/kg/day PO in two divided doses) with Praziquantel (50 mg/kg/day in 3 divided doses) for 10–14 days is recommended [57, 58]. Albendazole impairs glucose uptake by the larvae and adult stages, depletes glycogen stores, and decreases adenosine triphosphate (ATP) production, leading to parasite death [59, 60]. Praziquantel causes rapid, sustained muscular contraction and tegumental disruption, exposing the parasite antigens to the immune system [59, 60].

6.2 Anti-inflammatory drugs

The inflammatory response against parasites is a significant pathological mechanism seen in neurocysticercosis. Anti-inflammatory treatment is indicated for parenchymal neurocysticercosis with Vesicular neurocysticercosis, solitary cysticercus granuloma, or cysticercotic encephalitis, and all cases of extra-parenchymal neurocysticercosis. Corticosteroids are the anti-inflammatory agents of choice, recommended in patients with different forms of neurocysticercosis [57, 58].

Some corticosteroids in use include Prednisone, Prednisolone, methylprednisolone, and dexamethasone. High intravenous doses (e.g., dexamethasone 0.2–0.4 mg/kg/day) are used in significant inflammatory responses, and the dosage is adjusted based on the size and number of parasites. The corticosteroids are gradually tapered off after the end of the cysticidal treatment or as long as inflammation persists [61]. For children and adolescents, dexamethasone dosage is 0.1 to 0.2 mg/kg/dose PO daily in oral solution, while for adults, it is 6 to 8 mg PO daily in 3 divided doses. Prednisolone and prednisone are also prescribed at 1 to 2 mg/kg/dose PO daily [57].

Other drugs used in managing neurocysticercosis include Anti-Epileptic Drugs such as carbamazepine, phenytoin, phenobarbital, and valproic acid, as epilepsy is a major symptom of neurocysticercosis. The treatment of epilepsy in neurocysticercosis follows the standard management for epilepsy from other causes [59].

6.3 Surgical management

Surgery is reserved for selected cases, playing a minor role in the overall management since most cases can be effectively managed with antiparasitic and anti-inflammatory drugs [60, 62]. Indications for surgical treatment include extra-parenchymal neurocysticercosis with intraventricular cysts, hydrocephalus due to racemose cysts, or hydrocephalus due to ependymitis caused by neurocysticercosis. Surgical intervention is also considered for intramedullary and extramedullary spinal cysticercosis, large parenchymal colloidal cysts, subarachnoid racemose cysts causing mass effect, confirmation of the diagnosis of an atypical Solitary Cysticercus Granuloma, or in the case of surgery for intractable epilepsy associated with neurocysticercosis [63].

Surgical excision of cysts is the recommended treatment for intraventricular neurocysticercosis, especially lateral and third ventricular cysts. Endoscopic excision is minimally invasive, reducing the risk of complications associated with open craniotomy and minimising brain manipulation. The procedure involves placing a single burr hole in the pre-coronal region for access, grasping the cyst with forceps, and removing the entire scope assembly through the burr hole to prevent cyst loss or rupture in the ventricle [62, 63].

For managing hydrocephalus due to neurocysticercosis, surgical interventions such as fenestration of the anterior wall of the third ventricle and ventriculo-peritoneal shunt placement are considered. Hydrocephalus in neurocysticercosis arises from inflammation and mechanical obstruction from cysts or scars, affecting cerebrospinal fluid flow. Surgical excision of cysts usually relieves obstruction, but inflammatory reactions may persist, necessitating a ventriculo-peritoneal shunt to alleviate raised intracranial pressure and associated symptoms [59].

An alternative for managing hydrocephalus in neurocysticercosis is Endoscopic Third Ventriculostomy (ETV), providing an alternative route for cerebrospinal fluid flow directly from the third ventricle to the subarachnoid space, bypassing the fourth ventricle [64]. Combining cyst removal and ETV is less invasive than conventional craniotomies and avoids shunt-related complications [65].

7. Challenges in management

7.1 Drug resistance

The management of neurocysticercosis involves addressing various factors, such as the severity of symptoms, extent of cyst involvement, stage of cyst degeneration, and accompanying inflammation, while also considering potential future complications. Treatment typically includes the administration of anthelmintic medications, such as albendazole and praziquantel, alongside anti-epileptic drugs to manage seizures and corticosteroids to reduce inflammation. Surgical procedures may be necessary for cases resistant to conventional treatment methods. While some treatments lack robust randomised studies, anecdotal evidence supports the use of anthelmintics with corticosteroids for viable cysts. The emergence of drug resistance remains a significant concern in the management of neurocysticercosis. However, reports of drug resistance in neurocysticercosis have not been widely reported. Resistance to first-line drugs of choice like albendazole is therefore subject to ongoing research.

7.2 Surgical complications

Surgical intervention plays a crucial role in managing neurocysticercosis, particularly in cases of intraventricular cysts or giant cysts unresponsive to medical treatment. The shift towards endoscopic procedures, performed through a single burr hole, has become preferable due to its minimally invasive nature [1]. Experienced surgeons can achieve good outcomes with minimal side effects, and concerns about anaphylactic reactions to cyst rupture during surgery have not been substantiated [66]. The complications usually seen in patients with neurocysticercosis are common to other neurosurgical procedures, such as wound infection, fistula formation, and reported cases of intraoperative or postoperative haemorrhage. Ventricular bleeding can be seen after neuroendoscopy. Rupture of interventricular or cisternal cysticercus during surgery is not associated with disease dissemination [1, 66].

The management of hydrocephalus stemming from subarachnoid neurocysticercosis often necessitates CSF drainage or shunt placement. Ventriculocisternostomy with third ventricle fenestration offers a potential alternative, potentially averting the need for a shunt device and improving prognosis. Common complications associated with shunts, such as malfunction or infection, contribute to morbidity. Surgical complications leading to patient mortality correlate with the frequency of shunt revisions, although corticosteroids may mitigate the risk of shunt dysfunction [67].

The management of large cysts within the lateral fissure is a topic of debate, typically necessitating surgical intervention when conservative treatments prove unsuccessful. Surgical resection may be considered following ineffective medical management. Overall, surgical management tends to yield positive outcomes in most cases [66]. Surgeons play a crucial role in assessing the patient's clinical and radiographic features, customising the surgical approach to the specific characteristics and location of the cyst.

8. Advancements in research

8.1 Emerging diagnostic technologies

Confirming neurocysticercosis (NCC) histologically is often not feasible, necessitating reliance on neuroimaging and immunological tests. Despite advancements in these diagnostic methods, identifying neurocysticercosis remains challenging due to the limited specificity of clinical and neuroimaging findings and the less-than-ideal predictive values of immunodiagnostic tests, particularly in regions where the disease is endemic [67]. This diagnostic challenge has, therefore, necessitated the need to develop universal diagnostic criteria for neurocysticercosis.

In 1993, criteria were proposed and later validated in a 1997 study involving 401 patients with seizures and a solitary brain mass on CT scans. In 2001, an international expert group introduced neurocysticercosis diagnostic criteria. Despite some criticism, these criteria remain essential for clinicians worldwide when dealing with suspected NCC cases [62]. In 2017, Del Brutto et al. updated the diagnostic criteria for NCC, emphasising neuroimaging to reduce false positives in endemic regions and enhance detection in non-endemic areas where NCC is often overlooked [1, 18]. The revised criteria state that definitive NCC diagnosis requires visible tapeworm scolex on neuroimaging. However, challenges such as limited access to neuroimaging, radiologist training issues, and high imaging costs pose obstacles, particularly in developing countries.

Simple, affordable, and efficient diagnostic tools are required to detect infections and at-risk populations. Research indicates the possibility of isolating *T. solium* DNA from patients' urine, validated by positive Enzyme-linked immunoelectrotransfer blot (EITB) outcomes for anti-*T. solium* antibodies in individuals with subarachnoid and viable parenchymal cysts [67]. Using portable fluorescent sensors, capable of detecting antibodies and providing results for later examination on mobile devices, offers significant benefits in diagnosis and surveillance. Nonetheless, the sensitivity of urine tests is contingent upon the infection load. Similar to serological tests, they cannot pinpoint the location of cysts, whether in the central nervous system (CNS) or elsewhere in the body.

The real-time quantitative polymerase chain reaction (qPCR) test, targeting the repetitive Tsol13 sequence in the *T. solium* genome, demonstrates high sensitivity and specificity for Neurocysticercosis (NCC). This test serves as a marker for "cure" in cerebrospinal fluid (CSF) and offers a definitive diagnosis of NCC from plasma samples. Notably, all 18 CSF samples from patients with active NCC tested positive for *T. solium* DNA using the TsolR13 qPCR method [18]. Ongoing advances in neuroimaging are enhancing the early diagnosis and treatment of NCC. In a population study in Mexico, 9.1% of 155 asymptomatic, healthy patients revealed calcified lesions through MRI scanning. The approval of a portable MRI machine by the Food and Drug Administration (FDA) opens possibilities for increased accessibility to MRIs in hospitals and clinics, especially in Low- and Middle-Income Countries (LMIC) [68].

8.2 Novel treatment approaches

The search for innovative drug targets in treating neurocysticercosis and taeniasis is essential, considering the absence of recent clinical trials establishing specific indications, doses, and treatment durations for antihelminthic drugs. Despite debates on the safety and usefulness of anticysticercal treatment, there is a lack of vaccines or new drugs in the pipeline for clinical trials. Exploring tapeworm-specific detoxification pathways, non-canonical heat shock proteins, and their uniquely tailored proteome and metabolism could offer promising avenues for future drug intervention studies in neurocysticercosis [40].

Genome sequencing and mapping of parasitic tapeworms have unveiled approximately 250 to 300 novel protein kinases. These kinases, integral to major metabolic pathways of the parasite, emerge as potential targets. Notably, the mitogen-activated protein kinase (MAPK) family, including evolutionarily conserved extracellular signal-regulated kinases (ERK 1/2), plays a role in oestrogen-dependent reproduction of helminth parasites. Although the exact involvement of ERK 1/2 in host–parasite interaction remains unclear, the demonstrated role of an ERK-like protein suggests it could be considered a target for antihelminthic drug design [69].

In the same vein, sequences associated with a progesterone receptor have been detected in *T. solium* through RT-PCR and Western blotting, and an mRNA with sequence similarity to an oestrogen receptor has been demonstrated [69]. If steroidal hormone receptors exist in Taenia cysticerci, oestrogen receptor antagonists could significantly affect parasite transmission and development. Exploring the cysticidal effects of tamoxifen in *T. solium* may contribute to developing novel therapeutic agents for controlling cysticercosis in humans and livestock in future studies.

Antioxidant enzymes are vital for shielding parasites from host-induced oxidative stress (ROS) and are integral to numerous physiological functions. These enzymes, utilised by parasites for immune evasion, have been investigated in *T. solium*. The crystal structure of recombinant *T. solium* Cu/Zn-SOD was this organism's first reported protein structure. *T. solium* expresses cytosolic Cu, Zn superoxide dismutase, a 2-Cys peroxiredoxin, and two glutathione transferase isoforms, all proven to protect mice against cysticercosis [70]. Their presence throughout developmental and adult stages highlights the pivotal role of antioxidant enzymes in *T. solium* physiology, suggesting potential for novel drug development.

Yan et al. [70] conducted a study identifying 197 novel proteases in *T. solium*, belonging to 37 families [69, 70]. These proteases were classified based on the active site amino acid residue into categories like aspartic, cysteine, serine, metallo-serine, and threonine proteases. This contrasts with a previous study [71] identifying only three putative proteases in *T. solium* [71]. The newly discovered proteases have potential implications for drug development, as they are believed to play crucial roles in various aspects of the parasite's biology and interaction with the host immune system. Further exploration in this field is warranted.

9. Future prospects

9.1 Potential vaccines

Vaccination is one of the most effective methods of treating various parasitic and infectious diseases and has successfully prevented major epidemics worldwide.

Vaccines have been developed for infectious diseases such as malaria and typhoid, aiding in their treatment. In Addition, potential vaccines have also been developed for achieving herd immunity against pandemic diseases such as Ebola and coronavirus. No vaccines have been developed for treating neurocysticercosis or used in various clinical trials. However, some vaccines have been developed for pigs, which are being used in preclinical trials to pre-eliminate the parasite by preventing the transmission of the parasite from pigs to man since pigs are known to be an intermediate host of the diseases. Various vaccines, such as the recombinant oncosphere antigen, SP3VAC, pcDNA 3-B, and HP6/TSOL18, have been used in preclinical trials.

Recombinant oncosphere antigens are proteins cloned from Taenia solium oncosphere mRNA used to diagnose and manage Taenia solium-related diseases such as taeniasis and cysticercosis [72]. It has been found to be used as a vaccine through the development of proteins such as TSOL16, TSOL18, TSOL45-1A, and TSOL45-1B. these proteins have been used in various preclinical trials in pigs to evaluate their efficacy in protecting pigs against porcine cysticercosis (PCC). Of these vaccines, TSOL18 has been identified as the most effective candidate for protecting Pigs against PCC with a protection rate of 99.5% [1]. TSOL18, also known as Cysvax is a novel vaccine that was developed by Indian Immunological Limited and GALVmed and has been commercially available for sale and distribution in India since its formal licencing in 2016 [73]. Before it is licencing, it has been evaluated in various studies. For instance, Flisser et al [74] conducted a study evaluating the prevention of Pigs from PCC by vaccinating them with recombinant antigens TSOL18 and TSOL45-1A [74]. The study, which was conducted in Mexico and Cameroon showed a 100% protection rate from PCC through the use of these recombinant antigens. Other studies have also evaluated the combination of Cysvax with oxfendazole in the vaccination of pigs in Cameroon, Nepal, Uganda, and Tanzania, with a protection rate of>99% in these locations [75–78].

SP3VAC is a synthetic vaccine composed of three peptides (GK1, KETc1, and KETc12) expressed in taenia solium larva and adult stages. This vaccine was developed and evaluated in pigs in Mexico by Huerta et al., [79]. Results from the study showed a reduction in the prevalence of cysticercosis by 52.6% and helped protect against PCC by 98.7%. Results from a further evaluation by Sciutto et al. in 2007 also supported the efficacy of SP3VAC on the protective effects of the vaccine against PCC [80]. However, the study concluded that a single vaccination dose is ineffective in preventing the transmission of taenia solium in endemic regions [80]. Other clinical trials have also shown the efficacy of SP3VAC in the vaccination of pigs though there are limited clinical trials conducted presently on the use of this vaccine in the last decade [80–82].

Other vaccines, such as pcDNA 3-B, and HP6/TSOL18 have been used in some studies to vaccinate pigs. A notable example is the study by Guo in 2007, which used pcDNA3-B, a DNA vaccine, in contrast to the common mRNA vaccines that are currently widely used [83]. This vaccine was developed by integrating Taenia solium B antigen with the pcDNA3.1 plasmid. Immunisation of the pigs with this vaccine showed a 92.6% protection rate, showing the effectiveness of this vaccine [84]. No studies have been conducted using this vaccine to date. HP6/TSOL18 is also an effective vaccine for protecting pigs against PCC. Just like the pcDNA-3B, this vaccine has also been evaluated in only one study to date, which was conducted by Parkhouse in 2008, [84]. However, further improvements in the vaccine from an intramuscular administration to an oral administration were shown in a study conducted by Monreal-Escalante et al., [85]. The study also showed its potential as an effective vaccine against PCC.

9.2 Collaborative research initiatives

Collaborative research initiatives, whether locally or internationally, have been significant in managing a disease since, through proper clinical research, novel initiatives for the diagnosis and treatment of diseases can be generated. In addition, Challenges facing the management of a disease can also be identified with proper recommendations to tackle the challenges provided. International collaborative research has also helped improve the stage of scientific research in low-income countries Regarding neurocysticercosis, there have been up to 7860 papers published from 1928 up till 2021, with a rate of 200 papers per year since 2010 [86]. Most of the literature published on neurocysticercosis is case studies, while the least are systematic reviews. The USA stands as the country that produces the highest number of publications on neurocysticercosis to date. Many publications are also produced by endemic regions such as India, Peru, and Brazil [85].

The level of collaborative research initiatives locally is high while the level of international collaboration is uneven, with large countries such as India and Brazil having 9.9 and 18.7% in international collaborations, while low-income countries like Peru, Tanzania, and Kenya showing heavy international collaboration in 80% of their papers generated from these countries [87] income countries (HICs) and low- and middle-income countries (LMICs).

In addition to diagnosing and treating the disease, collaborative research should focus more on developing vaccines to eliminate the parasite in humans. More focus should also be placed on vaccines such as pcDNA-18 and HP6/TSOL18, as they can potentially be a vaccine source for humans. A planetary and one health approach is also a significant area of focus for collaborative research through the dynamics of transmission of the disease between humans, animals, and the environment. This approach involves the integration of human, animal, and environmental health, which will enable the generation and implementation of policies that will help prevent the transmission rate of the parasite [87].

10. Conclusion

This exploration of neurocysticercosis has uncovered critical insights into its complexities and offered a roadmap for future research and intervention. The understanding of *T. solium*'s intricate life cycle, particularly its neurological aspects, emphasises the need for a holistic approach considering both human and porcine dimensions. The global prevalence, shaped by diverse socioeconomic, cultural, and dietary factors, underscores the necessity for targeted interventions tailored to specific regions.

Diagnostic challenges persist, urging the continuous development of advanced tools such as CT, MRI scans, and serological tests. Treatment strategies, though in place, face challenges of drug resistance and surgical complications, necessitating ongoing research into innovative solutions. The significance of a One Health approach cannot be overstated, emphasising collaborative efforts across human, animal, and environmental health.

Socioeconomic impacts and ethical considerations highlight the broader implications of neurocysticercosis on communities, urging research to delve into economic burdens, productivity loss, and social stigmatisation. Integrating technology, particularly telemedicine, stands as a promising avenue for improving access to healthcare, especially in underserved regions.

Capacity building and training programs emerge as pivotal components, empowering healthcare workers and community health workers for more effective disease control. The collaboration of diverse stakeholders, including healthcare professionals, veterinarians, environmental scientists, and policymakers, is essential for a comprehensive and sustainable approach.

In envisioning the future of neurocysticercosis research, addressing these dimensions will not only enhance our understanding of the disease but also contribute to the development of practical, culturally sensitive, and globally applicable strategies for prevention, diagnosis, and treatment. As the scientific community collectively advances towards these goals, the potential for meaningful global health impact in the realm of neurocysticercosis becomes increasingly tangible.

List of abbreviations

NCC	neurocysticercosis
CT	computed tomography
MRI	magnetic resonance imaging
CNS	central nervous system
LMIC	low- and middle-income countries
FDA	food and drug administration
qPCR	quantitative polymerase chain reaction
CSF	cerebrospinal fluid
MAPK	mitogen-activated protein kinase
ERK	extracellular signal-regulated kinase
ROS	reactive oxygen species
EITB	enzyme-linked immunoelectrotransfer blot
SP3VAC	synthetic vaccine composed of three peptides (GK1, KETc1, and KETc12)
PCC	porcine cysticercosis

Author details

Nicholas Aderinto[1*], Gbolahan Olatunji[2], Emmanuel Kokori[2], Ismaila Ajayi Yusuf[3], Chimezirim Ezeano[4], Muili Abdulbasit[1] and Timilehin Isarinade[2]

1 Internal Medicine Department, LAUTECH Teaching Hospital, Ogbomoso, Nigeria

2 Department of Medicine and Surgery, University of Ilorin, Ilorin, Nigeria

3 Department of Medicine and Surgery, Obafemi Awolowo University Teaching Hospital, Ife, Nigeria

4 University of North Texas, Health Science Center, Fort Worth, Texas, United States

*Address all correspondence to: nicholasoluwaseyi6@gmail.com

References

[1] Butala C, Brook TM, Majekodunmi AO, Welburn SC. Neurocysticercosis: Current perspectives on diagnosis and management. Frontiers in Veterinary Science. 2021;**8**:2-3. DOI: 10.3389/fvets.2021.615703

[2] Del Brutto OH. Human neurocysticercosis: An overview. Pathogens. 2022;**11**(10):5. DOI: 10.3390/pathogens11101212

[3] Garcia HH, Nash TE, Del Brutto OH. Clinical symptoms, diagnosis, and treatment of neurocysticercosis. The Lancet Neurology. 2014;**13**(12):1202. DOI: 10.1016/S1474-4422(14)70094-8

[4] Sarria Estrada S, Frascheri Verzelli L, Siurana Montilva S, Auger Acosta C, Rovira Cañellas A. Neurocisticercosis. Hallazgos radiológicos [imaging findings in neurocysticercosis]. Radiología. 2013;**55**(2):130-141. DOI: 10.1016/j.rx.2011.11.009

[5] Guzman C, Garcia HH, Cysticercosis Working Group in Peru. Current diagnostic criteria for neurocysticercosis. Research and Reports in Tropical Medicine. 2021;**12**:197-203. DOI: 10.2147/RRTM.S285393

[6] Carmen-Orozco RP, Dávila-Villacorta DG, Delgado-Kamiche AD, Celiz RH, Trompeter G, Sutherland G, et al. Changes in inflammatory gene expression in brain tissue adjacent and distant to a viable cyst in a rat model for neurocysticercosis. PLoS Neglected Tropical Diseases. 2021;**15**(4):e0009295. DOI: 10.1371/journal.pntd.0009295

[7] Ung L, Stothard JR, Phalkey R, Azman AS, Chodosh J, Hanage WP, et al. Towards global control of parasitic diseases in the Covid-19 era: One health and the future of multisectoral global health governance. Advances in Parasitology. 2021;**114**:1-26. DOI: 10.1016/bs.apar.2021.08.007

[8] Molyneux DH, Dean L, Adekeye O, Stothard JR, Theobald S. The changing global landscape of health and disease: Addressing challenges and opportunities for sustaining progress towards control and elimination of neglected tropical diseases (NTDs). Parasitology. 2018;**145**(13):1647-1654. DOI: 10.1017/S0031182018000069

[9] Takayanagui OM, Haes TM. Update on the diagnosis and management of neurocysticercosis. Arquivos de Neuro-Psiquiatria. 2022;**80**(5 Suppl. 1):296-306. DOI: 10.1590/0004-282X-ANP-2022-S115

[10] Takayanagui OM, Odashima NS, Bonato PS, Lima JE, Lanchote VL. Medical management of neurocysticercosis. Expert Opinion on Pharmacotherapy. 2011;**12**(18):2845-2856. DOI: 10.1517/14656566.2011.634801

[11] WHO Guidelines on Management of Taenia Solium Neurocysticercosis [Internet]. Geneva: World Health Organization; 2021. Available from: https://www.ncbi.nlm.nih.gov/books/NBK573853/

[12] Prodjinotho UF, Lema J, Lacorcia M, Schmidt V, Vejzagic N, Sikasunge C, et al. Host immune responses during Taenia solium neurocysticercosis infection and treatment. PLoS Neglected Tropical Diseases. 2020;**14**(4):e0008005. DOI: 10.1371/journal.pntd.0008005

[13] Schmidt V, O'Hara MC, Ngowi B, Herbinger KH, Noh J, Wilkins PP, et al. Taenia solium cysticercosis and taeniasis in urban settings: Epidemiological

evidence from a health-center based study among people with epilepsy in Dar es Salaam, Tanzania. PLoS Neglected Tropical Diseases. 2019;**13**(12):e0007751. DOI: 10.1371/journal.pntd.0007751

[14] World Health Organization. Neurocysticercosis affects around 50 million people worldwide and is a major cause of epilepsy and seizures. Available from: https://www.who.int/news-room/fact-sheets/detail/taeniasis-cysticercosis

[15] Ta R, Blond BN. The prevalence of and contributors to neurocysticercosis in endemic regions. Journal of the Neurological Sciences. 2022;**441**:120393. DOI: 10.1016/j.jns.2022.120393

[16] Moyano LM, O'Neal SE, Ayvar V, Gonzalvez G, Gamboa R, Vilchez P, et al. High prevalence of asymptomatic neurocysticercosis in an endemic rural Community in Peru. PLoS Neglected Tropical Diseases. 2016;**10**(12):e0005130. DOI: 10.1371/journal.pntd.0005130

[17] Bustos J, Gonzales I, Saavedra H, Handali S, Garcia HH, Cysticercosis Working Group in Peru. Neurocysticercosis. A frequent cause of seizures, epilepsy, and other neurological morbidity in most of the world. Journal of the Neurological Sciences. 2021;**427**:117527. DOI: 10.1016/j.jns.2021.117527

[18] O'Connell EM, Harrison S, Dahlstrom E, Nash T, Nutman TB. A novel, highly sensitive qPCR assay for the diagnosis of subarachnoid and ventricular neurocysticercosis and for assessing response to treatment. Clinical Infectious Diseases. 2019;**70**:1875-1881. DOI: 10.1093/cid/ciz541

[19] Centers for Disease Control and Prevention (CDC). Cysticercosis. DPDx – Laboratory Identification of Parasites of Public Health Concern; 2024. Available from: https://www.cdc.gov/dpdx/cysticercosis/index.html

[20] Verastegui M, Gilman RH, Arana Y, Barber D, Velásquez J, Farfán M, et al. Taenia solium oncosphere adhesion to intestinal epithelial and Chinese hamster ovary cells in vitro. Infection and Immunity. 2007;**75**(11):5158-5166. DOI: 10.1128/IAI.01175-06

[21] Garcia HH, Gonzalez AE, Gilman RH. Taenia solium cysticercosis and its impact in neurological disease. Clinical Microbiology Reviews. 2020;**33**(3):e00085-e00019. DOI: 10.1128/CMR.00085-19

[22] MSD Manuals. Taenia solium (Pork Tapeworm) Infection and Cysticercosis. Available from: https://www.msdmanuals.com/professional/infectious-diseases/cestodes-tapeworms/taenia-solium-pork-tapeworm-infection-and-cysticercosis [Accessed: 2024, January 19]

[23] Western College of Veterinary Medicine (WCVM). Taenia solium and Cysticercus cellulosae. Available from: https://wcvm.usask.ca/learnaboutparasites/parasites/taenia-solium-and-cysticercus-cellulosae.php [Accessed: 2024, January 19]

[24] Alroy KA, Gilman RH. 130 – Tapeworm infections. In: Ryan ET, Hill DR, Solomon T, Aronson NE, Endy TP, editors. Hunter's Tropical Medicine and Emerging Infectious Diseases. 10th ed. Congo: Elsevier; 2020. pp. 932-940. ISBN 9780323555128. DOI: 10.1016/B978-0-323-55512-8.00130-7

[25] Castillo G, Fustamante L, Delgado-Kamiche AD, Camen-Orozco RP, Clark T, Bernal E, et al. Understanding the pathogenic mechanisms and therapeutic effects in neurocysticercosis. Brain Pathology. 2024;**3**:e13237. DOI: 10.1111/bpa.13237 [Epub ahead of print]

[26] CFSPH – Center for Food Security and Public Health, Iowa State University. Taenia. Center for Food Security and Public Health, Iowa State University. Available from: https://www.cfsph.iastate.edu/Factsheets/pdfs/taenia.pdf [Accessed: January 19, 2024]

[27] Carpio A. Neurocysticercosis: An update. The Lancet Infectious Diseases. 2002;**2**(12):751-762

[28] Carmen-Orozco RP, Dávila-Villacorta DG, Cauna Y, Bernal-Teran EG, Bitterfeld L, Sutherland GL, et al. Blood–brain barrier disruption and angiogenesis in a rat model for neurocysticercosis. Journal of Neuroscience Research. 2019;**97**(2):137-148

[29] Kumar A, Singh S, Singh VK, Chaurasia RN. Epidemiology and management of neurocysticercosis: An update. In: Viral, Parasitic, Bacterial, and Fungal Infections. Rwanda: Academic Press; 2023. pp. 375-381

[30] Restrepo BI, Alvarez JI, Castaño JA, Arias LF, Restrepo M, Trujillo J, et al. Brain granulomas in neurocysticercosis patients are associated with a Th1 and Th2 profile. Infection and Immunity. 2001;**69**(7):4554-4560

[31] Nash TE, Garcia HH. Diagnosis and treatment of neurocysticercosis. Nature Reviews Neurology. 2011;**7**(10):584-594

[32] García HH, Evans CA, Nash TE, Takayanagui OM, White AC Jr, Botero D, et al. Current consensus guidelines for treatment of neurocysticercosis. Clinical Microbiology Reviews. 2002;**15**(4):747-756

[33] Jewell PD, Abraham A, Schmidt V, Buell KG, Bustos JA, Garcia HH, et al. Neurocysticercosis and HIV/AIDS co-infection: A scoping review. Tropical Medicine & International Health. 2021;**26**(10):1140-1152

[34] García HH, Del Brutto OH. Imaging findings in neurocysticercosis. Acta Tropica. 2003;**87**(1):71-78. DOI: 10.1016/s0001-706x(03)00057-3

[35] Del Brutto OH, Rajshekhar V, White AC Jr, Tsang VC, Nash TE, Takayanagui OM, et al. Proposed diagnostic criteria for neurocysticercosis. Neurology. 2001;**57**(2):177-183. DOI: 10.1212/wnl.57.2.177

[36] Garcia HH, Del Brutto OH, Nash TE, White AC Jr, Tsang VCW, Gilman RH. New concepts in the diagnosis and management of neurocysticercosis (Taenia solium). American Journal of Tropical Medicine and Hygiene. 2005;**72**(1):3-9

[37] George U, Bansal G, Rathore S. MR spectroscopy aids diagnosis in subarachnoid space cysticercosis. Neurology India. 2010;**58**(6):957, 10.4103/0028-3886.73763-958

[38] Del Brutto OH, Wadia NH, Dumas M, Cruz M, Tsang VC, Schantz PM. Proposal of diagnostic criteria for human cysticercosis and neurocysticercosis. Journal of the Neurological Sciences. 1996;**142**(1-2):1-6

[39] Del Brutto OH, Rajshekhar V, White AC Jr, Tsang VC, Nash TE, Takayanagui OM, et al. Proposed diagnostic criteria for neurocysticercosis. Neurology. 2001;**57**(2):177-183

[40] Del Brutto O, Nash T, White A, Rajshekhar V, Wilkins P, Singh G, et al. Revised diagnostic criteria for neurocysticercosis. Journal of the Neurological Sciences. 2017;**372**:202-210. DOI: 10.1016/j.jns.2016.11.045

[41] Scheel CM, Khan A, Hancock K, Garcia HH, Gonzalez AE, Gilman RH, et al. Serodiagnosis of neurocysticercosis using synthetic 8-kD proteins:

Comparison of assay formats. The American Journal of Tropical Medicine and Hygiene. 2005;**73**(4):771-776

[42] Handali S, Klarman M, Gaspard AN, Noh J, Lee YM, Rodriguez S, et al. Multiantigen print immunoassay for comparison of diagnostic antigens for Taenia solium cysticercosis and taeniasis. Clinical and Vaccine Immunology: CVI. 2010;**17**(1):68-72. DOI: 10.1128/CVI.00339-09

[43] Rodriguez S, Dorny P, Tsang VC, Pretell EJ, Brandt J, Lescano AG, et al. Detection of Taenia solium antigens and anti-T. Solium antibodies in paired serum and cerebrospinal fluid samples from patients with intraparenchymal or extraparenchymal neurocysticercosis. The Journal of Infectious Diseases. 2009;**199**(9):1345-1352. DOI: 10.1086/597757

[44] Bobes RJ, Hernández M, Márquez C, Fragoso G, García E, Parkhouse RM, et al. Subarachnoidal and intraventricular human neurocysticercosis: Application of an antigen detection assay for the diagnosis and follow-up. Tropical Medicine & International Health. 2006;**11**(6):943-950. DOI: 10.1111/j.1365-3156.2006.01642.x

[45] Rodriguez S, Wilkins P, Dorny P. Immunological and molecular diagnosis of cysticercosis. Pathogens and Global Health. 2012;**106**(5):286-298. DOI: 10.1179/2047773212Y.0000000048

[46] Schantz PM, Tsang VC, Maddison SE. Serodiagnosis of neurocysticercosis. Reviews of Infectious Diseases. 1988;**10**(6):1231-1233

[47] Tsang VCW, Brand JA, Boyer AE. An enzyme-linked immunoelectrotransfer blot assay and glycoprotein antigens for diagnosing human cysticercosis (Taenia solium). Journal of Infectious Diseases. 1989;**159**(1):50-59

[48] Hancock K, Pattabhi S, Greene RM, Yushak ML, Williams F, Khan A, et al. Characterization and cloning of GP50, a Taenia solium antigen diagnostic for cysticercosis. Molecular and Biochemical Parasitology. 2004;**133**(1):115-124. DOI: 10.1016/j.molbiopara.2003.10.001. Erratum in: Mol Biochem Parasitol. 2004;134(2):285

[49] Hernández-González A, Noh J, Perteguer MJ, Gárate T, Handali S. Comparison of T24H-his, GST-T24H and GST-Ts8B2 recombinant antigens in western blot, ELISA and multiplex bead-based assay for diagnosis of neurocysticercosis. Parasites & Vectors. 2017;**10**(1):237. DOI: 10.1186/s13071-017-2160-2

[50] Hancock K, Khan A, Williams FB, Yushak ML, Pattabhi S, Noh J, et al. Characterization of the 8-kilodalton antigens of Taenia solium metacestodes and evaluation of their use in an enzyme-linked immunosorbent assay for serodiagnosis. Journal of Clinical Microbiology. 2003;**41**(6):2577-2586. DOI: 10.1128/JCM.41.6.2577-2586.2003

[51] Bueno EC, Vaz AJ, Machado LD, Livramento JA. Neurocysticercosis: Detection of IgG, IgA and IgE antibodies in cerebrospinal fluid, serum and saliva samples by ELISA with Taenia solium and Taenia crassiceps antigens. Arquivos de Neuro-Psiquiatria. 2000;**58**(1):18-24. DOI: 10.1590/s0004-282x2000000100003

[52] Harrison LJ, Joshua GW, Wright SH, Parkhouse RM. Specific detection of circulating surface/secreted glycoproteins of viable cysticerci in Taenia saginata cysticercosis. Parasite Immunology. 1989;**11**(4):351-370. DOI: 10.1111/j.1365-3024.1989.tb00673.x

[53] Brandt JR, Geerts S, De Deken R, Kumar V, Ceulemans F, Brijs L, et al.

A monoclonal antibody-based ELISA for the detection of circulating excretory-secretory antigens in Taenia saginata cysticercosis. International Journal for Parasitology. 1992;**22**(4):471-477. DOI: 10.1016/0020-7519(92)90148-e

[54] Castillo Y, Rodriguez S, García HH, Brandt J, Van Hul A, Silva M, et al. Urine antigen detection for the diagnosis of human neurocysticercosis. The American Journal of Tropical Medicine and Hygiene. 2009;**80**(3):379-383

[55] Fleury A, Gomez T, Alvarez I, Meza D, Huerta M, Chavarria A, et al. High prevalence of calcified silent neurocysticercosis in a rural village of Mexico. Neuroepidemiology. 2003;**22**(2):139-145. DOI: 10.1159/000068748

[56] Siddiqua T, Habeeb A. Neurocysticercosis. Saudi Journal of Kidney Diseases and Transplantation. 2020;**31**(1):254. DOI: 10.4103/1319-2442.279948

[57] International Journal of Medical Science and Clinical Research Studies issn(print): 2767-8326, issn(online): 2767-8342 [Internet]. 2024. Available from: https://ijmscr.org/index.php/ijmscrs/article/view/1336/1122

[58] White AC, Coyle CM, Rajshekhar V, Singh G, Hauser WA, Mohanty A, et al. Diagnosis and treatment of neurocysticercosis: 2017 clinical practice guidelines by the Infectious Diseases Society of America (IDSA) and the American Society of Tropical Medicine and Hygiene (ASTMH). Clinical Infectious Diseases. 2018;**66**(8):10-11. DOI: 10.1093/cid/cix1084

[59] Hamamoto Filho PT, Rodríguez-Rivas R, Fleury A. Neurocysticercosis: A review into treatment options, indications, and their efficacy. Research and Reports in Tropical Medicine. 2022;**13**:67-79. DOI: 10.2147/rrtm.s375650

[60] Fleury A, Jung H, Cardenas G, Sciutto E. Medical treatment for neurocysticercosis: Drugs, indications and perspectives. Current Topics in Medicinal Chemistry. 2008;**8**(5):424-433. DOI: 10.2174/156802608783790811

[61] Hamamoto Filho PT, Fragoso G, Sciutto E, Fleury A. Inflammation in neurocysticercosis: Clinical relevance and impact on treatment decisions. Expert Review of Anti-Infective Therapy. 2021;**19**(12):1503-1518. DOI: 10.1080/14787210.2021.1912592

[62] Rajshekhar V. Surgical management of neurocysticercosis. International Journal of Surgery. 2010;**8**(2):100-104. DOI: 10.1016/j.ijsu.2009.12.006

[63] Coyle CM. Neurocysticercosis: An update. Current Infectious Disease Reports. 2014;**16**(11):21. DOI: 10.1007/s11908-014-0437-6

[64] Torres-Corzo JG, Tapia-Pérez JH, Vecchia RR-D, Chalita-Williams JC, Sánchez-Aguilar M, Sánchez-Rodríguez JJ. Endoscopic management of hydrocephalus due to neurocysticercosis. Clinical Neurology and Neurosurgery. 2010;**112**(1):11-16. DOI: 10.1016/j.clineuro.2009.08.022

[65] Suri A, Goel RK, Ahmad FU, Vellimana AK, Sharma BS, Mahapatra AK. Transventricular, transaqueductal scope-in-scope endoscopic excision of fourth ventricular neurocysticercosis: A series of 13 cases and a review. Journal of Neurosurgery: Pediatrics. 2008;**1**(1):35-39. DOI: 10.3171/ped-08/01/035

[66] Peralta I, Ramírez MDJE, Baldoncini M, Vicente D, Willingham AL,

Nurmukhametov R, et al. Surgical nuances of giant neurocysticercosis according to intracranial location in the southwest region of the Dominican Republic, presentation of cases, and literature review. Surgical Neurology International. 2023;**14**:242. Available from: https://surgicalneurologyint.com/wp-content/uploads/2023/07/12431/SNI-14-242.pdf

[67] Fogang Y, Sawadogo A, Camara M, Toffa D, Sow A, Mansour NDIAYEM, et al. Managing neurocysticercosis: Challenges and solutions. International Journal of General Medicine. 2015;**2**:333. DOI: 10.2147%2FIJGM.S73249

[68] Wald LL, McDaniel PC, Witzel T, Stockmann JP, Cooley CZ. Low-cost and portable MRI. Journal of Magnetic Resonance Imaging: JMRI. 2020;**52**(3):686-696. DOI: 10.1002/jmri.26942

[69] Ahmad R, Khan T, Ahmad B, Misra A, Balapure AK. Neurocysticercosis: A review on status in India, management, and current therapeutic interventions. Parasitology Research. 2016;**116**(1):21-33. DOI: 10.1007/s00436-016-5278-9

[70] Yan HB, Lou ZZ, Li L, Brindley PJ, Zheng Y, Luo X, et al. Genome-wide analysis of regulatory proteases sequences identified through bioinformatics data mining in Taenia solium. BMC Genomics. 2014;**15**(1):428

[71] Li AH, Moon SU, Park YK, Na B-K, Hwang MG, Oh CM, et al. Identification and characterization of a cathepsin L-like cysteine protease from Taenia solium metacestode. Veterinary Parasitology. 2006;**141**(3-4):251-259

[72] Hossain MS, Shabir S, Toye P, Thomas LF, Falcone FH. Insights into the diagnosis, vaccines, and control of Taenia solium, a zoonotic, neglected parasite. Parasites & Vectors. 2023;**16**(1):380. DOI: 10.1186/s13071-023-05989-6

[73] WHO. First ever licensed vaccine and anthelmintic against the major cause of epilepsy in the developing world (who.int) [Internet]. [Updated: 22 May 2017; Cited: January 15, 2024]. Available from: https://www.who.int/news/item/22-05-2017-first-ever-licensed-vaccine-and-anthelmintic-against-the-major-cause-of-epilepsy-in-the-developing-world

[74] Flisser A, Gauci CG, Zoli A, Martinez-Ocaña J, Garza-Rodriguez A, Dominguez-Alpizar JL, et al. Induction of protection against porcine cysticercosis by vaccination with recombinant oncosphere antigens. Infection and Immunity. 2004;**72**(9):5292-5297. DOI: 10.1128/IAI.72.9.5292-5297.2004

[75] Assana E, Kyngdon CT, Gauci CG, Geerts S, Dorny P, De Deken R, et al. Elimination of Taenia solium transmission to pigs in a field trial of the TSOL18 vaccine in Cameroon. International Journal for Parasitology. 2010;**40**(5):515-519. DOI: 10.1016/j.ijpara.2010.01.006

[76] Poudel I, Sah K, Subedi S, Kumar Singh D, Kushwaha P, Colston A, et al. Implementation of a practical and effective pilot intervention against transmission of Taenia solium by pigs in the Banke district of Nepal. PLoS Neglected Tropical Diseases. 2019;**13**(2):e0006838. DOI: 10.1371/journal.pntd.0006838

[77] Kabululu ML, Ngowi HA, Mlangwa JED, Mkupasi EM, Braae UC, Colston A, et al. TSOL18 vaccine and oxfendazole for control of Taenia solium cysticercosis in pigs: A field trial in endemic areas of Tanzania. PLoS Neglected Tropical Diseases. 2020;**14**(10):e0008785. DOI: 10.1371/journal.pntd.0008785

[78] Nsadha Z, Rutebarika C, Ayebazibwe C, Aloys B, Mwanja M, Poole EJ, et al. Control trial of porcine cysticercosis in Uganda using a combination of the TSOL18 vaccination and oxfendazole. Infectious Diseases of Poverty. 2021;**10**(1):34. DOI: 10.1186/s40249-021-00823-6

[79] Huerta M, de Aluja AS, Fragoso G, Toledo A, Villalobos N, Hernández M, et al. Synthetic peptide vaccine against Taenia solium pig cysticercosis: Successful vaccination in a controlled field trial in rural Mexico. Vaccine. 2001;**20**(1-2):262-266. DOI: 10.1016/s0264-410x(01)00249-3

[80] Sciutto E, Morales J, Martínez JJ, Toledo A, Villalobos MN, Cruz-Revilla C, et al. Further evaluation of the synthetic peptide vaccine S3Pvac against Taenia solium cysticercosis in pigs in an endemic town of Mexico. Parasitology. 2007;**134**(Pt 1):129-133. DOI: 10.1017/S0031182006001132. Epub 2006 Sep 4

[81] de Aluja AS, Villalobos NM, Nava G, Toledo A, Martínez JJ, Plancarte A, et al. Therapeutic capacity of the synthetic peptide-based vaccine against Taenia solium cysticercosis in pigs. Vaccine. 2005;**23**(31):4062-4069. DOI: 10.1016/j.vaccine.2004.11.076. Epub 2005 Jan 26

[82] Morales J, Martínez JJ, Manoutcharian K, Hernández M, Fleury A, Gevorkian G, et al. Inexpensive anti-cysticercosis vaccine: S3Pvac expressed in heat inactivated M13 filamentous phage proves effective against naturally acquired Taenia solium porcine cysticercosis. Vaccine. 2008;**26**(23):2899-2905. DOI: 10.1016/j.vaccine.2008.03.042. Epub 2008 Apr 10

[83] Guo A, Jin Z, Zheng Y, Hai G, Yuan G, Li H, et al. Induction of protection against porcine cysticercosis in growing pigs by DNA vaccination. Vaccine. 2007;**25**(1):170-175. DOI: 10.1016/j.vaccine.2006.03.073. Epub 2006 Apr 18

[84] Parkhouse RM, Bonay P, González LM, Ferrer E, Gárate T, Aguilar CM, et al. TSOL18/HP6-TSOL, an immunogenic Taenia solium oncospheral adhesion protein and potential protective antigen. Parasitology Research. 2008;**102**(5):921-926. DOI: 10.1007/s00436-007-0853-8. Epub 2008 Jan 24

[85] Monreal-Escalante E, Govea-Alonso DO, Hernández M, Cervantes J, Salazar-González JA, Romero-Maldonado A, et al. Towards the development of an oral vaccine against porcine cysticercosis: Expression of the protective HP6/TSOL18 antigen in transgenic carrots cells. Planta. 2016;**243**(3):675-685. DOI: 10.1007/s00425-015-2431-0. Epub 2015 Nov 27

[86] Gonzalez-Alcaide G, Sosa N, Shevy L, Belinchon-Romero I, Ramos-Rincon J-M. Global research on cysticercosis and neurocysticercosis: A bibliometric analysis. Frontiers in Veterinary Science. 2023;**10**:1156834. DOI: 10.3389/fvets.2023.1156834

[87] Graham ID, Kothari A, McCutcheon C. Integrated knowledge translation research network project leads. Moving knowledge into action for more effective practice, programmes and policy: Protocol for a research programme on integrated knowledge translation. Implementation Science. 2018;**13**:22. DOI: 10.1186/s13012-017-0700-y

Chapter 9

Zoonotic Risk of *Cryptosporidium spp*. Prevention with One Health Approach in Indonesia

Wiwien S. Utami

Abstract

An important part of the One Health approach to preventing *Cryptosporidium spp*. infection is to better understand the environmental, epidemiologic, and aetiologic factors associated with *Cryptosporidium* infection to formulate better risk management. The future One Health strategy aims to integrate multidisciplinary knowledge and coordinate actions to create global synergies that benefit all aspects of human, animal, and environmental health (the One Health Triad). This multidisciplinary approach recognizes the complexity of the ecosystems in which humans and animals coexist. To prevent disease transmission to humans, it is necessary to control and eliminate disease in animals. This is not only to protect human health but also to protect animal health and welfare, maintain food security, and reduce poverty.

Keywords: *Cryptosporidium* spp., One Health approach, zoonotic, parasite, Indonesia

1. Introduction

Cryptosporidiosis is an infection of the small intestine caused by intracellular unicellular organisms, *Cryptosporidium spp.*, infecting microvillous epithelial cells in the gastrointestinal and respiratory tract of vertebrate animals [1]. Cryptosporidiosis, one of the neglected zoonotic diseases, is a disease whose transmission depends on interactions between humans and domestic animals or surrounding wildlife reservoirs [2]. Oocysts, the infective stage of *Cryptosporidium*, are environmentally resistant, especially *Cryptosporidium parvum*, which is widely distributed and can be transmitted to humans through direct contact with animals *via* oocyst contamination of water and food. Transmission between animals and humans does not occur to the same extent either in the wild or in some more favorable environments, such as intensive and confined animal farms, where animals are more isolated from humans or have been conditioned [3]. Although they do not spread rapidly at a global scale and are limited by ecological boundaries, the disease can be fatal if not treated early or properly. These diseases tend to be missed by doctors and other health-care providers and are not regularly screened, resulting in underdiagnosis and underreporting [4]. The underreporting makes it difficult to estimate the true burden of the disease, so published studies tend to be conservative or cited broadly [5]. Consequently, there is a lack of accountability for these zoonotic diseases at provincial, national, and even regional levels and a lack of priority for control in human and animal health [6]. Eventually, these diseases may impact animal health and productivity and may cause animal deaths. Thus, there are double burdens on human and animal health in dealing with these issues [7].

An important part of the One Health concept for the prevention of *Cryptosporidium* infection is a better understanding of the environmental, epidemiological, and etiological factors associated with *Cryptosporidium* infection to formulate better risk management [8]. The future One Health strategy aims to integrate multidisciplinary knowledge, and coordinate interventions, to create global synergies that serve all aspects of health care for humans, animals, and the environment (One Health Triad) [9]. This multidisciplinary approach takes into account the complexity of ecosystems where humans and animals coexist. To prevent disease transmission in humans, it is necessary to control and eliminate disease in animals. This is not only to protect public health but also to protect the health and improve animal welfare, maintain food security, and reduce poverty.

2. *Cryptosporidium* spp.

Cryptosporidiosis is a small intestinal infection caused by intracellular protozoa, *Cryptosporidium* spp., which infect microvillous epithelial cells of vertebrate gastrointestinal and respiratory tracts. It causes chronic diarrhea in children, adults, AIDS patients, and other immunocompromised individuals. The oocysts, the infective stage of *Cryptosporidium*, are known to be environmentally resistant and widely distributed. They can be transmitted to humans through direct contact with animals by contamination of water and food with oocysts and can cause outbreaks in various locations [10]. Common symptoms of cryptosporidiosis are sometimes underdiagnosed, leading to suboptimal treatment and prevention efforts [11]. Cryptosporidiosis is self-limiting, localized to the intestinal tract, and relatively resistant to reinfection in immunocompetent individuals. In patients with impaired cellular immune response (e.g., AIDS, malnourishment, and CD40-CD154 system deficiency), *Cryptosporidium* spp. often leads to persistent or chronic diarrhea, and it is not uncommon for the infection to reach the bile ducts, which is potentially life-threatening and is known to contribute to poorly absorbed antivirals and treatment failure in HIV [12].

Understanding the epidemiology of human and environmental cryptosporidiosis is critical to preventing and controlling the disease. There are also several factors that promote the transmission of *Cryptosporidium* infections, such as rapid modernization, exponential population growth, increased population movement, and higher rates of HIV/AIDS [13]. Cryptosporidiosis epidemics are linked to lack of clean water, poor sanitation, overcrowded housing, many animals in the environment at risk of water contaminated by infected human or animal fecal matter, proximity to rivers or farms, flooded housing, season, nutrition, drinking water from lakes or swimming pools, poor diapering, unsanitary practices in nurseries, exposure to sick people in hospitals, and exposure to infected animals in zoos, farms, or veterinary hospitals. The increase in the means of transportation, both within and between countries, and the development of tourism in developing countries have also increased the potential for the spread of several infectious diseases, including cryptosporidiosis [10].

In recent years, more research has focused on the high prevalence of *Cryptosporidium* infections in farms and the role of these animals in the risk of zoonotic transmission of the parasite either directly or indirectly through water or food, such as contaminated vegetables and fruits through aboveground fertilization or irrigation with contaminated water [14]. *Cryptosporidium* oocysts in livestock products such as milk, eggs, and meat have also been found in several cases. Livestock appears to be a source of transmission in outbreaks occurring in several countries. On the other hand, livestock living close to rivers may also be a potential source of transmission to the surrounding water. Animals suspected of harboring these pathogens are sometimes asymptomatic, even appearing healthy, without signs of illness or other symptoms indicating the presence of the pathogen. Transmission occurs through people touching, handling, feeding, or being around these animals or through contact with animals during birthing and cage cleaning or through contamination of clothing, shoes, cage floors, or other hygienic items [15].

The current methods of examination for the detection of these parasites in feces are still based on light microscopy or immunoassays, which have a low level of sensitivity and specificity. Molecular techniques, especially PCR-based genotyping techniques, aim to determine the coding genes and gene structure of *Cryptosporidium* isolates [16]. Molecular characterization provides useful information not only in the differentiation of genotypes/subgenotypes between isolates of different species strains but also in the knowledge of the coevolution and adaptation mechanisms of the host-parasite and the spread of the infection in the host population [17]. Similar to human and veterinary samples, water and environmental samples should also be tested for oocyst contamination using molecular techniques [18].

3. Zoonotic transmission of *Cryptosporidium* spp.

There have been many reports of outbreaks or cases of cryptosporidiosis in various countries. Children with a history of contact with cattle or goats are particularly susceptible. Recent genotyping studies have showed that only *C. parvum* is capable of zoonotic transmission but was found in several host species (humans, cattle, pigs, and goats) [19]. The high incidence of *C. parvum* in cattle and goats and the presence of large numbers of oocysts, especially in young animals, make these species very important sources of infection for environmental contamination with *Cryptosporidium* oocysts, which can spread to humans [20].

The genotyping and subtyping of parasites can be an effective added value for the surveillance and epidemiology of infectious diseases. Using the 18S rRNA gene is widely recommended as a target for screening *Cryptosporidium* from fecal and environmental samples due to the high copy number of sequences in the genome, thus increasing detection sensitivity [21]. Therefore, more comprehensive molecular epidemiological studies of genetic diversity, mode of transmission, and zoonotic potential should be performed in different host types (human, animal, and environment) [22]. Molecular screening techniques, such as polymerase chain reaction (PCR), are an important part of the One Health approach as they can facilitate the understanding of zoonotic transmission routes by identifying parasite species with a much higher degree of specificity than traditional microscopy [23]. Proper management of sources of infection, including animals, their housing, water sources, and the surrounding environment, can reduce the risk of zoonotic transmission [8].

The World Health Organization (WHO) states that except for emerging zoonoses such as SARS ,HPAI, and H5N1, most other zoonoses are not prioritized by national and international health systems. They are therefore referred to as Neglected Zoonotic Diseases (NZD) [24]. The morbidity and mortality associated with these neglected zoonotic diseases are difficult to assess in their entirety. Many of the neglected zoonoses are difficult to diagnose [25]. They are found in poor communities where surveillance and medical or veterinary care are inadequate. This leads to underreporting of the true prevalence of disease and does not receive the attention it deserves.

Research conducted in a community of cattle farmers in Sleman Regency Yogyakarta, Indonesia, demonstrated the transmission of *Cryptosporidium* spp. from animals to their owners through phylogenetic examination [26]. *Cryptosporidium* species were identified through PCR examination using specific primers, namely, Cr18S-S1: 5′TAAACGGTAGGGTATTGGCCT-3′ (forward) and Cry18S-AS1 3′-CAGAC TTGCCCTCCAATTGATA-5′ (reverse) with a target of 240 bp [27]. The results of the DNA electrophoresis were then sequenced according to the Sanger method. A phylogenetic analysis of *Cryptosporidium* in the 18S small subunit (SSU) rRNA gene was carried out to determine the genetic diversity and relationship between the human samples and several animal samples with other isolates from the gene banks as shown in **Figure 1**.

Phylogenetic analysis of human isolates revealed 21 human, six bovine, and seven goat isolates clustered with *Cryptosporidium parvum* and *Cryptosporidium hominis*.

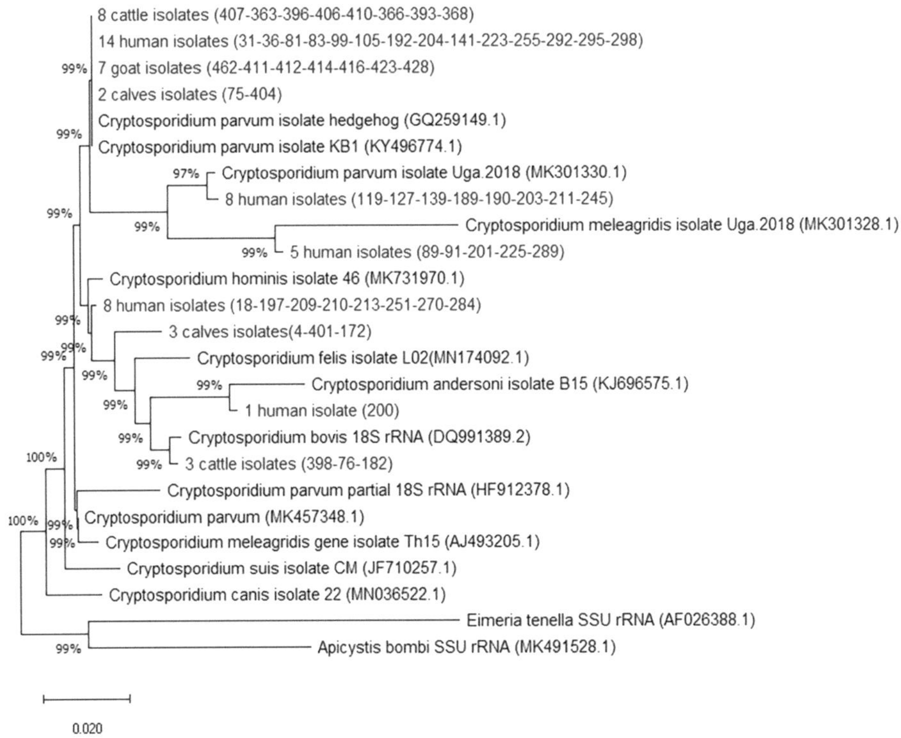

Figure 1.
Phylogenetic tree Cryptosporidium spp. from human and livestock isolates using the neighbor-joining method in the Mega X application, based on the 18S rRNA gene. Bootstrap analysis was performed with 1000 replications to assess the reliability of this phylogenetic tree.

In another branch, there were five human isolates and two bovine isolates that clustered with *Cryptosporidium meleagridis* but were still in the same clade as *Cryptosporidium parvum*. There were nine human isolates clustering with *Cryptosporidium hominis*, six bovine isolates clustering with *Cryptosporidium bovis*. On the other branch, two bovine and one human isolates clustered with *Cryptosporidium* andersoni. In this phylogenetic tree, species clustered very strongly, with high bootstrap values (99%).

Cluster groupings between human and animal species are shown in the phylogenetic tree above. This indicates that there is a relationship, or close relationship, between *Cryptosporidium* species in animals and that in humans. The relation may be due to ownership of the animals or due to environmental sources, such as cages owned by other people or water sources contaminated with feces from other infected animals. The transmission of infection from one animal to another is facilitated by the placement of cages in proximity in a group of animals. The results of this molecular analysis revealed zoonotic *Cryptosporidium* clusters of *Cryptosporidium* parvum, *Cryptosporidium* hominis, *Cryptosporidium* andersoni, *Cryptosporidium* bovis, and *Cryptosporidium* meleagridis species in the farming community in Mulati Sleman Regency, Yogyakarta. The clusters detected were from both animal and human samples, indicating close contact between animals and humans within the farm community. Thus, the presence of or some contact with animals (livestock) is essential for zoonotic disease transmission. Initiatives to control animal-associated zoonotic diseases are usually already in place at each farm site. However, a better understanding of the contact patterns of microorganism transmission from animals to humans is necessary for prevention and therefore deserves more attention.

In general, the results of this study indicate the possibility of transmission of *Cryptosporidium* infection from animals to humans (zoonosis) and/or from humans to humans (anthroponosis). Statistical analysis results indicate that livestock ownership plays a significant role in *Cryptosporidium* infection, especially when there is a history of diarrhea. *Cryptosporidium parvum*, *Cryptosporidium hominis*, *Cryptosporidium andersoni*, *Cryptosporidium bovis,* and *Cryptosporidium meleagridis* have been identified as zoonotic organisms in humans and animals. All cases of *Cryptosporidium* infection found in this study were asymptomatic in humans as they occurred in immunocompetent individuals; these results should raise our awareness of similar infections in immunocompromised individuals. It has the potential to cause an outbreak that threatens public health if not handled and managed appropriately. The lack of routine screening for *Cryptosporidium* at the first level of health care and the lack of specific and sensitive diagnostic tools to detect this oocyst parasite mean that cases of *Cryptosporidium* infection are still rarely found in Indonesia [28].

Bases encoding the 18S rRNA gene can be used to construct phylogenetic trees showing an organism's ancestry and relatedness [29]. In most genomes, multiple copies of the 18S rRNA bases are arranged in tandem on a single chromosome, and many of these occur many times due to frequent gene conversions. Sequence homogeneity among these simultaneously produced 18S rRNA copies is required for accurate inference of phylogenetic relationships. Some genomes have divergent copies of 18S rRNA distributed along the chromosome. As previously described, the diversity of *Cryptosporidium* species is also distinguished based on 18S rRNA gene phylogenetics [30]. Rooney explained that genetic variation in this 18S rDNA gene results from the evolutionary process of birth and death, where new genes arise through duplication and self-evolution and acquire new functions, become nonfunctional, or are deleted [31]. Due to the high number of copy sequences in the genome of the 18S rRNA gene, more than one species can be found in an individual, so it can be referred to as a mixed infection. Similarly, Kurniawan et al. [32] found single (*C. hominis, C. felis*, and *C. meleagridis*), double (*C. hominis* and *C. meleagridis*), and triple (*C. hominis, C. meleagridis*, and *C. parvum*) infections [32]. However, this mixed infection may result from failure to concentrate the fecal sample prior to DNA extraction. Morphological differentiation is still difficult, and species differences in this host can be determined only by PCR and sequencing. In general, the information provided by the identification of genotypes and subgenotypes of *Cryptosporidium* species in humans and animals in different geographical areas is useful for understanding the transmission patterns of the parasite and the zoonotic potential of animals in the population. Further comprehensive epidemiologic studies are needed to determine whether zoonotic transmission is closely linked to this immunocompromised population, given the significant prevalence of potentially zoonotic *C. parvum*. This is in line with the study by Iqbal et al. [33], where a more in-depth analysis of the level of genetic diversity of *Cryptosporidium* is required to determine a more comprehensive molecular epidemiology in Malaysia [33].

Detection of zoonotic genotypes of *Cryptosporidium* spp. allows the prevention of potential risks and consequences of zoonoses in immunocompetent human populations. Therefore, further investigations are needed, considering different spatiotemporal factors, using molecular diagnostic tools, and simultaneously assessing *Cryptosporidium spp.* genotypes in other domestic animals, water sources, and environments such as soil contaminated with animal or human waste. There is an urgent need for better diagnostic tools to identify *Cryptosporidium* infections [34]. Several studies point to the importance of health-care workers in rural areas or in close contact with at-risk animals being trained to recognize zoonotic diseases they encounter as well. Many studies have shown that misdiagnosis of *Cryptosporidium* infection results from misinterpreting microscopic findings. These errors lead to a differential diagnosis beyond the actual infection and may eventually lead to failed disease control efforts [35].

In terms of exposure to infected animals, farm workers are at increased risk of infection because they are the first to be exposed to infected animals and are therefore at higher risk of acquiring several zoonotic infections. Farm workers are exposed to these microorganisms daily in every aspect of their work. Direct contact with animals and animal butchering have been identified as the highest risk factors for *Cryptosporidium* infection [36]. For people who have occupational contact with livestock, the risk of becoming infected with *Cryptosporidium* oocysts can occur in any activity related to livestock, from handling, bathing, feeding, cleaning manure, and providing water to slaughterhouses. For farm family members who do not have contact with livestock, infection can be acquired through contact at home. Nonanimal workers are much less exposed to zoonotic agents than animal workers [11]. However, in developing countries, where people are exposed to animal infections either at work or at home, it is often impossible to distinguish the route of microbial transmission.

From an environmental perspective, optimizing the management of water sources, reclaimed water, and water for tourism must also be considered in efforts to prevent waterborne Cryptosporidiosis. The protection of water sources and swimming pools is an important element of cryptosporidiosis control, as contamination of drinking water and swimming pools is the primary mode of infection [37]. Primary prevention in the management of infections can be achieved only through a good understanding of transmission routes, sources of contamination (human and animal), disease prevalence in a population, and host risk factors. Although most of the sources of *Cryptosporidium* infection in this study population were due to contact with livestock because of living in farm communities, there is still a need for efforts in public health education and intervention. Health-care providers and the public need to be aware of the multiple modes of transmission of *Cryptosporidium* to prevent sporadic *Cryptosporidium* infections in asymptomatic individuals [38]. The fact that zoonotic properties of *Cryptosporidium* have been detected in both human and animal samples suggests that zoonotic transmission may be an important piece of information at this study site. Considering the risk factors that influence the transmission of Cryptosporidiosis in the livestock population, it seems that the zoonotic potential of this parasite needs to be further studied in other communities to formulate better strategies for the prevention of this infectious disease.

In addition, there remains a need to improve the compatibility of reporting systems for neglected diseases in humans and livestock to understand the burden of disease in an area. The results of this research need to be disseminated to the livestock population, as well as knowledge on how to avoid the spread of *Cryptosporidium* infection to other livestock or the surrounding population.

4. One Health approach

One Health is an approach, not a new discipline, highlighted as "the collaborative efforts of multiple disciplines - working at local, national and global levels - to achieve optimal health for humans, animals and the environment" [39]. Another definition of One Health is the effective application of interdisciplinary expertise to improve human, animal, and environmental health in the management of zoonoses and zoonotic emergencies that are complex and include prevention, surveillance, and response to zoonoses [40]. The One Health Initiative was launched in November 2009 by the One Health Commission, a national nonprofit partnership of the National Institutes of Health (NIH), Centers for Disease Control and Prevention (CDC), Food and Drug Administration (FDA), Department of Agriculture (USDA), and other global health agencies, and the Institute for Laboratory Animal Research, to identify the linkages between human, animal, and ecosystem health and to quantify the potential value of a One Health approach at the national and global levels [41].

One Health Concept (one health, one medical science, and one world) has the goal of reducing the risk of high-impact diseases in the animal-human ecosystem [42]. It is an approach to addressing complex challenges at the interface of animal, human, and environmental health, such as emergency pandemic diseases, the global food crisis, and climate change, through integrated and expanded multi-sectoral and multi-professional collaboration to improve long-term health and well-being [43].

Hippocrates, a Greek physicist, said that air, water, and place play an important role in public health, illustrating that environmental factors can affect human health and leading him to write: "The concept of public health is highly dependent on environmental health" [44]. This concept emphasizes that human health, animal health, and environmental health are interconnected. This suggests a coordinated, collaborative, transdisciplinary, and cross-sectoral approach to address potential and existing risks from the interface between animals, humans, and ecosystems [45].

Although this is not a new concept, the approach is increasingly being used to address health issues such as infectious diseases in developing countries, food and environmental safety, and chronic diseases [46]. One Health requires systems thinking, the ability to build successful multidisciplinary teams, and the leadership skills to coordinate effectively with stakeholders from a range of disciplines and sectors [47].

We know that there are many threats to our health status, both globally and locally. Cryptosporidiosis is currently very widespread globally, with high prevalence in several countries [48]. The disease could pose serious problems for Indonesia as well if it cannot effectively address the threat. *Cryptosporidium* is highly contagious, and only a few oocysts are needed to transmit the disease to a healthy person. Another factor that contributes to the transmission and spread of *Cryptosporidium* is the limited number of treatments available. The only drug approved by the US Food and Drug Administration (FDA) is nitazoxanide. However, nitazoxanide is moderately effective only in malnourished children and immunocompetent people and fails to treat immunocompromised people such as those living with HIV.

One Health, as defined by Schwabe [43], is a global strategy to improve health and well-being by reducing and preventing disease risks arising from interactions between people, animals, and their environment. An essential part of the One Health approach to preventing *Cryptosporidium* infection is to understand the environmental, epidemiological, and human factors associated with Cryptosporidium infection to formulate better risk management. The objectives of the approach focus on the prevention of cryptosporidiosis, including improved detection, diagnosis, and treatment; the importance of understanding zoonotic transmission; risk management; and better environmental stewardship. Global livestock trade, climate change, pathogen ecology, and bioterrorism are all interlinked threats that need to be addressed professionally using a One Health (OH) approach, where multidisciplinary teams work across disciplines and sectors to respond [49]. This requires engaging people who share the vision of improving health in Indonesia.

One Health is the unity of multiple practices working together locally, nationally, and globally to achieve optimal human, animal, and environmental health. Humans, animals, and the environment combine to form the One Health Triad as seen at **Figure 2** [50]. The One Health strategy aims to integrate multidisciplinary knowledge and coordinate actions to create global synergies that benefit all aspects of human, animal, and environmental health. This multidisciplinary approach recognizes the complexity of the ecosystem in which humans and animals coexist. Efforts to control disease in animals will be easy in humans. The goal is not only to protect human health but also to protect animal health and welfare, maintain food security, and reduce poverty [51].

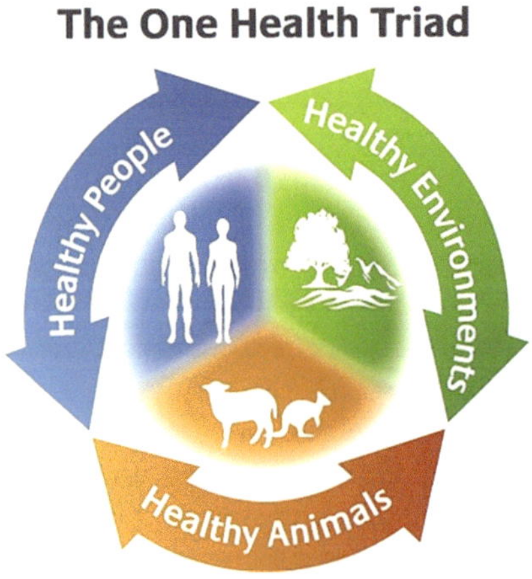

Figure 2.
The One Health Triad shows the interplay of health issues between wildlife, domestic animals, the environment, and human health that are interconnected [50].

5. One Health implementation in Indonesia

The interaction between livestock and humans is increasing due to the increase of basic human needs. In developing countries such as Indonesia, livestock play an important role in household welfare. Under certain conditions, livestock can serve to alleviate poverty [40]. Furthermore, interacting with animals also provides many benefits for children and adults, including reducing anxiety and lowering blood pressure [52]. Environmental degradation caused by land conversion, waste (domestic and industrial), and natural disasters are factors that increase vulnerability to disease. The world is facing an increasing threat of new infectious diseases, known as emerging infectious diseases (EIDs), 70% of which are zoonotic or transmitted from animals to humans and include bacteria, viruses, fungi, protozoa, and parasites [42]. In Southeast Asia, social and cultural practices combined with weak health infrastructure facilitate zoonoses to occur and spread. Southeast Asia has become a hotspot for the emergence of new infectious diseases (EIDs) due to significant changes in population growth and corresponding climatic conditions and abundant wildlife [53]. Due to the unpreparedness of the system to work synergistically, the outbreak of EIDs has caused multiple impacts and many casualties. World experts recommend One Health as a concept for addressing zoonotic threats [54].

One Health is a global strategy to expand interdisciplinary collaboration and communication in all aspects of health care for people, animals, and the environment. These strategies will advance 21st century health care by accelerating biomedical research discoveries, improving public health outcomes, rapidly expanding scientific knowledge, and improving medical education and clinical care. If properly implemented, this concept will help protect and save millions of lives in our present and future generations [55].

One Health has been implemented and applied in Indonesia. The implementation at the level of education in universities has been carried out in the form of training activities, workshops, seminars, and forms of cooperation that have been developed by several agencies from different sectors. There remains a need to improve and expand the understanding of the main concepts of One Health, the health pursued in the approach, and the actions broken down into several forms of intersectoral cooperation that can be applied, solved, and sustained for the welfare of human lives in relation to the national social governance system [40]. In Indonesia's One Health system, cross-sectoral roles still focus on health (physicians, veterinarians, public health, dentists, etc.). In the field, cross-sectoral roles should not stop at the concept, but should have directly implemented activities in a sustainable and integrated manner that are actively reported and published. In *Cryptosporidium* infection transmission, pathogenic *Cryptosporidium* oocysts affect animals and humans, where the parasite shares the same ecosystem for living and circulating. The efforts of one sector alone will not be enough to prevent or reduce the spread of *Cryptosporidium* infection. The concept of One Health or multi-sectoral approach in the management of *Cryptosporidium* infection, including the laboratory network, is expected to prevent or overcome the spread of *Cryptosporidium* infection [56].

The One Health approach in Indonesia has been advanced and is in the process of being prepared for the next stage of development. Seminars, trainings, and workshops in collaboration with health sectors, as well as incorporating One Health approach into health courses at each university, have been gradually implemented. There is a need to increase the understanding of One Health concept, starting from individual health, which focuses on health management in health sector, to One Health concept, which focuses on more complex individual health [57].

In order to develop an effective and integrated zoonosis prevention and control plan, the first step is the identification of potential zoonotic problems and knowledge gaps in specific areas and mapping of zoonotic diseases in Indonesia. For a more global understanding of knowledge gaps and research needs in zoonosis prevention and control, an expansion of surveillance methods is needed in Indonesia as part of an interdisciplinary and multi-sectoral strategic network on zoonoses [58].

Neglected zoonotic diseases (NZDs) are diseases that are a major cause of animal and human illness and death, especially among poor people living near animals, often in unsanitary conditions and with inadequate health services. The best way to combat these diseases is to manage the livestock reservoir because it is the most cost-effective. However, control and elimination of these diseases requires human intervention, increased public awareness to reduce human–animal contact, and/or modification of the environment to control the rate of spread of infection. To date, cryptosporidiosis has not been included in the 2019 WHO-OIE list of neglected zoonotic diseases, following anthrax, bovine tuberculosis (*Mycobacterium tuberculosis* complex), brucellosis, rabies, cysticercosis/taeniasis, echinococcosis, and trypanosomosis [24]. Similarly, in the list of strategic diseases in Indonesia, cryptosporidiosis is still not included as one of the potential epidemic diseases or strategic infectious animal diseases. So far, there have been many studies on cryptosporidiosis worldwide but not many in Indonesia [59]. It is time that more attention is paid to this disease in Indonesia, as it has a major impact when it breaks out.

Cryptosporidiosis, as one of the neglected zoonotic diseases, is a disease whose transmission is dependent on the interaction between humans and domestic animals or the wildlife reservoirs that surround them. Whether in the wild or in some more favorable environments, such as intensive and controlled animal production, where animals are more isolated from humans or are conditioned, transmission between animals and humans does not occur to the same degree. Although the disease does not spread rapidly on a global scale and is limited by ecological boundaries, it can be fatal without early or appropriate treatment. Neglected zoonotic diseases (NZDs) not only represent a significant burden to human health on a global scale but also place a significant financial burden on their owners in terms of livestock production. The One Health approach aims to reduce the economic losses caused by human-animal NZDs, in addition to controlling diseases caused by the interaction between people, animals, and their environment. There is a strong link between human health, livestock health, and household economic well-being in livestock-dependent communities. It is estimated that nearly a billion people depend on livestock for their livelihoods and nutrition [51]. However, the relationships between animal health and productivity and human health and well-being are complex, and a quantitative understanding of these relationships is important for poverty reduction and public health interventions through improved human and animal health.

Early warning systems for livestock diseases and prediction of their occurrence and spread to new areas are important requirements for the control of zoonoses, including cryptosporidiosis. This system is easier and more economical than dealing with the disease after it has spread. The prevention and control of zoonotic diseases is dependent on the early detection of the disease agents. The early detection of such agents plays an important role in the formulation of disease control policies, for prevention and mitigation. One of the pillars for early and rapid detection of these diseases is targeted surveillance of the environment and livestock at high risk of zoonotic infection. The presence of a well-equipped laboratory with qualified staff and the ability to detect zoonoses is very important in support of early disease

DOI: http://dx.doi.org/10.5772/intechopen.1004735

detection. Good communication with all stakeholders is essential to identify the needs for disease surveillance, epidemiology, and capacity building of the laboratory [60]. Detection and mapping of the distribution of the parasite can be accelerated by molecular characterization and visualization of different *Cryptosporidium* genotypes from all regions of Indonesia. Screening techniques can be developed by collaborating with several universities and the private sector in Indonesia. The strength of Indonesian laboratories in disease control and prevention will be demonstrated through bioinformatics reporting of *Cryptosporidium* infections.

In line with the One Health approach, synchronized surveillance with laboratory capacity building for detection and prevention of zoonoses will be implemented. This will include surveillance at the animal-human interface for early detection of *Cryptosporidium* infection. We can learn how zoonotic agents emerge and spread through the livestock-human interface by testing samples from infected livestock and comparing the results with similar surveillance of human and other livestock samples. This surveillance requires good community cooperation, especially farmer/livestock groups as main community, village or hamlet officials, local government, district or provincial health, and livestock services in coordination with the General Livestock and Health Agencies. The report will be used to prevent and control zoonotic cryptosporidiosis at national, provincial, and district/city levels.

6. Conclusions

A better understanding of the environmental, epidemiological, and etiological factors associated with Cryptosporidium infections is a future One Health strategy aimed at improving health outcomes for humans, animals, and the environment. This multidisciplinary approach considers the complexity of ecosystems where humans and animals live together to prevent and control disease transmission to humans. This is not only to protect human health but also to protect animal health and welfare, maintain food security, and reduce poverty.

Acknowledgements

The author is grateful to the supervisors and professors who have provided guidance in the completion of this doctoral study.

Conflict of interest

The authors declare no conflict of interest.

Author details

Wiwien S. Utami
Faculty of Medicine, Jember University, Jember, Indonesia

*Address all correspondence to: wiwien.dr@unej.ac.id

References

[1] CDC, "Parasites - Cryptosporidium (also known as 'Crypto') | Cryptosporidium | Parasites | CDC," Centers for Disease Control and Prevention, 2019. Available from: https://www.cdc.gov/parasites/crypto/ [Accessed: March 16, 2024]

[2] Enbom T, Suominen K, Laitinen S, Ollgren J, Autio T, Rimhanen-Finne R. Cryptosporidium parvum: An emerging occupational zoonosis in Finland. Acta Veterinaria Scandinavica. 2023;**65**(1):1-9. DOI: 10.1186/s13028-023-00684-z

[3] Gongal G, Ofrin RH, de Balogh K, Oh Y, Kugita H, Dukpa K. Operationalization of one health and tripartite collaboration in the Asia-Pacific region. WHO South-East Asia Journal of Public Health. 2020;**9**(1):21-25. DOI: 10.4103/2224-3151.282991

[4] Bamaiyi PH, Redhuan NEM. Prevalence and risk factors for cryptosporidiosis: A global, emerging, neglected zoonosis. Asian Biomedicine. 2016;**10**(4):309-325. DOI: 10.5372/1905-7415.1004.493

[5] Alexander CL, Currie S, Pollock K, Smith-Palmer A, Jones BL. An audit of cryptosporidium and Giardia detection in Scottish National Health Service Diagnostic Microbiology Laboratories. Epidemiology and Infection. 2017;**145**(8):1584-1590. DOI: 10.1017/S0950268817000462

[6] Innes EA, Chalmers RM, Wells B, Pawlowic MC. A one health approach to tackle cryptosporidiosis. Trends in Parasitology. 2020;**36**(3):290-303. DOI: 10.1016/j.pt.2019.12.016

[7] Welburn SC, Beange I, Ducrotoy MJ, Okello AL. The neglected zoonoses-the case for integrated control and advocacy. Clinical Microbiology and Infection. 2015;**21**(5):433-443. DOI: 10.1016/j.cmi.2015.04.011

[8] Ryan U, Zahedi A, Paparini A. Cryptosporidium in humans and animals—A one health approach to prophylaxis. Parasite Immunology. 2016;**38**(9):535-547. DOI: 10.1111/pim.12350

[9] Khan A, Abbas RZ, Aguilar-Marcelino L, Saeed NM, Younas M. One Health Triad, Volume 1. Pakistan: Unique Scientific Publishers, Pakistan, 2023. [Online]. Available from: https://uniquescientificpublishers.com/one-health-triad-volume-1

[10] Chalmers RM. Cryptosporidium. In: Microbiology of Waterborne Diseases. 2nd ed. Swansea, UK: Elsevier; 2014. pp. 287-326. DOI: 10.1016/B978-0-12-415846-7.00016-0

[11] Johansen H et al. Symptomatic and asymptomatic secondary transmission of Cryptosporidium parvum following two related outbreaks in schoolchildren. Epidemiology and Infection. 2014;**143**(08):1-8. DOI: 10.1017/S095026881400243X

[12] Utami WS, Murhandarwati EH, Artama WT, Kusnanto H. Cryptosporidium infection increases the risk for chronic diarrhea among people living with HIV in Southeast Asia: A systematic review and meta-analysis. Asia Pacific Journal of Public Health. 2020;**1**(11)1-11. DOI: 10.1177/1010539519895422

[13] Caccio SM, Putignani L. Epidemiology of Human Cryptosporidiosis. In: Cacciò SM,

Widmer G, editors. Cryptosporidium: Parasite and Disease. Rome, Italy. Berlin Heidelberg: Springer-Verlag; 2014. pp. 1-564. DOI: 10.1007/978-3-7091-1562-6

[14] Pumipuntu N, Piratae S. Cryptosporidiosis: A zoonotic disease concern. Veterinary World. 2018;**11**:681-686. DOI: 10.14202/vetworld.2018.681-686

[15] Brankston G, Boughen C, Ng V, Fisman DN, Sargeant JM, Greer AL. Assessing the impact of environmental exposures and cryptosporidium infection in cattle on human incidence of cryptosporidiosis in Southwestern Ontario. PLoS One. 2018;**13**(4):1-12

[16] Yu JR, Lee SU, Park WY. Comparative sensitivity of PCR primer sets for detection of Cryptosporidium parvum. The Korean Journal of Parasitology. 2009;**47**(3):293-297. DOI: 10.3347/kjp.2009.47.3.293

[17] Plutzer J, Karanis P. Genetic polymorphism in cryptosporidium species: An update. Veterinary Parasitology. 2009;**165**(3-4):187-199. DOI: 10.1016/j.vetpar.2009.07.003

[18] Swaffer BA, Vial HM, King BJ, Daly R, Frizenschaf J, Monis PT. Investigating source water Cryptosporidium concentration, species and infectivity rates during rainfall-runoff in a multi-use catchment. Water Research. 2014;**67**:310-320. DOI: 10.1016/j.watres.2014.08.055

[19] Adamska M. Molecular characterization of Cryptosporidium and Giardia occurring in natural water bodies in Poland. Parasitology Research. 2014;**114**(2):687-692. DOI: 10.1007/s00436-014-4234-9

[20] Amer S, Zidan S, Feng Y, Adamu H, Li N, Xiao L. Identity and public health potential of Cryptosporidium spp. in water buffalo calves in Egypt. Veterinary Parasitology. 2013;**191**(1-2):123-127. DOI: 10.1016/j.vetpar.2012.08.015

[21] Weigum SE, Castellanos-Gonzalez A, White AC, Richards-Kortum R. Amplification-free detection of *Cryptosporidium parvum* nucleic acids with the use of DNA/RNA-directed gold nanoparticle assemblies. The Journal of Parasitology. 2013;**99**(5):923-926. DOI: 10.1645/12-132.1

[22] Nguyen TT et al. Prevalence and molecular characterization of Cryptosporidum spp. and Giardia spp. in environmental samples in Hanam province, Vietnam. Food and Waterborne Parasitology. 2016;**3**:13-20. DOI: 10.1016/j.fawpar.2016.03.003

[23] Chalmers RM, Campbell BM, Crouch N, Charlett A, Davies AP. Comparison of diagnostic sensitivity and specificity of seven Cryptosporidium assays used in the UK. Journal of Medical Microbiology. 2011;**60**(11):1598-1604. DOI: 10.1099/jmm.0.034181-0

[24] WHO. The Control of Neglected Zoonotic Diseases: Community-Based Interventions for Prevention and Control. Department of Control of Neglected Tropical Diseases. Geneva, Switzerland. [Online]. 2010. Available from: http://www.who.int/neglected_diseases/zoonoses/en/

[25] WHO. Research Priorities for Zoonoses and Marginalized Infections, no. 971. Geneva, Switzerland: WHO Press; 2012

[26] Utami WS, Kusnanto H, Artama WT, Murhandarwati EEH. Potential Analysis of Transmission of Cryptosporidium Infection as a Zoonosis with the One Health Concept in Sleman Yogyakarta. Universitas Gadjah Mada Yogyakarta,

Indonesia. [Online]. 2020. Available from: http://etd.repository.ugm.ac.id/

[27] Zebardast N, Yeganeh F, Gharavi MJ, Abadi A, Seyyed Tabaei SJ, Haghighi A. Simultaneous detection and differentiation of *Entamoeba histolytica*, *E. dispar*, *E. moshkovskii*, *Giardia lamblia* and *Cryptosporidium* spp. in human fecal samples using multiplex PCR and qPCR-MCA. Acta Tropica. 2016;**162**:233-238. DOI: 10.1016/j.actatropica.2016.07.004

[28] Magi B, Canocchi V, Tordini G, Cellesi C, Barberi A. Cryptosporidium infection: Diagnostic techniques. Parasitology Research. 2006;**98**(2):150-152. DOI: 10.1007/s00436-005-0050-6

[29] Mammeri M et al. Molecular characterization of Cryptosporidium isolates from diarrheal dairy calves in France. Veterinary Parasitology: Regional Studies and Reports. 2019;**18**(July):100323. DOI: 10.1016/j.vprsr.2019.100323

[30] Stenger BLS et al. Highly divergent 18S rRNA gene paralogs in a Cryptosporidium genotype from eastern chipmunks (*Tamias striatus*). Infection, Genetics and Evolution. 2015. Available from: https://www.ncbi.nlm.nih.gov/pmc/articles/PMC4417453/pdf/nihms671733.pdf;**32**(June):113-123 [Accessed: November 15, 2017]

[31] Rooney AP. Mechanisms underlying the evolution and maintenance of functionally heterogeneous 18S rRNA genes in apicomplexans. Molecular Biology and Evolution. 2004;**21**(9):1704-1711. DOI: 10.1093/molbev/msh178

[32] Kurniawan A et al. Cryptosporidium species from human immunodeficiency infected patients with chronic diarrhea in Jakarta, Indonesia. Annals of Epidemiology. 2013;**23**(11):720-723. DOI: 10.1016/j.annepidem.2013.07.019

[33] Iqbal A, Sim BLH, Dixon BR, Surin J, Lim YAL. Molecular epidemiology of cryptosporidium in HIV/AIDS patients in Malaysia. Tropical Biomedicine. 2015;**32**(2):310-322

[34] Checkley W et al. A review of the global burden, novel diagnostics , therapeutics, and vaccine targets for cryptosporidium. The Lancet Infectious Diseases. 2015;**15**:85-94. DOI: 10.1016/S1473-3099(14)70772-8

[35] Elsafi SH, Al-Sheban SS, Al-Jubran KM, Abu Hassan MM, Al Zahrani EM. Comparison of Kinyoun's acid-fast and immunofluorescent methods detected an unprecedented occurrence of Cryptosporidium in the Eastern Region of Saudi Arabia. The Journal of Taibah University Medical Sciences. 2014;**9**(4):263-267. DOI: 10.1016/j.jtumed.2014.03.008

[36] Klous G, Huss A, Heederik DJJ, Coutinho RA. Human-livestock contacts and their relationship to transmission of zoonotic pathogens, a systematic review of literature. One Health. 2016;**2**:65-76. DOI: 10.1016/j.onehlt.2016.03.001

[37] Plutzer J, Karanis P. Neglected waterborne parasitic protozoa and their detection in water. Water Research. 2016;**101**:318-328. DOI: 10.1016/j.watres.2016.05.085

[38] Das K, Nair LV, Ghosal A, Sardar SK, Dutta S, Ganguly S. Genetic characterization reveals evidence for an association between water contamination and zoonotic transmission of a cryptosporidium sp. from dairy cattle in West Bengal, India. Food and Waterborne Parasitology. 2019;**17**:e00064. DOI: 10.1016/j.fawpar.2019.e00064

[39] Destoumieux-Garzón D et al. The one health concept: 10 years old and a

long road ahead. Frontiers in Veterinary Science. 2018;**5**(FEB):1-13. DOI: 10.3389/fvets.2018.00014

[40] Negara KSP et al. One health strategy in prevention and control of parasitic zoonosis globally and Indonesia-from theory to practice: A mini-review. Bali Medical Journal. 2022;**11**(3):1537-1542. DOI: 10.15562/bmj.v11i3.3632

[41] Mackenzie JS, Jeggo M. The one health approach—Why is it so important? Tropical Medicine and Infectious Disease. 2019;**4**(88):2-4. DOI: 10.3390/tropicalmed4020088

[42] Kelly TR et al. One Health proof of concept: Bringing a transdisciplinary approach to surveillance for zoonotic viruses at the human-wild animal interface. Preventive Veterinary Medicine. 2017;**137**:112-118. DOI: 10.1016/j.prevetmed.2016.11.023

[43] Zinsstag J, Mackenzie JS, Jeggo M, Heymann DL, Patz JA, Daszak P. Mainstreaming one Health. EcoHealth. 2012;**9**:107-110. DOI: 10.1007/s10393-012-0772-8

[44] Wilcox B, Jessop H. Ecology and Environmental Health, in Environmental health: from global to local. In: Frumkin H, editor. Vol. 2. no. 3. San Fransisco: Wiley Blackwell; 2007. pp. 316-318. DOI: 10.1080/17441690601109175

[45] Vesterinen HM et al. Strengthening multi-sectoral collaboration on critical health issues: One Health Systems Mapping and Analysis Resource Toolkit (OH-SMART) for operationalizing one Health. PLoS One. 2019;**14**(7):1-16. DOI: 10.1371/journal.pone.0219197

[46] Capps B, Lederman Z. One Health and paradigms of public biobanking. Journal of Medical Ethics. 2015;**41**:258-262. DOI: 10.1136/medethics-2013-101828

[47] Mersha C, Tewodros F. One Health one medicine one world: Co-joint of animal and human medicine with perspectives, a review. Veterinary World. 2012;**5**(4):238-243. DOI: 10.5455/vetworld.2012.238-243

[48] Koutsoumanis K et al. Public health risks associated with food-borne parasites. EFSA Journal. 2018;**16**(12):1-114. DOI: 10.2903/j.efsa.2018.5495

[49] G7 Germany. The Need for a One Health Approach to Zoonotic Diseases and Antimicrobial Resistance. Germany; 2022. DOI: 10.26164/leopoldina_04_00533

[50] Essack SY. Environment: The neglected component of the one Health triad. The Lancet Planetary Health. 2018;**2**(6):e238-e239. DOI: 10.1016/S2542-5196(18)30124-4

[51] Thumbi SM et al. Linking human health and livestock health: A 'one-Health' platform for integrated analysis of human Health, livestock Health, and economic welfare in livestock dependent communities. PLoS One. 2015;**10**(3):1-19. DOI: 10.1371/journal.pone.0120761

[52] Hale CR et al. Estimates of enteric illness attributable to contact with animals and their environments in the United States. Clinical Infectious Diseases. 2012;**54**(Suppl):5. DOI: 10.1093/cid/cis051

[53] Lim YAL, Vythilingam I. Parasites and their vectors: A special focus on Southeast Asia. Vienna: Springer Vienna; 2013. DOI: 10.1007/978-3-7091-1553-4

[54] WHO. The control of neglected zoonotic diseases, from advocacy to action. WHO Conference Report. 2014

[55] Kelly TR et al. Implementing One Health approaches to confront emerging and re-emerging zoonotic disease threats: Lessons from PREDICT. One Health Outlook. 2020;**2**(1):1-7. DOI: 10.1186/s42522-019-0007-9

[56] Wang X et al. Using a one health approach to prioritize zoonotic diseases in China, 2019. PLoS One. 2021;**16**(11):1-13. DOI: 10.1371/journal.pone.0259706

[57] Mackenzie JS, Richt JA. One Health: The Human-Animal-Environment Interfaces in Emerging Infectious Diseases. Vol. 366. Berlin, Heidelberg: Springer Berlin Heidelberg; 2013. DOI: 10.1007/978-3-642-35846-3

[58] Artama WT. Prioritization and Mapping of Zoonotic Diseases in Indonesia. In: MSU International Conference on animal health in AEC. Aug 2016. pp. 2-3

[59] Savioli L, Smith H, Thompson A. Giardia and cryptosporidium join the 'neglected diseases initiative'. Trends in Parasitology. 2006;**22**(5):203-208. DOI: 10.1016/j.pt.2006.02.015

[60] Mazet JAK, Uhart MM, Keyyu JD. Stakeholders in one health. Revue Scientifique et Technique/ Office International des Épizooties. 2014;**33**(2):443-452. DOI: 10.20506/rst.33.2.2295

Chapter 10

Trophically Transmitted Parasites and Their Responses to Microbial Pathogens and Consumed Plastic Contaminants

Kate L. Sheehan, Sonja Barber, Ryan F. Hechinger, Brian S. Dorr and Douglas Causey

Abstract

Trophically transmitted parasites, which move from one host to the next through host feeding activities, are subject to direct and indirect stressors within their hosts and the surrounding ecosystem. Infection success can be disrupted by host defenses and environmental conditions that exceed the tolerances of the parasites or their hosts. These interruptions can be caused by various factors, including host-derived antagonists, alterations in the host's environment, exposure to toxic molecules, and disruption to the host's microbial communities. Here, we present novel findings on the responses of intestinal helminth infracommunities to stressors associated with shifts in the microbiome due to bacterial infection and under a range of conditions where microplastics were consumed.

Keywords: helminths, disease, microplastics, avian botulism, land use

1. Introduction

1.1 Helminths are ubiquitous and important

Parasitism is one of the most common ways that organisms acquire critical resources. While the exact numbers are not fully resolved, several studies [1, 2] suggest that for every type of vertebrate host (free-living organisms), one or more species of parasitic helminths occur, and this only counts parasites of three phyla. Despite its commonness, parasitism remains an underexplored trophic strategy that may shape direct and indirect interactions among free-living organisms and other symbionts. Moreover, parasites are not passive players in this dynamic; they respond to the behaviors of their hosts that introduce other symbionts and foreign substances to their sites of infection, particularly the gastrointestinal tract (GIT).

The ecological consequences of parasitism include impacts on biodiversity through modifications of community structure, genetic diversity, and trait frequency distributions [3]. Further, parasites can influence niche development and host specialization by altering the behaviors of intermediate hosts and modulating trophic interaction strengths between predators and prey [4]. Because trophically transmitted parasites exploit predator-prey interactions, these parasites can be useful ecological indicators [5, 6]. For instance, Kuris et al. [7] used parasites to infer that shortfin mako sharks and sperm whales are common predators of oarfish, a teleost that is rarely observed in the wild and has no previously documented predators. The utility of parasites in shedding light on host interactions is, thus, impactful at scales that range from cellular processes to predator-prey interactions within ecosystems and beyond. Alterations to parasite community composition and structure can have nuanced yet sweeping consequences on individuals, populations, communities, and ecosystems.

Losses in parasite diversity can have major implications on overall biodiversity, considering that around half of Earth's animals are parasitic [1]. Losses to parasite diversity result from intentional anthropogenic actions designed to eliminate human and veterinary diseases but also stem from losses in host diversity that occur from changing distributions, densities, and the carrying capacities of hosts' habitats [8, 9]. As parasite communities respond to host distributions, their infections can adapt to new surroundings, sometimes becoming more threatening and sometimes rendered benign [10].

Trophically transmitted parasites will only infect hosts that have consumed them, and thus, can be used to learn about shifting diets in their hosts. For example, altered frequencies of the echinostomatid *Drepanocephalus auritus* in Double-crested Cormorants indicate the extent to which the trematode's intermediate host (catfish) [11] are included or excluded from a bird's diet [6, 12]. In some cases, these altered feeding habits occur as hosts migrate through areas where the parasite is absent [13] because the intermediate host is locally rare due to invasions or extirpations [14] or because the feeding preferences of individual hosts lead to niche partitioning and differentiation of parasite infracommunities [15]. Similarly, when intermediate host populations are threatened by anthropogenic landscape alterations, parasite populations with complex life cycles can be reduced or eliminated [16].

1.2 Parasites live in ever-changing conditions

Although parasitism costs the host, the severity and type of those consequences occur along a spectrum. Deadly outbreaks can occur when endemic pathogens mutate, as occurred with the Zika virus in an avian outbreak from 2014 to 2016 [17]. The host-parasite relationship becomes lethal when a parasite's survival depends on the host's death. Likewise, when direct contact is not needed because vectors or other transport agents spread propagules, deadly diseases can persist unchecked [18]. However, many such relationships are not sustainable through evolutionary time. Highly virulent diseases often remove the genes of high susceptibility from host populations, leaving a larger proportion of tolerant or resistant individuals [19]. Consequently, virulence in some contagions is reduced as the host-parasite interaction evolves [18, 20]. Benign infections are widespread for typical parasites infecting definitive hosts, as symbiont fitness increases with host longevity.

In established relationships between hosts and parasites, the host can tolerate some parasite load without experiencing detrimental impact [21]. This is likely more of a reflection of the faculties of parasites that manipulate host immune function and evade detection and immune responses. However, when parasites use cellular commodities produced by the host, the immune system can be activated by danger-associated molecular patterns (DAMPs) that occur when host tissue is damaged [22]. The innate and adaptive immune systems can eliminate parasitic propagules, but many parasites are well-defended and highly evolved to escape host defenses [23, 24]. Additionally, host chronic immune responses can be energetically costly, disrupting tissues with systemic inflammation and inducing lethal health problems like tumorigenesis, fibrosis, and sepsis [25]. Because animal predators cannot eliminate all infectious agents within their prey, they are exposed repeatedly to trophically transmitted parasites while feeding. Because immune responses are not feasible solutions to parasite avoidance, definitive hosts often tolerate infections and isolate damaged tissues rather than defend against parasites [26]. This tolerance and stability can change when climatic, environmental, and biotic conditions shift. Anthropogenic changes are currently the greatest drivers of change affecting local and global environments.

With an estimated 45% of the Earth's habitable land used for agriculture, the widespread replacement of diverse communities with monocultures has important implications [27]. The expansion of agriculture pasture and turf at the expense of previously diverse communities profoundly impacts the forage base, feeding behavior, and the transfer of nutrients and energy in these systems. Agriculture as a primary land cover can prompt some avian species to adjust their migration patterns, impacting their regional abundances [28, 29]. In turn, ecosystem alteration, extensive retooling of landscapes for agriculture, and consequent changes in energy and nutrient transfer can alter parasite communities. Some of these changes could harm host organisms or agriculture [30]; however, the full extent of large-scale ecosystem change caused by agriculture on organisms and parasite communities remains unknown. One challenge for elucidating the impacts of landscape change on specific taxonomic groups, such as birds, arises from the diverse trophic positions occupied within the class Aves. Comparing bird species with varying dietary preferences, such as those consuming plants, freshwater invertebrates, marine invertebrates, freshwater fishes, marine fishes, and combinations across different ranges and seasons, presents analytical complexity. The dynamic nature of dietary needs and prey availability further complicates the assessment of avian feeding behaviors. An established approach to categorically assess these organisms involves evaluating their trophic position by analyzing stable isotope concentrations of elements like Carbon and Nitrogen.

Many elements can vary in their number of neutrons, affecting their atoms' isotopic weight. Lighter isotopes move more freely in biological processes and chemical reactions, while heavier isotopes accumulate in tissues during slow metabolic processes [31]. The fractionation of heavy and light isotopes in organisms' tissues correlates with the biology of the organism. For example, plants using the C_3 photosystem cycle tend to have a higher accumulation of the heavy carbon isotope (C^{13}) compared to those using the C_4 photosystem, making it possible to differentiate between basal photosynthetic groups and those from which higher organisms derive [32]. Similarly, $Nitrogen^{15}$, being heavier than N^{14}, tends to accumulate in higher trophic level organisms due to its slower metabolic processing, representing a form of bioaccumulation [31]. Thus, we can learn about the implications of ecosystem change to hosts and parasites with stable isotope concentrations. Human-made products can also disturb parasite communities. Anthropogenic waste management introduces pollutants and other contaminants into the environment, affecting food webs. Plastic debris is a recently emerged concern, posing physical and chemical threats to wildlife, agriculture, and human health [33].

1.3 Helminths and contaminants

Parasites have long been recognized as valuable bioindicators for habitat and host disruption [34–36]. Unfortunately, the responses that different parasite taxa exhibit vary with the type of stressor [37, 38]. As biomarkers, monogeneans and acanthocephalans have been sensitive to changing concentrations of dissolved oxygen, fecal coliform, and total ammonia nitrogen in water [39]. Some trematodes and nematodes increase in prevalence when hosts are exposed to heavy metal contaminants [34], and reductions in acanthocephalans are documented in fishes downstream of pulp mill discharges [40]. However, some groups, like cestodes, tend to increase or decrease depending on the combination of contaminants [35].

Beyond the direct effects of contaminants on helminths *in situ*, polluted systems can also disrupt the life cycle of parasites. When these interferences include reduced densities or richness of obligate or facultative hosts, the cycle can contract to levels where it is no longer supported [41]. For example, the tapeworm *Bothriocephalus acheilognathi* has a 2-host life cycle that includes a copepod (*Cyclops strenuus*) and a freshwater fish. When exposed to cadmium pollution, copepod populations decline (especially when copepods are parasitized with tapeworms: [42]), and infections in the fish hosts become rare. This is problematic in highly dynamic and stochastic systems, where temporary removal of hosts via migration or extirpation could eliminate the parasite from the system or alter its host specificity and virulence [43].

Contaminants can also modulate the trophic interactions of organisms by changing their behaviors, physical conditions, and crypsis [44]. For example, fishes exposed to microplastic contaminants were more difficult to capture by a simulated predator than controls [45]. Contrastingly, Zebra Finches exposed to fluoxetine reduced avoidance of high-risk locations for predation and freezing behavior in the presence of a simulated predator, increasing the likelihood of predation [46]. The system-wide consequences of these altered trophic interactions can modify the transfer of energy and cycling of nutrients, indicators of ecological integrity [47].

Considering the migratory nature of many bird host species, there is an increased risk of their exposure to threats at large spatial and climactic scales [48]. Climate change contributes to the altered distributions of organisms as abiotic conditions vary spatially, and biotic communities respond to them. Within these new climate regimes, all organisms have the potential to respond to changed conditions, and the presence of additional contaminants can further modify the impacts that organisms experience. Of particular concern in contamination science is the added presence of plastics that represent persistent chemical compounds and durable physical composites that enter food webs [49].

Marine debris impacts the environment, wildlife, and human communities, especially in remote islands and coastal areas. These areas have experienced environmental degradation due to the accumulation of marine debris on their shorelines [50]. This issue interests community members who rely on subsistence species, such as seabirds and marine mammals, which can ingest or become entangled in marine debris [51–53].

Plastic debris does not degrade; it only gets smaller [54]. Some of the smallest components, microplastics (1–10 mm) and nanoplastics (<1 mm), are increasingly seen as serious contaminants in marine ecosystems. They have been implicated in altering physiological processes in the organisms that come into contact with them [55–57]. Furthermore, micro- and nano-plastics affect parasite presence [58, 59] and host-parasite interactions [60, 61] in marine phytoplankton [62], invertebrates [63], and vertebrates [57, 64]. Overall, it seems that micro- and nano-plastics have harmful effects on the interactions between living and non-living elements in host-parasite systems at all levels of the food chain. Therefore, the implications of plastic contamination on helminth communities occur at both large and small scales. In addition to helminths, the distributions of other symbiotic organisms, such as bacteria, also respond to human-caused environmental changes, climate change, and contamination.

1.4 Microbe-helminth interactions

The host microbiome is crucial in resistance to parasitic infections. It harbors symbiotic organisms, particularly mutualistic bacteria, pivotal for combating parasitic threats through various mechanisms such as antibiotic production, enhanced digestion efficiency, and pathogen resistance [65, 66]. These bacteria, specialized and sensitive to specific environmental conditions, are subject to influences from abiotic factors like the microclimate and pH of the infection site and biotic factors such as the host's taxa and diet [67, 68].

Extensively studied, GIT microbiome composition varies among individuals and is shaped by sex, migration status, age, and the host's physiological condition, including nutrition, stress hormones, and parasitic infections [69, 70]. Under normal circumstances, a delicate balance exists among microbial mutualists and commensals, ensuring sustained symbiotic benefits. Disruptions, like the reduction or loss of these beneficial microbes, may lead to dysbiosis, favoring colonization by other pathogens and exogenous microbes, thereby jeopardizing host health [71–73].

The microbiome extends its influence beyond the GIT to other host compartments, engaging in microbial exchanges between the skin, blood, and vectors, facilitating pathogen dissemination [74, 75]. Notably, helminthic parasites and microbial symbionts share infection sites and immune evasion strategies, with interactions shaping host defenses and microbial richness [76, 77]. While complimentary associations between microbes and helminths are well-documented, antagonistic dynamics underscore the complexity of these relationships [77, 78].

Mouse studies have further elucidated the intricate interplay between helminths and the gut microbiota, demonstrating how host defenses are modulated in response to infection and affect digestion efficiency and fecal composition [79, 80]. Perturbing the microbial community through dysbiosis or specific bacterial triggers can impede parasite colonization pathways, underscoring the interconnectedness of host-microbe-parasite dynamics and ecosystem health [81, 82]. Moreover, microbial metabolic reactions can activate virulence factors in pathogenic bacteria, impacting community structure and ecosystem resilience, thus highlighting the broader implications of microbial dysbiosis beyond host-parasite interactions [83, 84]. Understanding these interactions offers insights into managing host-parasite dynamics and underscores the broader ecological consequences of microbial disruptions.

While fewer instances document reductions of helminths by bacteria [78], the absence of *Escherichia coli* and *Salmonella typhimurium*, or dysbiosis that impedes their function, reduces the ability of nematodes like *Trichuris muris* to colonize a host successfully. *E. coli* and *S. typhimurium* are triggers that initiate the opening of *T. muris* eggs in the host intestine [81, 85]. Thus, treatments that disrupt the microbial community can lead to various pathways where parasites are reduced or eliminated from hosts [82, 86].

Here, we present findings from multiple bird collections in which avian hosts were examined for gastrointestinal helminths and ingestion of plastics. Some of the birds were sourced from an outbreak of Avian Botulism, where it is believed that the hosts perished due to botulinum neurotoxin (BoNT) poisoning and experienced distinct shifts in their surficial microbial communities. Although all the birds in the collection are waterbirds, they represent various taxonomic and trophic groups. As such, many birds were also analyzed for stable isotope concentrations. This allowed us to assess the effects of two stressors on the infracommunities of their internal parasitic helminths: contamination by microplastics and pathogenic bacteria capable of causing dysbiosis of the GIT.

2. Empirical evidence and hypothesis testing

2.1 Methodologies

Since 2015, we have simultaneously assessed the GITs for trophically transmitted parasites and consumed plastics of 26 species (n = 124 for whole birds and another 241 GITs for a total of 366 birds). All birds were collected on the water, at roost sites over water, or soon after death from natural causes, like Avian Botulism. Whole carcass assessments (n = 102) included quantitative necropsy, where morphometric weights of each primary organ system were measured and evaluated for condition. Although several organ systems besides the GIT were assessed, we focus on the helminth parasites of the gut here. Because the sources of birds varied in time and space, the handling of carcasses varied by agency, and the condition of GITs or their contents varied by project, we do not attempt to make conclusions regarding individual parasite species but instead use the community composition (=infracommunity) of each bird, using parasite morphotypes as operational "species." These morphotypes were based on general morphological characteristics and were consistent at the host species level.

Most of the whole birds were sourced from natural populations of seabirds in the Western Aleutian Islands in cooperation with the U.S. Fish and Wildlife Service. We shot these birds on the water, froze them within 1 hour of collection, and wrapped them in aluminum foil to ensure minimal contact and contamination of plastics. We took body measurements and qualitatively assessed body condition [87], washed the external surfaces with soap and water, and retained the resulting "ectowash" (containing ectoparasites) before opening the birds for qualitative necropsy [88]. We sampled liver tissue during necropsy for stable isotope measurements and various tissues for plastic congener quantification. For these 124 samples, we compare the host trophic position with parasite metrics and the frequencies of consumed plastics and their chemical congeners.

Within the whole bird samples, we had a subset (n = 21) associated with a die-off event on Middleton Island, Alaska, in the summer of 2021. Black-legged Kittiwakes (*Rissa tridactyla*: BLKI) (n = 21) and Glaucous-winged Gulls (*Larus glaucescens*: GWGU) (n = 2), were frozen within hours of death and later were also fully processed with quantitative necropsy, gut parasitology, and stable isotope analyses. Further, we performed microbial assessments of the parasites from the ectowashes (lice, mites, ticks, and fleas) of the BLKI to learn whether there were differences between their microbiomes and those of the same species from the 2016 Aleutian Island collection [89].

In addition to the whole-body assessments, we include host data collected by the U.S. Department of Agriculture, Animal Plant Health Inspection Service, Wildlife

Services, National Wildlife Research Center (NWRC) on commercial aquaculture facilities or at roost sites near aquaculture. The first set of samples (n = 136) consisted of two bird species, Double-crested Cormorants (*Nannopterum auritum*) and Lesser Scaup (*Aythya affinis*), foraging on baitfish aquaculture farms in Arkansas and roosting near catfish aquaculture ponds in Mississippi in 2016 and 2017. These birds were shot in the field, individually wrapped and placed on ice, and transported to an NWRC lab for necropsy within 24 hours of collection. We emptied the gut contents into warm saline and transferred them into formalin, and liver tissue samples were taken for stable isotope analyses [12, 90]. The second sample set consisted of seven waterbird species (N = 105) shot on shrimp aquaculture farms in Alabama and Florida in 2020 and 2021. Gut contents were processed similarly to the former group, except half of the samples were preserved in ethanol and the other half in 10% buffered formalin.

Parasite analyses following quantitative necropsy were separated by the anatomical regions of the digestive system: the esophagus, stomach/gizzard, duodenum, jejunum, ileum, colon, and cloaca. For these assessments, we could evaluate the co-infections of parasites and infer the preferential infection sites for many parasites. In contrast, in gut content analyses from birds processed from aquaculture collections, all GIT sections were combined into a single sample. We could not ascertain infection localities beyond upper and lower GIT. While assessing digestate from samples, we scrutinized the liquid diluted with 0.04% saline (Instant Ocean) in square, gridded sorting under 4–40× total magnification (stereoscope). Any parasites or plastics were removed, placed into 9-well borosilicate glass plates, sorted into morphologically distinct groupings (i.e., "morphospecies"), and preserved in either 10% buffered formalin for long-term preservation or 90% ethanol for DNA conservation. Each morphospecies was counted for abundance estimates and plastic type (fiber, shard, etc.) was enumerated and recorded.

Data from each project were combined into a database where each row pertained to a given morphospecies present in the GIT. When assessments had previously split components of the GIT into several sections (n = 124), we summed the counts of each morphospecies to calculate a total infrapopulation for each bird. In addition, we summed the number of plastics found within each organ, when applicable, and for birds where we measured them, we included mean stable isotope values for each species, as well as mean plastic chemical congener concentrations.

We extracted the microbiome of diseased BLKI samples using a combination of 2.3 and 0.5 mm silica beads for homogenization. DNA extraction followed the Qiagen DNeasy Blood and Tissue Kit protocol with an extended 36-hour incubation period at 56°C [91]. 16S metagenomic sequencing was conducted on the Illumina MiSeq platform using standard Illumina primers for the hypervariable region V3-V4. Data processing occurred in QIIME2, denoising sequences with DADA2, and filtering based on quality scores and expected errors for chloroplasts, mitochondria, and unclassified sequences. Sequences were clustered to 99% similarity, and taxonomy was assigned using a combination of the Silva 138 and GreenGenes databases, resolving discrepancies in favor of higher confidence assignments [92–95].

We used a sampling depth of 29k for the core metrics function in QIIME2 to analyze the microbial community composition. The Jaccard dissimilarity matrix was exported to R and assessed with Canonical Analyses of Principal Coordinates (CAP: vegan). The CAPs were constrained separately by helminthic parasite assemblage, host plastic consumption, and year. P-values were based on PERMANOVA with 999 permutations of each variable to determine statistical significance and the R^2 values indicate the variation attributable to that environmental variable.

2.2 Ecological differentiation of hosts

Using δC[13] and δN[15] isotopic ratios of the 11 assessed bird species, we grouped the hosts into five distinct trophic clusters (K-means clusters based on Principal Components, **Figure 1**). Two singleton clusters contain species that are high-order predators yet feed in distinctly different habitats: Double-crested Cormorants, piscivorous birds that breed primarily in freshwater habitats but also feed in coastal habitats during non-breeding seasons, and the Northern Fulmar (*Fulmarus glacialis*), a highly marine species that breeds on oceanic islands. While these species appear to share a similar trophic level, suggesting a highly piscivorous diet, the habitats in which they occur provide sufficient separation in trophic ordinate space, separating them through cluster analysis. The remaining three groups (**Figure 2**) include bird species that persist in low-to-intermediate trophic levels.

The invertebrate-specialist group (cluster 2) spans habitat types and includes freshwater and marine specialists. This group contains Lesser Scaup, a ubiquitous species that can consume a range of prey from plant seeds and small invertebrates to small fishes; the Crested Auklet (*Aethia cristatella*), a consumer of marine/pelagic arthropods and sometimes small fish; and the Horned Puffin (*Fratercula corniculatus*), a frequent consumer of small fishes, all of which might share similar trophic positions with predatory invertebrates in freshwater systems.

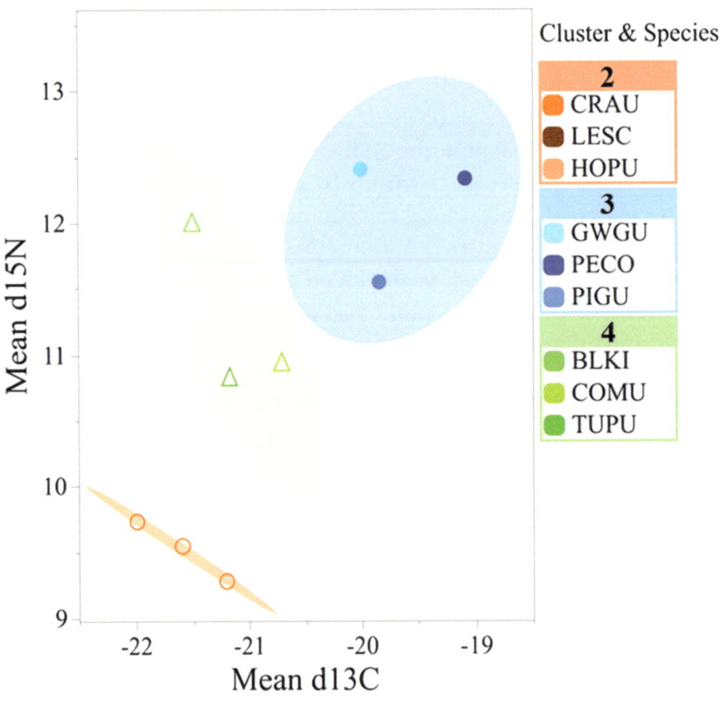

Figure 1.
Of the five clusters identified from distinct heavy nitrogen and carbon isotope concentrations, three multi-species clusters could be differentiated. These groups included invertebrate consumers (2: orange), coastal predators (4: green), and offshore predators (3: blue). BLKI = Black-legged Kittiwake, COMU = Common Murre, CRAU = Crested Auklet, GWGU = Glaucous-winged Gull, HOPU = Horned Puffin, LESC = Lesser Scaup, PECO = Pelagic Cormorant, PIGU = Pigeon Guillemot, TUPU = Tufted Puffin.

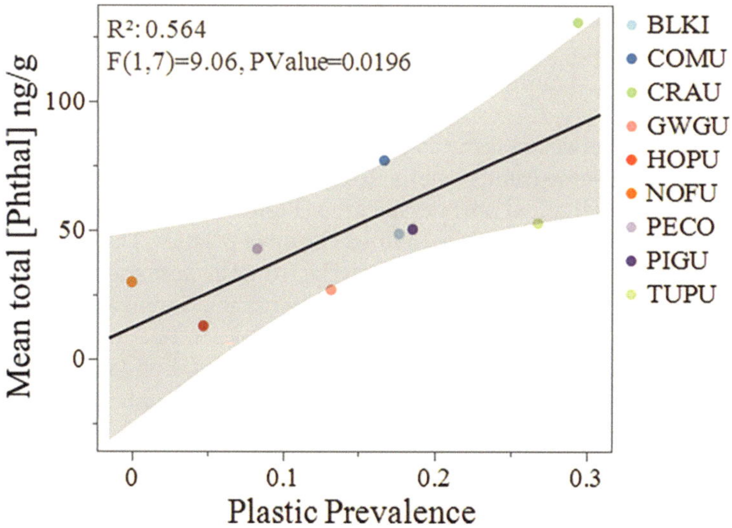

Figure 2.
Mean concentrations of total phthalates and the plastic prevalence (proportion of birds with plastic in gastrointestinal tract) of nine species of seabirds (colored by American Ornithological Union code) with sample sizes of 3 or more individuals. BLKI = Black-legged Kittiwake, COMU = Common Murre, CRAU = Crested Auklet, GWGU = Glaucous-winged Gull, HOPU = Horned Puffin, NOFU = Norther Fulmar, PECO = Pelagic Cormorant, PIGU = Pigeon Guillemot, TUPU = Tufted Puffin.

The coastal-specialist group (cluster 3) includes bird species that breed and forage near coastlines or shallow marine communities. It includes Pelagic Cormorants (*Urile pelagicus*), Pigeon Guillemots (*Cepphus columba*), and Glaucous-winged Gulls. While cormorants are often considered fish specialists (like the Double-crested Cormorant above), feeding on small coastal fish can shift their isotopic signatures to be similar to those of trophic generalists and coastal predators like gulls and guillemots [31].

The coastal-pelagic group (cluster 4) consists of species that typically feed in areas beyond the continental shelf, where certain groups of organisms (such as Gastropoda) are largely absent. By feeding on small pelagic fishes, krill, and intraguild predators of these prey, the isotope similarities indicate that Tufted Puffin (*Fratercula cirrhata*), Common Murre (*Uria aalge*), and Black-Legged Kittiwakes belong to a similar trophic guild. Despite all being waterbirds, their varied diets and geographic ranges make them valuable bioindicators for other avian groups at similar trophic levels.

2.3 Trends of plastic contamination in hosts

Some correlations between plastic abundances and their congeners were detected within the isotopic trophic groupings. Considering mean values for tissue total phthalates for each species where they were measured (n = 9 species, 110 hosts), as plastic consumption increased, so did phthalate concentrations (**Figure 2**). Within the trophic clusters of this sample set, plastic consumption increased in the invertebrate-consumers group (cluster 2), as did the concentration of DEHP, a plastic phthalate congener. This contaminant also increased in the coastal generalist/piscivore group, although the relative frequencies of plastics consumed were consistent. The offshore piscivorous birds showed consistent patterns for plastic frequencies (count), and the amount of plastic ingested by these birds was consistent with the

DEHP plastic congener concentration in their muscle tissues. These results agree with previous works of plastic phthalate congeners of the same species [54], where the foraging strategy explained more variance in congener concentrations than geographic locality, size, or sex.

The relationship between plastic consumption and parasites has yet to be fully resolved [58, 94], yet some trends emerge from the entire dataset evaluated here (n = 356). From the individual host perspective (**Figure 3**), those that contained more helminths (higher intensities) also contained the most plastics. Thus, these trends appear among individuals and species. Similarly, from the host species' perspective (**Figure 4**), we find that waterbirds that harbor higher maximum abundances of parasites also contain higher abundances of consumed plastics. Further, the maximum species richness of helminths increased with parasite load (abundance) and plastic frequencies at the host species level (**Figure 5**). The causality associated with this correlation has yet to be established, and it is unclear whether species that interact with higher frequencies of parasites also interact with more plastic debris. These are important considerations for future exploration, as contaminants and parasites can alter the probability of consumption for intermediate hosts [95], and whether they have confounding, additive, or synergistic effects on definitive host plastic consumption remains unknown.

As hosts migrate, they move from one foraging location to another and are exposed to differential compositions of infectious agents and contaminants. Double-crested Cormorants and Lesser Scaup collected in 2016 and 2017 were documented as consistently consuming microplastics; however, the prevalence of microplastics in

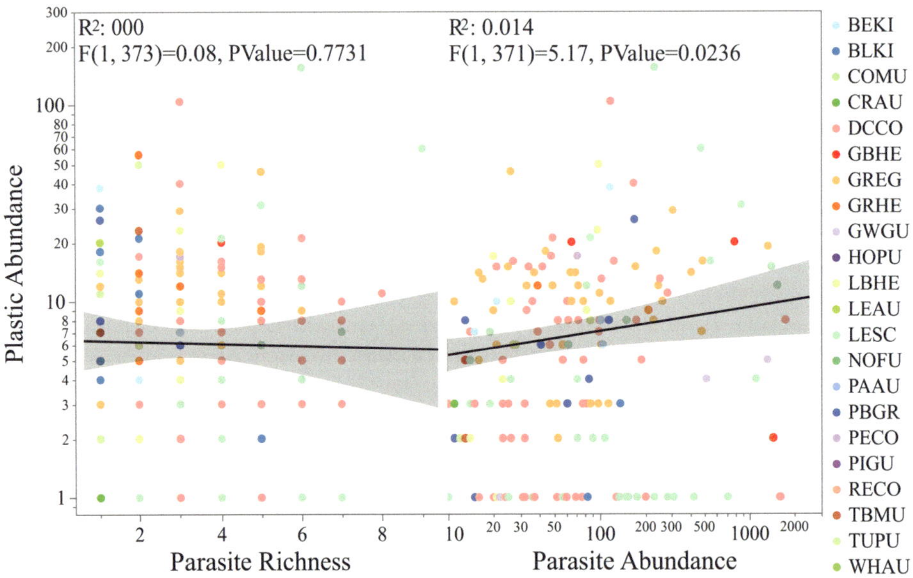

Figure 3.
Species richness (left) and count data (right) for gut helminth infracommunities and consumed plastic microfibers for individuals from 22 species of waterbirds (colored by American Ornithological Union code). BEKI = Belted Kingfisher, BLKI = Black-legged Kittiwake, COMU = Common Murre, CRAU = Crested Auklet, DCCO = Double-crested Cormorant, GBHE = Great Blue Heron, GREG = Great Egret, GRHE = Green Heron, GWGU = Glaucous-winged Gull, HOPU = Horned Puffin, LBHE = Little Blue Heron, LEAU = Least Auklet, LESC = Lesser Scaup, NOFU = Northern Fulmar, PAAU = Parakeet Auklet, PBGR = Pied-billed Grebe, PECO = Pelagic Cormorant, PIGU = Pigeon Guillemot, RECO = Red-faced Cormorant, TBMU = Thick-billed Murre, TUPU = Tufted Puffin, WHAU = Whiskered Auklet.

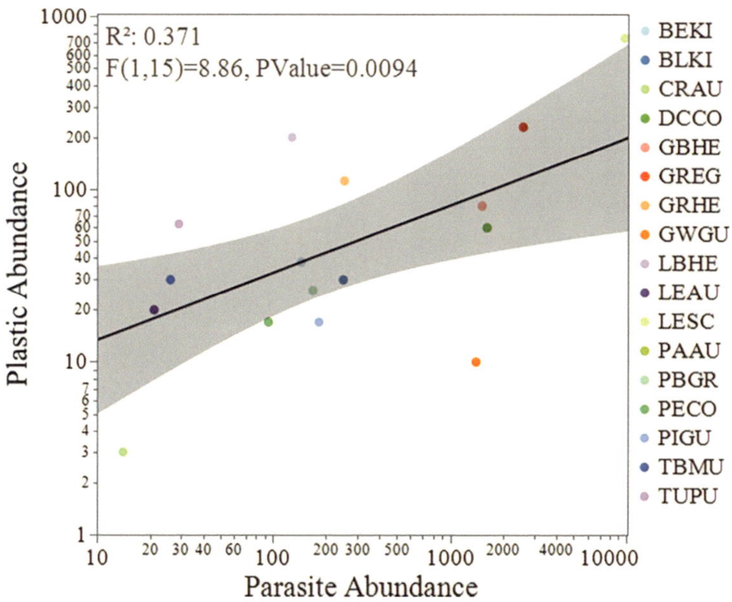

Figure 4.
Count data for gut helminth infracommunities and consumed plastic microfibers for 18 species of waterbirds (colored by American Ornithological Union code) with sample sizes of 3 or more hosts. BEKI = Belted Kingfisher, BLKI = Black-legged Kittiwake, COMU = Common Murre, CRAU = Crested Auklet, DCCO = Double-crested Cormorant, GBHE = Great Blue Heron, GREG = Great Egret, GWGU = Glaucous-winged Gull, HOPU = Horned Puffin, LBHE = Little Blue Heron, LEAU = Least Auklet, LESC = Lesser Scaup, PAAU = Parakeet Auklet, PBGR = Pied-billed Grebe, PECO = Pelagic Cormorant, PIGU = Pigeon Guillemot, TBMU = Thick-billed Murre, TUPU = Tufted Puffin.

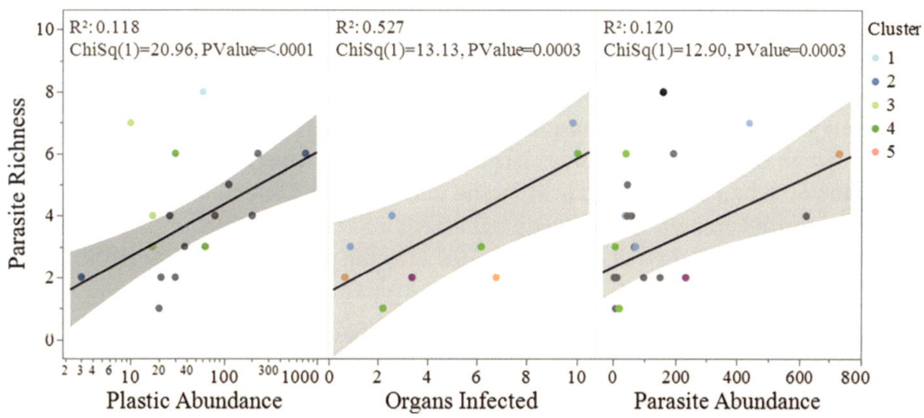

Figure 5.
The maximum species richness of intestinal helminths reported for a waterbird species compared to plastic frequencies (left = count of plastics for a species: middle = mean count of plastics within an organ) and total parasite intensity (load). Bird species are colored based on trophic cluster: large piscivores (1: black), invertebrate consumers (2: orange), coastal predators (4: green), and offshore predators (3: blue), offshore small piscivores (5: red).

our samples differed seasonally and by species (**Figure 6**). These birds were arriving in their southern non-breeding territories and using baitfish and catfish aquaculture facilities to feed opportunistically. In some instances, birds continued southward after stopping at the fishponds. In other instances, individual birds apparently alternated

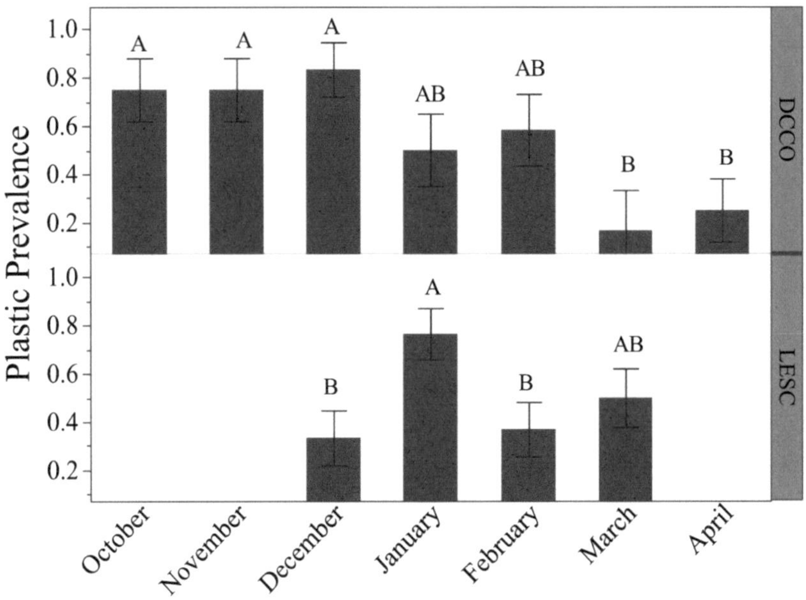

Figure 6.
Monthly frequencies of plastics combined by month over 2 collections (2016–2018) of Double-crested Cormorants (DCCO) and Lesser Scaup (LESC) during the non-breeding seasons in Arkansas and Mississippi, USA.

between inland and more coastal foraging habitats [96]. We observe higher frequencies of plastics in the GIT of cormorants as they arrived on the ponds from northern and southern trips, whereas just before leaving for their northern breeding grounds, fewer individuals contained plastics (R^2 = 0.20, df = 6, F = 3.02, p = 0.0109), but the plastic load did not differ (p = 0.3558).

Scaup showed a peak of plastic prevalence in January (R^2 = 0.111, df = 3, F = 2.846, p = 0.044); however, with only 4 months of collection data to compare (n = 71), we do not suggest that a seasonal change can be readily recognized from this analysis. Further, given that there are likely shifts in the loads of microplastic contaminants depending on when and where a host is, the individual and species-level trends we report above are compelling. As the distributions and collection times of the aggregated datasets represent what should amount to a considerable variation within a host, even moderate trends are telling of large-scale trends.

2.4 Impacts of bacterial dysbiosis on helminth communities

Birds associated with the summer 2021 die-off event on Middleton Island, Alaska, were infected with the pathogenic *C. botulinum*/phage combination, resulting in intoxication with BoNT/C. We note that none of the birds assessed here were directly tested for the toxin. However, following several tests, other birds from the die-off were found to contain the neurotoxin and were absent of any other disease agents and toxins [97]. As such, we consider the birds from Middleton as "diseased" birds and those we compare them to from the Western Aleutian Islands as "healthy" because there was no die-off occurring at those locations during that summer collection. The geographic distance between our two sites is more than 2000 km, and this, too, has the potential to influence the trophic interactions that a host experiences, whether that be from different prey populations, vectors, or pathogens present in the Pacific/Beringean oceanic realm (Aleutian samples) and those in the Gulf of Alaska (Middleton Island samples). Here, we present comparisons of the microbial and helminth communities of diseased and healthy birds from those collections.

We processed birds for the Middleton-Aleutian comparisons for C^{13} and N^{15}. We found slight differences in isotopic signatures between kittiwakes and gulls but pronounced shifts in the signatures between the two seabird collections (**Figure 7**). Whether dysbiosis in the microbial community is influenced by *C. botulinum* infection or local microbe community contributions has yet to be definitively addressed; however, there appears to be distinct differentiation of isotopic signatures between both species and possibly health status.

The endoparasites and plastics consumed by this subset of birds also differed based on location/year/disease status (**Figure 8**). Kittiwakes (hereafter BLKI, n = 42) from the Middleton Island die-off in 2021 contained larger counts (R^2 = 0.16, df = 1, p = 0.0216) and types (R^2 = 0.32, df = 1, p = 0.0008) of parasites; however, the number of organs infected within the GIT was lower (R^2 = 0.72, df = 1, p < 0.0001). Conversely, diseased birds contained fewer plastic particles when compared to healthy conspecifics collected from the western Aleutian Islands in 2016. With a smaller sample size (n = 12), Glaucus-winged Gulls exhibited similar parasite frequencies (p = 0.340), richness (p = 0.166), and plastic frequencies (0.680). However, like the BLKI, parasites were distributed among more organs in healthy birds compared to diseased conspecifics from the Middleton disease event (R^2 = 0.95, df = 1, p < 0.0001).

In addition to differences in the endoparasite communities of birds associated with a die-off event, similar trends in ectoparasite ecological metrics occurred in these birds [89]. Moreover, differences occurred in the microbiome of these hosts based on ecological metrics (alpha, beta, and gamma diversity) for BLKI [89].

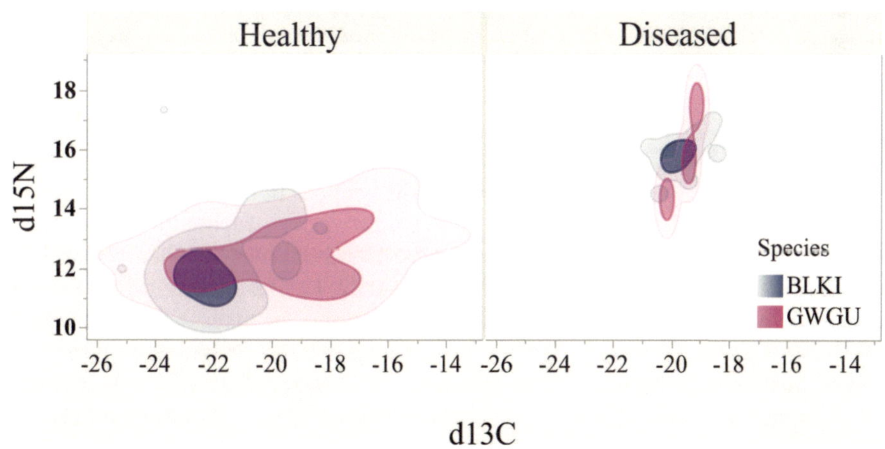

Figure 7.
Stable isotopic heat maps indicating the trophic position of Black-legged Kittiwakes (BLKI) and Glaucus-winged Gulls (GWGU) for birds collected during non-die-off conditions ("Healthy") between 2009 and 2019 from the western Aleutian Islands and birds of the same species collected during a presumed Avian Botulism outbreak on Middleton Island in 2021 ("Diseased").

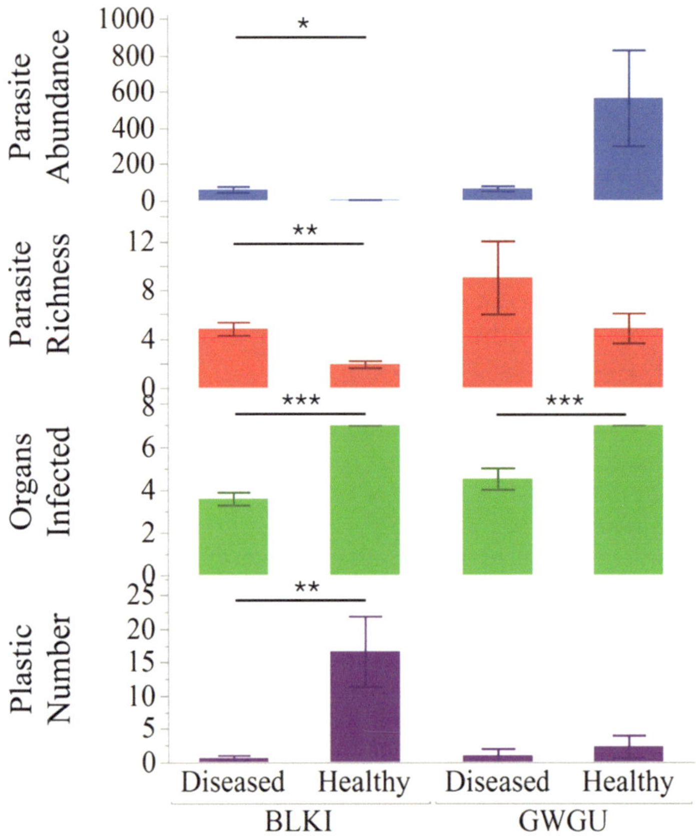

Figure 8.
Frequencies of parasites and plastics in two species of seabirds (Black-legged Kittiwakes [BLKI] and Glaucus-winged Gulls [GWGU]) from a die-off event in 2021 on Middleton Island (diseased) and the western Aleutian Island (healthy) of Alaksa. Metrics include the number of parasites found in a host (abundance), the number of parasite species in a host (richness), the mean number of host organs that were infected, and the frequency of consumed plastics observed (plastic number). Lines above paired bars indicate significant differences at 0.05 (*), 0.001 (**) and <0.0001 (***).

Although the microbial communities were based on each bird's ectoparasites and surficial symbionts, we document marginal differences in microbial composition based on Constrained Analysis of Principal Coordinates informed by helminth communities and year (**Figure 9**). We found differences between healthy and diseased birds (p = 0.046; R^2 = 0.67; CAP 1 = −0.32, CAP 2 = −0.58); however, we cannot conclusively say whether geographic, temporal, or disease status differences drove these differences. Further, no parasite metrics provided explanatory power of host separation in ordinate space (p = 0.298). Similarly, plastic ingestion did not impact the surficial microbial communities of the birds assessed here (p = 0.283).

Helminthic communities can drive microbial community alterations [83–85], so the interplay between microbial responses to helminthic parasites and helminths' responses to microbial pathogens remains to be elucidated. This will likely require laboratory experiments where helminth and pathogen infection dynamics can be controlled.

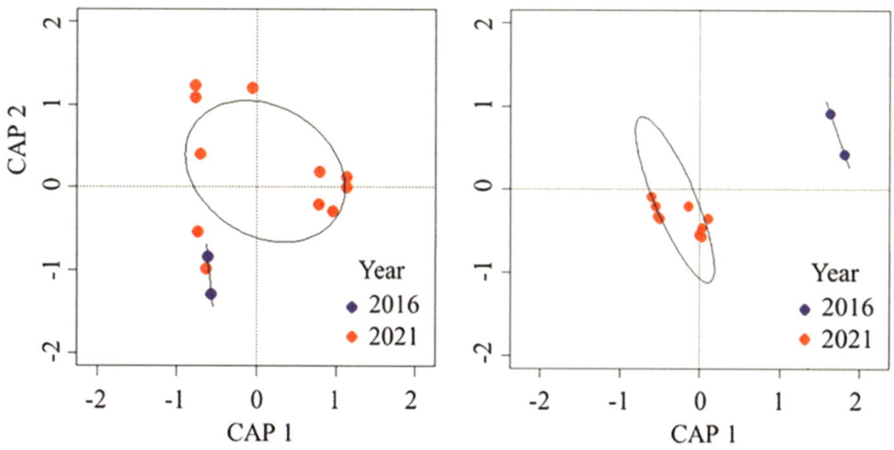

Figure 9.
Ordination plot based on principle coordinates analysis of microbial communities of Black-legged Kittiwakes from a collection of birds taken in the Western Aleutian Islands in 2016 (blue) and a presumed Avian Botulism outbreak in the Gulf of Alaska in 2021 (red). Metadata for evaluation of ordinate separation based on parasite infracommunity compositions (left) and consumed microplastic frequencies (right).

3. Conclusions

The utility of endoparasites as ecological indicators for host foraging behavior allows researchers and managers to understand the consequences of land use change, expanding reaches of plastic contamination, and expanding ranges of pathogens like *C. botulinum*.

When assessing the complete suite of waterbirds included in these analyses, we found that the infracommunities of birds varied by location (**Figure 8**), season (**Figure 6**), and, most importantly, bird species (**Figures 2–5**). As waterbird hosts are also recognized as sentinels of ecosystem change [49], the prospect of parasite assessments to more fully evaluate alterations in trophic structure is compelling. Further, the differentiation resolution observed here confirms the utility of parasite intracommunity assessments in the niche divergences of birds that forage in similar habitats and at similar trophic levels (**Figure 5**).

Previous works demonstrate that trophic strategies can correlate with plastic contamination [54]; however, many of those studies report macroplastics as opposed to microplastics evaluated here and did not find that phthalate concentrations correlated with increased plastics consumption. Here, we provide evidence that this is the case so long as microplastics are also considered, as plastic consumption increased, so did phthalate concentrations in tissues, especially total phthalates and DEHP.

While the contaminant concentrations in host tissues were not reflected in parasite infracommunity metrics, plastic frequencies did correspond with higher intensities. However, causality between parasite burden and plastic consumption remains unclear. There is the potential for parasitized intermediate hosts to have an increased probability of plastic exposure or entanglement. Likewise, it could be that intermediate hosts interacting with plastic are more susceptible to parasitic infection. Further experimentation would help understand the dynamic relationships.

It is necessary for the prosperity and security of human populations to consider the impact of land use change and contamination from anthropogenic waste products, such as single-use plastics, on natural systems and organisms. We have discovered a notable positive correlation between parasites and plastic frequencies and have found that aquaculture facilities appear to be sinks rather than sources of plastic contamination. The interaction of human-created stressors on organisms and their symbionts undoubtedly responds to changes in these systems. There is an urgent need for highly replicated and robust research to determine their consequences.

Birds from Middleton Island, affected by a 2021 die-off, likely due to *C. botulinum*/phage exposure, had distinct parasite communities compared to healthy birds from the Western Aleutian Islands. Geographic distance between sites may affect trophic interactions, and the isotopic signatures of birds from the die-off suggest a substantial shift and contraction of dietary niche breadth in the diseased hosts. Middleton birds had more parasites but fewer plastics in their GI tracts than healthy Aleutian birds. Ectoparasite metrics and microbial diversity varied between diseased and healthy birds, possibly influenced by helminth communities. Further study is needed to understand microbial responses to helminths and vice versa.

The Bering Sea region faces numerous environmental threats impacting its health and the sustainability of its communities and fisheries, from global climate change to marine debris pollution. Bering Sea communities are working to maintain a healthy ecosystem in many ways, including taking leadership actions to clean up marine debris. Efforts to manage this ecosystem would be informed by a better understanding of the ecological and physiological relationships of seabirds with their prey, their parasites, and plastic contaminants.

Acknowledgements

We express our sincere gratitude to the decade of training and funding contributions that helped make the development and execution of these ideas possible. Agencies that contributed financial and additional resources include the National Science Foundation (USA), the U.S. Department of Agriculture/Animal Plant Health Inspection Service/Wildlife Services/National Wildlife Research Center (NWRC), and the National Oceanographic and Atmospheric Association. Institutional contributions include Frostburg State University, University of Alaska Anchorage, University of California, San Diego (UCSD) and Santa Barbara, Scripps Institute of Oceanography, University of Georgia Southeastern Cooperative for Wildlife Health Service, and Clemson University. We also thank collaborators at the New England and Cape Wildlife Centers for their expertise and donation of specimens.

Specimens were collected under permits ADFG 16-096, 17-093, 18-100, 19-152, 22-101; USFWS MB 795841; and IACUC protocols 1216862, 1216863, 1721620, 1721621.

Funding for specimen collection and processing came, in part, from NSF EEID (OCE-1115965), the Southern Regional Aquaculture Center Grant number 2016-38500-25752 from the U.S. Department of Agriculture National Institute of Food and Agriculture, a Frontiers of Innovation Scholars Program grant from UCSD, a 2022-2023 Research Publication Grant in Engineering, Medicine, and Science from the American Association of University Women, and cooperative agreements with the U.S. Department of Agriculture, Animal Plant Health Inspection Service, Wildlife Services, National Wildlife Research Center 17-7428-1326-CA and 18-7428-1326-CA.

Thanks

We thank the dozens of university students and technicians who assisted in processing samples, data entry, diet analysis, and parasitology for the hundreds of birds included in our analyses. In particular, Dr. Veronica Padula's hard work in tissue assessments for plastic congeners is most appreciated.

Author details

Kate L. Sheehan[1,2,3*], Sonja Barber[1], Ryan F. Hechinger[2], Brian S. Dorr[4] and Douglas Causey[3]

1 Frostburg State University, Frostburg, Maryland, United States of America

2 Scripps Institute of Oceanography, University of San Diego, California, United States of America

3 University of Alaska, Anchorage, Alaska, United States of America

4 U.S. Department of Agriculture, Animal Plant Health Inspection Service, Wildlife Services, National Wildlife Research Center, Starkville, Mississippi, United States of America

*Address all correspondence to: klsheehan@frostburg.edu

References

[1] Dobson A, Lafferty KD, Kuris AM, Hechinger RF, Jetz W. Homage to Linnaeus: How many parasites? How many hosts? PNAS. 2008;**105**(S1):11482-11489. DOI: 10.1073/pnas.0803232105

[2] Carlson CJ, Dallas TA, Alexander LW, Phelan AL, Phillips AJ. What would it take to describe the global diversity of parasites? Proceedings of the Royal Society B: Biological Sciences. 2020;**287**:20201941. DOI: 10.1098/rspb.2020.1841

[3] Franier A, McKie BG, Amundsen PA, Knudsen R, Lafferty KD. Parasitism and the biodiversity-functioning relationship. Trends in Ecology & Evolution. 2018;**33**:260-268. DOI: 10.1016/j.tree.2018.01.011

[4] Britton RJ, Andreou D. Parasitism as a driver of trophic niche specialisation. Trends in Parasitology. 2016;**32**:437-445. DOI: 10.1016/j.pt.2016.02.007

[5] Gardner SL, Campbell ML. Parasites as probes for biodiversity. The Journal of Parasitology. 1992;**78**(4):596-600

[6] Sheehan KL, Tonkyn DW, Yarrow G, Johnson RJ. Parasite assemblages of double-crested cormorants as indicators of host populations and migration behavior. Ecological Indicators. 2016;**67**:497-503. DOI: 10.1016/j.ecolind.2016.03.008

[7] Kuris AM, Jaramillo AG, McGlaughlin JP, Weinstein SP, Garcia-Vedrenne AE, Polnar GO Jr, et al. Monsters of the sea serpent: Parasites of an oarfish *Regalecus russellii*. The Journal of Parasitology. 2015;**101**:41-44. DOI: 10.1645/14-581.1

[8] Koh LP, Dunn RR, Sodhi NS, Colwell RK, Proctor HC, Smith VS. Species coextinctions and the biodiversity crisis. Science. 2024;**305**:1632. DOI: 10.1126/science.1101101

[9] van Dijk J, De Baets K. Biodiversity and host-parasite (co)extinction. In: De Baets K, Huntley JW, editors. The Evolution and Fossil Record of Parasitism: Topics in Geobiology. Vol. 50. Cham: Springer; 2021. DOI: 10.1007/978-3-030-52233-9_3

[10] Ishtiaq F, Renner SC. Bird migration and vector-borne parasite transmission. In: Santiago-Alarcon D, Marzal A, editors. Avian Malaria and Related Parasites in the Tropics. Cham: Springer; 2020. DOI: 10.1007/978-3-030-51633-8_16

[11] Kudlai O, Kostadinova A, Pulis EE, Tckach VV. A new species of Drepanocephalus Dietz 1090 (Digenea: Echinstomatidae) from the double-crested cormorant *Phalacrocorax auritus* (lesson) (Aves: Phalacrocoraacidae) in North America. Systematic Parasitology. 2015;**90**:321-330. DOI: 10.1007/s11230-015-9550-7

[12] Sheehan KL, Dorr BS, Clements SA, Christie TW, Hanson-Dorr KC, Davis RSA, et al. Predicting consistent foraging ecologies of migrating waterbirds: Using stable isotope and parasite measurements as indicators of landscape use. Ecological Indicators. 2022;**140**:109038. DOI: 10.1016/j.ecolind.2022.109038

[13] Doughherty ER, Carlson CJ, Bueno VM, Burgio KR, Cizauskas CA, Clements CF, et al. Paradigms for parasite conservation. Conservation Biology. 2016;**30**:724-733. Available from: https://www.jstor.org/stable/24761033

[14] Farrell MJ, Stephens PR, Berrang-Ford L, Gittleman JL, Davies TJ. The path to host extinction can lead to loss of generalist parasites. The Journal of Animal Ecology. 2015;**84**:978-984. DOI: 10.1111/1365-2656.12342

[15] Lyndon AR, Kennedy CR. Colonisation and extinction in relation to competition and resource partitioning in acanthocephalans of freshwater fishes of the British Isles. Folia Parasitologica. 2001;**48**:37-46

[16] Lafferty KD, Kuris AM. Parasitism and environmental disturbances. In: Thomas F, Renaud F, Guegan J-F, editors. Parasitism and Ecosystems (Oxford, 2005; online edn, Oxford Academic, 1 Sept. 2007). DOI: 10.1093/acprof:oso/9780198529873.003.0008

[17] Collette NM, Lao VHI, Weilhammer DR, Zingg B, Cohen SD, Hwang M, et al. Single amino acid mutations affect Zika virus replication in vitro and virulence in vivo. Viruses. 2020;**12**:1295. DOI: 10.3390/v12111295

[18] Ewald PW. The evolution of virulence. Scientific American. 1993;**268**(86-88):90-93. Available from: https://www.jstor.org/stable/10.2307/24941444

[19] Fofana AM, Hurford A. Parasite-induced shifts in host movement may explain the transient coexistence of high- and low-pathogenic disease strains. Journal of Evolutionary Biology. 2022;**35**:1072-1086. DOI: 10.1111/jeb.14053

[20] Singh P, Best A. Simultaneous evolution of host resistance and tolerance to parasitism. Journal of Evolutionary Biology. 2021;**34**:1932-1943. DOI: 10.1111/jeb.13947

[21] Hechinger RF, Sheehan KL, Turner AV. Metabolic theory of ecology successfully predicts distinct scaling of ectoparasite load on hosts. Proceedings of the Royal Society B: Biological Sciences. 2019;**286**:20191777. DOI: 10.1098/rspb.2019.1777

[22] Ianiro GA, Porcari IS, Masucci L, Sanguinetti M, Perno CF, Gasbarrini A, et al. How the gut parasitome affects human health. Therapeutic Advances in Gastroenterology. 2022;**15**:1-15. DOI: 10.1177/175628482210915

[23] Chulanetra M, Chaicumpa W. Revisiting the mechanisms of immune evasion employed by human parasites. Frontiers in Cellular and Infection Microbiology. 2021;**11**:701215. DOI: 10.3389/fcimb.2021.702125

[24] Shukla R, Soni J, Kumar A, Pandey R. Uncovering the diversity of pathogenic invaders: Insights into protozoa fungi and worm infections. Frontiers in Microbiology. 2024;**15**:1374438. DOI: 10.3389/fmicb.2024.1374438

[25] Pawelec G, Goldeck D, Derhovanessian E. Inflammation, aging, and chronic disease. Current Opinion in Immunology. 2014;**29**:23-28. DOI: 10.1016/j.coi.2014.03.007

[26] King IL, Li Y. Host-parasite interactions promote disease tolerance to intestinal helminth infection. Frontiers in Immunology. 2018;**9**:1-10. DOI: 10.3389/fimmu.2018.02128

[27] Ritchie H, Roser M. Half of the World's Habitable Land Is Used for Agriculture [Internet]. 2019. Available from: https://ourworldindata.org/global-land-for-agriculture [Accessed: May 3, 2024]

[28] Burr PC, Dorr BS, Avery LJ, Street GM, Strickland BK. Long term changes in aquaculture influence migration regional abundance and

distribution of an avian species. PLoS ONE. 2023;**18**:e0284265. DOI: 10.1371/journal.pone.0284265

[29] Glahn JF, Tobin ME, Harrel JB. Possible effects of catfish exploitation on overwinter body condition of double-crested cormorants. In: Symposium on Double-Crested Cormorants: Population Status and Management Issues in the Midwest. 1997. p. 11. Available from: https://digitalcommons.unl.edu/nwrccormorants/11

[30] Wise DJ, Hanson TR, Tucker CS. Farm-level economic impacts of Bolbophorus infections of channel catfish. North American Journal of Aquaculture. 2008;**70**:382-383. DOI: 10.1577/A07-089.1

[31] Shipley ON, Matich P. Studying animal niches using bulk isotope ratios. Oecologia. 2020;**193**:27-51. Available from: https://www.jstor.org/stable/10.2307/48696064

[32] Ubierna N, Holloway-Phillips MM, Wingate L, Ogee J, Busch FA, Farquhar GD. Using carbon stable isotopes to study C3 and C4 photosynthesis: Models and calculations. In: Covshoff S, editor. Photosynthesis . Methods in Molecular Biology. New York, NY: Humana; 2024. p. 2790. DOI: 10.1007/978-1-0716-3790-6_10

[33] Awuchi CG, Awuchi CG. Impacts of plastic pollution on the sustainability of seafood value chain and human health. International Journal of Advanced Academic Research. 2019;**5**:46-138

[34] Marcogliese DJ, Brambilla LG, Gagne F, Gendron AD. Join effects of parasitism and pollution on oxidative stress biomarkers in yellow perch *Perca flacescens*. Diseases of Aquatic Organisms. 2005;**63**:77-84

[35] Sures BM, Selbach NC, Macroglieses DJ. Parasite responses to pollution: What we know and where we go in 'Environmental Parasitology'. Parasites & Vectors. 2017;**10**:65. DOI: 10.1186/s13071-017-2001-3

[36] Sures B, Nachev M, Schwelm J, Grabner D, Selbach C. Environmental parasitology: Stressor effects on aquatic parasites. Trends in Parasitology. 2023;**39**:461-474. DOI: 10.1016/j.pt.2023.03.005

[37] Overstreet RM. Parasitological data as monitors of environmental health. Parasitologica. 1997;**59**:169-175

[38] Vidal-Martinez VM, Pech D, Sures B, Purucher T, Poulin R. Can parasites really reveal environmental impact? Trends in Parasitology. 2009;**26**:44-51. DOI: 10.1016/j.pt.2009.11.001

[39] ACF L, Roumbedakis K, Bereta JGS Jr, APO N, Petrucio MM, Martins ML. Fish parasites as indicators of organic pollution in southern Brazil. Journal of Helminthology. 2018;**92**:322-331. DOI: 10.1017/S0022149X17000414

[40] Billard SM, Khan RA. Chronic stress in cunner *Tautogolabrus adspersus* exposed to municipal and industrial effluents. Ecotoxicology and Environmental Safety. 2003;**55**:9-18. DOI: 10.1016/S0147-6513(02)00090-8

[41] Cohen S, Gianaros PJ, Manuck SB. A stage model of stress and disease. Perspectives on Psychological Science. 2016;**11**:456-463. DOI: 10.1177/1745691616646305

[42] Khalil M, Furness DN, Zholobenko V, Hoole D. Effect of tapeworm parasitism on cadmium toxicity in the bioindicator copepod, *Cyclops strenuous*. Ecological Indicators.

2014;**37**:21-26. DOI: 10.1016/j.ecolind.2013.09.033

[43] Farrell MJ, Park AW, Cressler CE, Dallas T, Huang S, Mideo N, et al. The ghost of hosts past: Impacts of host extinction on parasite specificity. Philosophical Transactions of the Royal Society B. 2021;**376**:20200351. DOI: 10.1098/rstb.2020.0351

[44] Kobiela ME, Cristol DA, Swaddle JP. Risk-taking behaviours in zebra finches affected by mercury exposure. Animal Behaviour. 2015;**103**:153-160. DOI: 10.1016/j.anbehav.2015.02.024

[45] McHale ME, Sheehan KL. Bioaccumulation transfer and impacts of microplastics on wild animals in aquatic food webs. Journal of Environmental Exposure Assessment. 2024;**3**:15, 1-20. DOI: 10.20517/jeea.2023.49. ISSN 2771-5949 (in-press Online)

[46] Martin JM, Saarista M, Bertram MG, Lewis PJ, Coggan TL, Clarke BO, et al. The psychoactive pollutant fluoxetine compromises antipredator behaviour in fish. Environmental Pollution. 2017;**222**:592-599. DOI: 10.1016/j.envpol.2016.10.010

[47] DeAngelis DL. Dynamics of Nutrient Cycling and Food Webs. Suffolk: Chapman and Hall, Springer Media; 2012. 288 pp. DOI: 10.1007/978-94-011-2342-6

[48] Seewagen CL. The threat of global mercury pollution to bird migration: Potential mechanisms and current evidence. Ecotoxicology. 2020;**29**:1254-1267. DOI: 10.1007/s10646-018-1971-z

[49] Wilcox C, Sebille EV, Hardesty BD. Threat of plastic pollution to seabirds is global pervasive and increasing. PNAS. 2015;**112**:11899-11904. DOI: 10.1073/pnas.1502108112

[50] Padula V, Beaudreau AH, Causey D, Divine LM, Merculieff M. Including local voices in marine debris conversations to advance environmental justice for island and coastal communities: Perspectives from St. Paul Island, Alaska. Facets. 2023;**8**:0047. DOI: 10.1139/facets-2023-0047

[51] Gagne TO, Johnson EM, Hyrenbach DD, Hagemann ME, Bass OL, MacDonald M, et al. Coupled trophic and contaminant analysis in seabirds through space and time. Environmental Research Communications. 2019;**1**:111006. DOI: 10.1088/2515-7620/ab4921

[52] Fossi MM, Coppola D, Baini M, Giannetti M, Guerranti C, Marsili L, et al. Large filter feeding marine organisms as indicators of microplastic in the pelagic environment: The case studies of the Mediterranean basking shark (*Cetorhinus maximus*) and fin whale (*Balaenoptera physalus*). Marine Environmental Research. 2014;**100**:17-24. DOI: 10.1016/j.marenvres.2014.02.002

[53] Gall SC, Thompson RC. The impact of debris on marine life. Marine Pollution Bulletin. 2015;**92**:170-179. DOI: 10.1016/j.marpolbul.2014.12.041

[54] Padula V, Beaudreau AH, Hagedorn B, Causey D. Plastic-derived contaminants in Aleutian archipelago seabirds with varied foraging strategies. Marine Pollution Bulletin. 2020;**158**:111435. DOI: 10.1016/j.marpolbul.2020.111435

[55] Causey D, Padula VM. Phthalates in western Aleutian Island seabirds. McGraw-Hill AccessScience. 2015;**2015**:YB150685. DOI: 10.1036/1097-8542.YB150685

[56] Rodríguez AF, Carrasco RMN, Chiaradia A. Seabird plastic ingestion differs among collection methods:

Examples from the short-tailed shearwater. Environmental Pollution. 2018;**243**:1750-1757. DOI: 10.1016/j.envpol.2018.09.007

[57] Schwantes U. Impact of anthropogenous environmental factors on the marine ecosystem of trophically transmitted helminths and hosting seabirds: Focus on North Atlantic North Sea Baltic and the Arctic seas. Helminthologia. 2023;**60**:300-326. DOI: 10.2478/helm-2023-0034

[58] Zhang EM, Rueda KL, Rochman C, VanWormer E, Moore J, Shapiro K. Association of zoonotic protozoan parasites with microplastics in seawater and implications for human and wildlife health. Scientific Reports. 2022;**12**:6532. DOI: 10.1038/s41598-022-10485-5

[59] Mavrianos S, Manzi F, Agha R, Azoubib N, Schampera C, Wolinskaya J. Nanoplastics modulate the outcome of a zooplankton-microplastic interaction. Freshwater Biology. 2023;**68**:847-859. DOI: 1111/fwb.14068

[60] Buss NB, Sander JJ. Effects of polyester microplastic fiber contamination on amphibian-trematode interactions. Environmental Toxicology and Chemistry. 2021;**41**:869-879. DOI: 10.1002/etc.5035

[61] Balsdon MKC, Koprivnika J. Effects of microplastics and nanoplastics on host–parasite interactions in aquatic environments. Oecologia. 2024;**204**:413-425. DOI: 10.1007/s00442-023-05502-x

[62] Schampera C, Wolinska J, Bachelier JB, Machado A, Rosal R, González-Pleiter M, et al. Exposure to nanoplastics affects the outcome of infectious disease in phytoplankton. Environmental Pollution. 2021;**277**:116781. DOI: 10.1016/j.envpol.2021.116781

[63] Li M, Ha B, Li Y, Vrieling K, Fu Z, Yu Q, et al. Toxicological impacts of microplastics on virulence reproduction and physiological process of entomopathogenic nematodes. Ecotoxicology and Environmental Safety. 2024;**273**:116153. DOI: 10.1016/j.ecoenv.2024.116153

[64] Hernandez-Milian GA, Lusher S, MacGabban ER. Microplastics in grey seal (*Halichoerus grypus*) intestines: Are they associated with parasite aggregations? Marine Pollution Bulletin. 2019;**146**:349-354. DOI: 10.1016/j.marpolbul.2019.06.014

[65] Soler JJ, Martin-Vivldi M, Peralta-Sanchez JM, Ruiz-Rodriguez M. Antibiotic-producing bacteria as a possible defense of birds against pathogenic microorganisms. The Open Ornithology Journal. 2010;**3**:93-100. DOI: 10.2174/1874453201003010093

[66] Holzapfel WH, Haberer P, Snel J, Schillinger U, Huis in't Veld JH. Overview of gut flora and probiotics. International Journal of Food Microbiology. 1998;**41**:85-101. DOI: 10.1016/s0168-1605(98)00044-0

[67] Pearce DS, Hoover BA, Jennings S, Nevitt GA, Docherty KM. Morphological and genetic factors shape the microbiome of a seabird species (*Oceanodroma leucorhoa*) more than environmental and social factors. Microbiome. 2017;**5**:1-16. DOI: 10.1186/s40168-017-0365-4

[68] Stevens CE, Hume ID. Contributions of microbes in vertebrate gastrointestinal tract to production and conservation of nutrients. Physiological Reviews. 1998;**78**:394-419

[69] Grond K, Sandercock B, Jumpponen A, Zeglin LH. The avian gut microbiota: Community physiology and

function in wild birds. Journal of Avian Biology. 2018;**49**:e01788. DOI: 10.1111/jav.01788

[70] Hird SM, Sanchez C, Carstens BC, Brumfield RT. Comparative gut microbiota of 59 neotropical bird species. Frontiers in Microbiology. 2015;**6**:01403. DOI: 10.3389/fmicb.2015.01403

[71] Kamada N, Chen G, Inohara N, Nunez G. Control of pathogens and pathobionts by the gut microbiota. Nature Immunology. 2023;**14**:685-690. DOI: 10.1038/ni.2608

[72] Lloyd-Price J, Abu-Ali G, Huttenhower C. The healthy human microbiome. Genome Medicine. 2016;**8**:51. DOI: 10.1186/s13073-016-0307-y

[73] Bien J, Palagani V, Bozko P. The intestinal microbiota of dysbiosis and *Clostridium difficile* infection: Is there a relationship with inflammatory bowel disease? Therapeutic Advances in Gastroenterology. 2023;**6**:53-68. DOI: 10.1177/1756283X12454590

[74] Narasimhan S, Swei A, Abouneameh S, Pal U, Pedra JHF, Fikrig E. Grappling with the tick microbiome. Trends in Parasitology. 2021;**37**:722-733. DOI: 10.1016/j.pt.2021.04.004

[75] Glowska E, Filutowska ZK, Dabert M, Gerth M. Microbial composition of enigmatic bird parasites: *Wolbachia* and *Spiroplasma* are the most important bacterial associates of quill mites (Acariformes: Syringophilidae). Microbiology. 2020;**9**:e964. DOI: 10.1002/mbo3.964

[76] Reynolds LA, Finlay BB, Maizels RM. Cohabitation in the intestine: Interactions among helminth parasites bacterial microbiota and host immunity. Journal of Immunology. 2015;**195**:4059-4066. DOI: 10.4049/jimmunol.1501432

[77] Jenkins TP, Rathnayaka Y, Perera PK, Peachey LE, Nolan MJ, Krause L, et al. Infections by human gastrointestinal helminths are associated with changes in faecal microbiota diversity and composition. PLoS ONE. 2017;**12**:e0184719. DOI: 10.1371/journal.pone.0184719

[78] Zaiss MM, Harris NL. Interactions between the intestinal microbiomed and helminth parasites. Parasite Immunology. 2016;**S38**:5-11. DOI: 10.1111/pim.12274

[79] D'Elia R, DeSchoolmeester ML, Zeef LA, Wright SH, Pemberton AD, Else KJ. Expulsion of *Trichuris muris* is associated with increased expression of angiogenin 4 in the gut and increased acidity of mucins within the goblet cell. BMC Genomics. 2009;**10**:492. DOI: 10.1186/1471-2164-10-492

[80] Long SR, Lanter BB, Pazos MA, Mou H, Barrios J, Su CW, et al. Intestinal helminth infection enhances bacteria-induced recruitment of neutrophils to the airspace. Scientific Reports. 2019;**9**:15703. DOI: 10.1038/s41598-019-51991-3

[81] Hayes KS, Bancroft AJ, Goldrick M, Portsmouth C, Roberts IS, Grencis RK. Exploitation of the intestinal microflora by the parasitic nematode *Trichuris muris*. Science. 2010;**328**:1391-1394. DOI: 10.1126/science. 1187703

[82] Stensvold CR, van der Giezen M. Associations between gut microbiota and common luminal intestinal parasites. Trends in Parasitology. 2018;**34**:369-377. DOI: 10.1016/j.pt.2018.02.004

[83] Sabotic J, Kos J. Microbial and fungal protease inhibitors—Current

and potential applications. Applied Microbiology and Biotechnology. 2012;**93**:1351-1375. DOI: 10.1007/s00253-011-3834-x

[84] Blair P, Diemert D. Update on prevention and treatment of intestinal helminth infections. Current Infectious Disease Reports. 2015;**17**:12. DOI: 10.1007/s11908-015-0465-x

[85] Glendenning L, Nausch N, Free A, Taylor DW, Mutapi F. The microbiota and helminths: Sharing the same niche in the human host. Parasitology. 2014;**141**:1255-1271. DOI: 10.1017/S0031182014000699

[86] Sharpton TJ, Combrink L, Arnold HK, Gaulke CA, Kent M. Harnessing the gut microbiome in the fight against anthelminthic drug resistance. Current Opinion in Microbiology. 2020;**53**:26-34. DOI: 10.1016/j.mib.2020.01.017

[87] van Franeker J. Save the North Sea Fulmar-Litter-EcoQO manual part 1: Collection and dissection procedures. In: Alterra Rapport No. 672. Wageningen Netherlands: Alterra; 2004. 38 pp. Available from: https://library.wur.nl/WebQuery/wurpubs/fulltext/40451

[88] Work TM. Avian Necropsy Manual for Biologists in Remote Refuges. Honolulu, Hawaii, USA: USGS Hawaii; 2003. ISBN 13: 9781479138890

[89] Barber S, Puthoff D, Nazar S, Causey D, Hechinger RF, Sheehan KL. Shifts of Black-legged Kittiwake symbiotic communities during an Avian Botulism outbreak. Comparative Parasitology. 2024. (in-review)

[90] Amacker CA. Avian predation on low-salinity shrimp aquaculture [thesis]. Auburn, Alabama: Auburn University; 2023. Available from: https://etd.auburn.edu//handle/10415/8850

[91] Paquin P, Vink CJ. Testing compatibility between molecular and morphological techniques for arthropod systematics and minimally destructive DNA extraction method that preserves morphological integrity and the effect of lactic acid on DNA quality. Journal of Insect Conservation. 2009;**13**:453-457. DOI: 0.1007/s10841-008-9183-0

[92] McDonald D, Price MN, Goodrich J, Nawrocki EP, DeSantis TZ, Probst A, et al. An improved Greengenes taxonomy with explicit ranks for ecological and evolutionary analysis of bacteria and archaea. The ISME Journal. 2012;**6**:610-618. DOI: 10.1038/ismej.2011.139

[93] Quast C, Pruesse E, Yilmaz P, Gerken J, Schweer T, Yarza P, et al. The SILVA ribsosomal RNA gene database project: Improved data processing and web-based tools. Nucleic Acids Research. 2013;**41**:D590-D596. DOI: 10.1093/nar/gks1219

[94] Ormsby MJ, Akinbobola A, Quilliam RS. Plastic pollution and fungal protozoan and helminth pathogens—A neglected environmental and public health issue? Science of the Total Environment. 2003;**882**:163093. DOI: 10.1016/j.scitotenv.2023.163093

[95] Lafferty KD, Morris AK. Altered behavior of parasitized killifish increases susceptibility to predation by bird final hosts. Ecology. 2006;**77**:1390-1397. DOI: 10.2307/2265536

[96] Clements S, Dorr B, Davis J, Luke R, Engle C, Hanson-Dorr K, et al. Diets of scaup occupying baitfish and sportfish farms in Eastern Arkansas. Food Webs. 2020;**23**:e00141. DOI: 10.1016/j.fooweb.2020.e00141

[97] Schoen S, Tremblay F, Bodenstein B, Sheehan K, et al. Ecosystem Status Report 2021: Gulf of Alaska. Stock Assessment and Fishery Evaluation Report. Anchorage, AK: North Pacific Fishery Management Council; 2021. 269 pp. Available from:https://apps-afsc.fisheries.noaa.gov/refm/docs/2021/GOAecosys.pdf

Chapter 11

Major Parasites in Fish Affecting Public Health

Said Dahani and Rachid Khatouf

Abstract

In Morocco, the fishing sector plays a crucial socio-economic role and constitutes one of the cornerstones of the country's economy. However, the role of these products in transmitting parasitic diseases to humans has been acknowledged. The issue of parasites in fish holds significant importance in terms of health, socio-economics, media coverage, and environmental impact. The primary parasites found in fish include nematodes (*Anisakis*), cestodes (*Gymnorhynchus gigas*), protozoa, and isopods. Anisakids take the lead in terms of prevalence in certain fish species, causing the anisakiasis disease in humans. Preventing these diseases in humans relies on actively searching for parasites in fish that are visibly parasitized before their commercialization in the market. Mastering the hazard of "parasites in fish" for humans is a shared responsibility between fishing industry professionals and the relevant health authorities.

Keywords: *Anisakis*, control, fish, hazard, Morocco, parasites

1. Introduction

The fishing sector plays a crucial socio-economic role in Morocco and constitutes one of the pillars of the national economy. However, the role of these products in transmitting parasitic diseases to humans has been recognized. To date, the consumption of raw fish is increasingly widespread globally, which represents an emerging risks for consumers. Indeed, the role of fish products in transmitting parasitic diseases to humans is well-established. They may contain parasites, including those from the Anisakidae family, which is most implicated in human infestations, primarily with two genera: *Anisakis* and *Pseudoterranova*.

Parasites are naturally present in fish of all species worldwide. Specifically, Anisakidae circulate in the marine ecosystem, using marine mammals, birds, or fish as definitive hosts. Through the consumption of raw, undercooked, or inadequately processed fish, humans become accidental hosts. Nevertheless, the ingested Anisakidae cannot reach the adult stage in humans.

2. Replace main parasites of fishery products

Like any animal species, fish and cephalopods (mollusks) are susceptible to parasites. These parasites are naturally present in the marine environment, fish and cephalopods are part of their life cycle. Among them, the Anisakidae family (*Anisakis* and *Pseudoterranova*) poses a hazard to consumer health and can be responsible for anisakidosis in humans.

2.1 Anisakids

Zoonoses account for approximately 75% of emerging diseases. The increasing attention to foodborne zoonoses is the result of two main factors. The first is the rising prevalence of these diseases linked to changes in dietary habits, an increasing rate of international travel, trade exchanges, as well as cultural and demographic changes. The second factor is related to improved diagnostic capabilities through advanced techniques and a higher number of instrumental investigations [1].

However, parasitic zoonoses remain insufficiently studied because their actual and potential economic and health impact are not well unknown. Any infestation caused by nematode larvae belonging to various genera of the Anisakidae family is called anisakidosis, which manifests as either acute or chronic gastric or intestinal forms after several hours to several days, months, or even years post-infestation. The most common Anisakids in humans are *Pseudoterranova*, such as *Pseudoterranova decipiens*, and Anisakis simplex, the latter can also induce allergic problems. Moreover, some 33 allergens of *Anisakis simplex* are thermostable, increasing the allergic risk for consumers. Allergies can result in hives, itching, angioedema, bronchospasm, or, more rarely, anaphylactic shock. Other less common Anisakids in humans, *Contracaecum* spp., which can pose public health issues but remain very rare. Hysterothylacium spp. does not cause any public health problems as it is destroyed at a temperature of 37°C. However, like other genera, its presence in fish can lead to rejection by the consumer.

Indeed, anisakidosis has around 20,000 reported cases to date, with the vast majority (90%) in Japan. Human anisakidosis is usually more common than human pseudoterranovosis in Japan and Europe, although in North America, Pseudoterranova spp. is the most frequent. Cases of human pseudoterranovosis have been reported in Chile and Peru [2].

2.1.1 Morphology

For the classification and differentiation of various genera within the Anisakidae family, criteria such as the morphology of excretory and digestive systems, as well as the sexual organ (spicule), are used [2]. However, the similarity and the morphological resemblance of these worms, including size, shape, differences between males and females, the presence or not of the cuticular striations on the body, as well as the shape of the head and tail, unfortunately complicate their identification [3].

2.1.1.1 Anisakis

The name Anisakis is composed of "anis-" (a Greek prefix meaning different) and "akis" (Greek for spine or spicule). The worms belonging to the genus *Anisakis* are usually found in herring, which serves as the paratenic host, and in whales, which are the definitive hosts.

Anisakis, being nematodes, are unsegmented roundworms with a thick cuticle, ranging in color from light white to yellowish, measuring 2 to 6 cm in length and a few millimeters in diameter. The cuticle is characterized by large, irregular, and discontinuous transverse grooves across the body, with fine parallel ridges between the grooves. On a live larva, a visible white portion of 2 mm in length corresponds to the esophageal ventricle. At the other end, there is a triangular penetration tooth, next to which is the excretory pore followed by the excretory canal.

The larva has a ring-shaped nervous system. Regarding internal morphology, the larva possesses a complete digestive system consisting of a trilabiate mouth (one dorsal and two subventral), an esophagus with two parts (an anterior muscular and a posterior glandular), ending in the anus. The excretory system terminates in ventro-lateral lips, and numerous peri-anal papillae are present. There is no cecum or esophageal appendix [4].

The L3 larva found in fish can measure from 9 to 39 mm in length. Whitish in color, it may be coiled and encysted. Most L3 larvae are located in the body cavity, on the liver, and on the wall of the digestive tract, and less commonly, in the flesh of the fish (**Figure 1**).

2.1.1.2 Pseudoterranova

Worms of the genus *Pseudoterranova* are also known as codworms or sealworms. The L3 larvae of these worms are typically found in the flesh of fish and less commonly in the visceral cavity. The larvae found in fish measure approximately 9 to 58 mm in length and can have a whitish-cream, yellow-brown, or reddish-brown color. They are coiled within irregularly shaped cysts. Morphologically, they are characterized by the presence of an anterior boring tooth near the excretory pore. The esophagus consists of a relatively long proventriculus and a ventricle. The intestine, located immediately behind the ventricle, extends forward as a cecum (retrograde) and narrows backward to enter the rectum, which opens at the anus. The posterior end of the larva bears a small spine called the mucron [5].

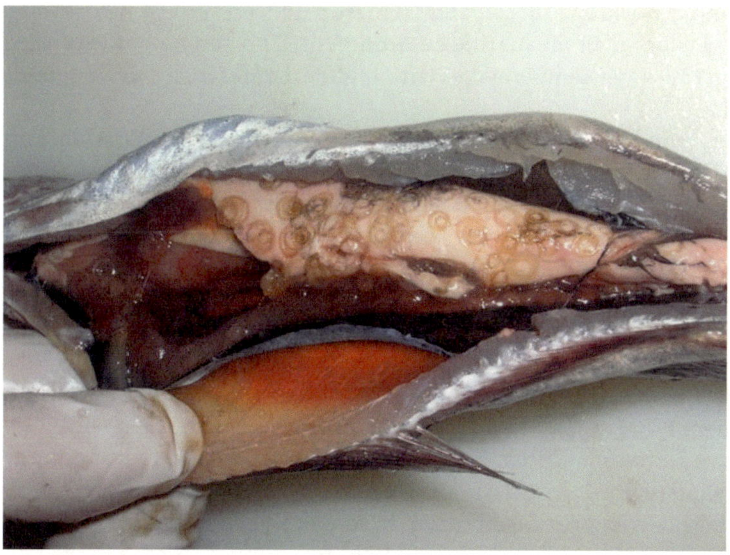

Figure 1.
Larva of Anisakis spp. in Silver scabbardfish.

2.1.1.3 Contracaecum

The worms belonging to the *Contracaecum* spp. genus are whitish-yellow to greenish, and sometimes tinged with red. They have a length of 1.5 to 28.1 mm and a width of 0.13 to 1.18 mm. In adults, males measure between 15 and 70 mm in length and 0.8 to 1.5 mm in width, while females measure between 15 and 90 mm in length and 0.8 to 2 mm in width. The larvae have a pointed tail without a mucron. The excretory pore opens between the two subventral lips. The piercing tooth is small. The esophageal appendix is longer than the cecal appendix. The caudal papillae consist of 2 pairs subventrally and 2 to 3 pairs sublaterally [6–8].

2.1.1.4 Hysterothylacium

Worms belonging to the genus *Hysterothylacium* spp. are Anisakidae with a whitish to gray and highly active larva. The larva has a length of 1.5 to 2.5 mm, and the female can reach 8 cm. They have fish as definitive hosts, with the same individual hosting both larval and adult forms. *Hysterothylacium* does not pose health problems for humans as they are killed at low temperatures. They are very active at 10°C but die at 30°C. The survival of these larvae requires a low temperature [2].

The nematode is characterized by a three-lipped head, each with a pair of triangular ridges, and the presence of semi-interlabia and cervical wings. The worm also has a cuticle with fine transverse striations, an anterior cecum and an esophageal ventricle with a posterior appendix; the appendix and cecum are roughly equal in size, the excretory pore is located at the level of the neural ring, the tail has a terminal "cactus," and the male spicules are approximately equal in size [9].

2.1.2 Life cycle

The Anisakidae have a heteroxenous life cycle (**Figure 2**). Unembryonated eggs of Anisakidae are excreted with the feces of the definitive host into the marine environment. The larvae L1, L2, and L3 mature within the egg before hatching into free-living L3 larvae in the marine environment. The hatching rate of the larvae depends on the water temperature, with higher temperatures leading to faster hatching [10].

The free-living L3 larvae are more often ingested by crustaceans (shrimp, crab, amphipod, krill, etc.), intermediate hosts. Fish and cephalopods then act as paratenic hosts by feeding on the infected crustaceans. If a fish or mollusk carrying L3 larvae is ingested by another non-definitive predator fish, the capsules containing Anisakidae larvae are digested, and the larvae encyst again in this new host, which, in turn, plays the role of a paratenic host. This is crucial from an epidemiological and food safety perspective as larvae can be transferred from one fish to another, leading to an accumulation of these parasites throughout the food chain. Some Anisakidae migrate from the digestive tract to the body cavity and reach various organs. Definitive hosts for the genera *Pseudoterranova* and *Anisakis* are marine mammals, while *Contracaecum* also includes piscivorous birds. *Hysterothylacium* has predator fish as definitive hosts.

After being ingested by this definitive host, L3 develops into L4, L5, and then reaches adulthood and sexual maturity. In some cases, L3 does not progress to the adult stage and causes definitive eosinophilic granulomas, as seen in the *Balaena mysticetus* [11].

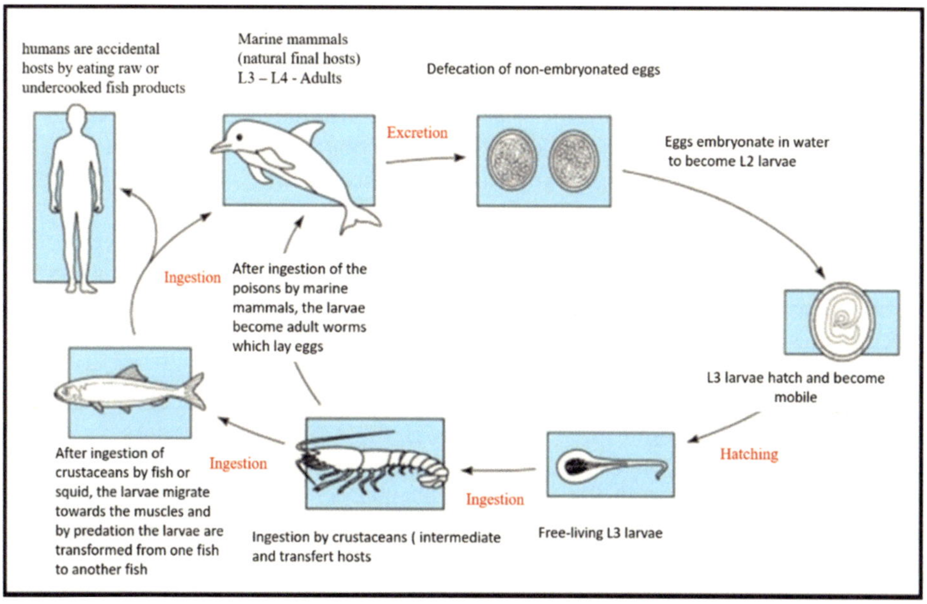

Figure 2.
Anisakis life cycle [2].

Humans are accidental hosts that do not allow the normal development of the larva. Infection occurs through the ingestion of L3 larvae present in raw or undercooked fish. These larvae can cause two types of pathologies: digestive and allergic [10].

Other accidental hosts have been mentioned in the literature, including mammals such as bears, monkeys, dogs [12], cats, raccoons [13], birds, amphibians, and reptiles such as turtles [14], and crocodiles [15].

2.1.3 Impact of Anisakidae on public health

The first case of Anisakid disease was described in 1876 by Leuckart [16]; however, the disease was not widely recognized until the 1960. The larva was identified as *A. simplex* at the 3rd larval stage. Since that time, numerous cases of this zoonotic infestation have been described in other countries, such as Japan where the consumption of raw fish is common. Over 20,000 cases of anisakiasis had been reported worldwide by EFSA on 2010, with the highest prevalence (over 90%) coming from Japan, reporting an annual rate of 2000 to 3000 cases of anisakiasis. The adoption of diverse cuisines worldwide, the development of better diagnostic tools, and an improved understanding of Anisakis and its infestation have led to a significant increase in the reporting of anisakiasis cases. Among other countries where anisakiasis cases have been reported are Korea, China, Malaysia, Taiwan, the UK, Australia, Spain, Italy, France, Germany, Denmark, Norway, Croatia, the USA, South America, Egypt, South Africa, indicating the presence of anisakiasis on every continent except Antarctica.

A strong tradition of consuming raw or undercooked fish, through traditional recipes such as "ceviche" in South America, marinated anchovies in Spain, and raw fish prepared in traditional Japanese dishes like "sushi" and "sashimi," coupled with an exponential increase in the number of restaurants worldwide, are the major risk factors for the spread of anisakiasis [17].

2.1.3.1 Pathogenic power

Humans are accidental hosts of the Anisakis parasite. Infestation occurs through the consumption of fish and marine crustaceans contaminated with third-stage larvae. Two main mechanisms are believed to be responsible for anisakiasis: allergic reactions and direct tissue damage resulting from the penetration of larvae into the site of the target organ [2].

The survival duration of Anisakis in humans is very short, and they are typically expelled or destroyed within a few days or weeks. However, a few hours after ingesting this parasite through an infested fish, the worm burrows into the human intestinal wall, causing an acute and transient infection with symptoms such as abdominal pain, vomiting, or diarrhea. The invasion of the intestinal wall by the parasite sometimes leads to the development of a granuloma or perforation, causing direct tissue damage.

The part of the gastrointestinal tract in which the Anisakis larva lodges, and the type of Anisakis spp. ingested, largely determine the clinical manifestations of observed anisakiasis. Penetration of the gastric mucosa leads to inflammation, giving rise to some of the symptoms. Anisakis can cause gastrointestinal infections, which can be classified into acute, chronic, ectopic, or allergic reactions [17].

2.1.3.2 Gastric form

In gastric anisakiasis, a predilection for penetration into the greater curvature of the stomach has been suggested. The larva burrows into the walls of the stomach. Typically, significant edema of the gastric mucosa around the penetration site is observed through endoscopy. The typical clinical presentation is often reported as acute and severe epigastric pain, nausea, vomiting, mild fever, excessive salivation, and heartburn occurring a few hours after the consumption of infected fish, with symptoms developing within 12 hours [8].

2.1.3.3 Intestinal form

Intestinal anisakiasis presents with non-specific clinical features such as nausea, vomiting, or diarrhea, typically developing 1 to 5 days after the consumption of infected fish. It is known to take more time for symptoms of intestinal anisakiasis to manifest as the incubation period is longer (3 to 72 hours). However, it has been recognized that patients are often misdiagnosed with other diseases such as intestinal inflammation, intestinal obstruction, ulcer, acute appendicitis, diverticulitis, mad cow disease, etc. [6].

2.1.3.4 Allergic reaction

In all cases, the body responds to the intrusion of the parasite with an eosinophil-mediated immune reaction. When the parasite lodges in the organism, it secretes biochemical substances foreign to the immune system, triggering the migration of eosinophils towards the parasite, forming a granuloma around it and isolating it from the organism. This immune response is responsible for the inflammatory reaction in the host, manifested by hives, rhinitis, bronchoconstriction, coughing, asthma, conjunctivitis, contact dermatitis, gastrointestinal symptoms (epigastric pain and nausea), intestinal edema, and potentially anaphylactic shock [2].

2.2 *Gymnorhynchus gigas*

Pomfret, among the most consumed fish by humans worldwide, exhibits a high level of parasitism by *Gymnorhynchus gigas*. However, since it is not transmissible to humans, and its potential relevance to human health has not been questioned, and it poses no hazard to consumers, it is noteworthy that this parasite, despite its abundance in nature, has not been studied to date [18].

2.2.1 Morphology

Gymnorhynchus gigas is a flatworm visible to the naked eye. When young, it is dark white, almost transparent, and as it ages, it becomes larger, with its color shifting towards yellowish-white and becoming more opaque. *G. gigas* consists of three distinct parts:

- Anterior or cephalic part: It contains the scolex, usually invaginated, measuring approximately 11 × 1.9–2 mm. It has four botryoids at the apical end and four proboscides enclosed in a sheath that can be reversible from the scolex, containing hooks at the end of the stalk.

- Central part: Formed by an ovoid vesicle, about 12 × 12 cm in diameter.

- Caudal part: Its length and width are highly variable, sometimes measuring up to 1 m long. It performs complex convolutions within the fish's musculature, making the parasite difficult to remove in its entirety (**Figure 3**) [18].

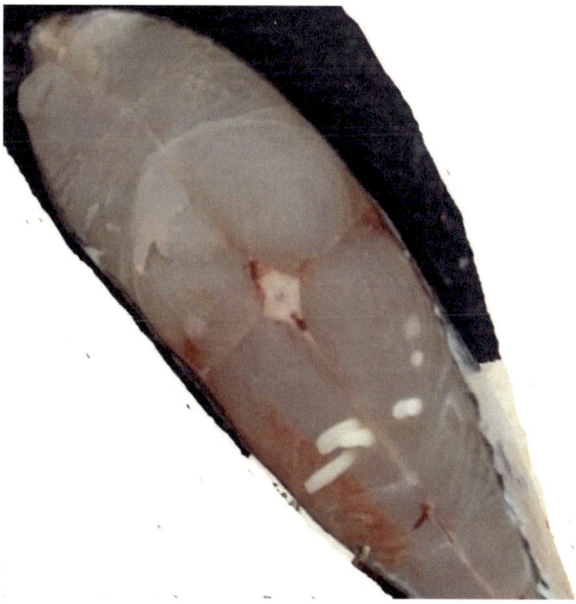

Figure 3.
Larva of Gymnorhynchus gigas in Pomfret.

2.2.2 Life cycle

Life cycle involving at least two hosts. Fish can serve as final or intermediate hosts for these tapeworms, which are oviparous, and their eggs are transmitted in the feces of the final host. The eggs hatch in water to release free-swimming larvae, propelled by cilia. In the order Trypanorhyncha, these larvae are called coracidium and must be ingested by a suitable invertebrate intermediate host, typically a crustacean, mollusk, clupeid, or scombrid. The tapeworm larva penetrates through the intestinal wall of the host and undergoes a transformation process in the abdominal cavity to the procercoid stage, capable of infecting the fish host. If the procercoid is ingested by a suitable fish host, it penetrates the intestinal wall and encysts in the viscera or musculature, where it develops into the plerocercoid stage.

Fish in which a plerocercoid stage is formed act as second intermediate hosts, such as teleosts. The life cycle completes when an infected fish is eaten by a definitive host, which is an elasmobranch (rays and sharks), in whose intestine the tapeworm develops to maturity.

The plerocercoids of *Gymnorhynchus gigas* are often found in the musculature of the Ray's bream (*Brama raii*), causing a mass invasion in the fish muscles. The mode of infection appears to be either through the fish's skin or by ingesting zooplankton or parasitized crustaceans [19].

2.2.3 Health aspect

The parasite *Gymnorhynchus gigas* is capable of causing significant changes in the musculature. These changes are sometimes visible in freshly caught fish, appearing as grayish spots that become more evident when the parasite is in the superficial layers of the musculature, closer to the skin. The muscle tissue around the parasite may have a yellowish color compared to the pinkish-white color of healthy muscle and histologically shows interstitial myositis. The parasite itself and these lesions are likely to reduce the shelf life and assessment of fish inspection, directly affecting organoleptic characteristics; the muscle is less firm, and analytical parameters (chemical and microbiological) used for freshness evaluation are indirectly disrupted [20].

This parasite contributes to the fish's unpleasant taste and poses an economic issue by being a reason for rejecting Moroccan fish intended for export.

2.3 Protozoa

Protozoa are commonly encountered in fish, with major groups including ciliates, flagellates, microsporidia, and myxosporidia. They can accumulate in large numbers in fish, leading to weight loss, debilitation, and mortality. Ciliates and flagellates have direct life cycles and particularly affect fish populations raised in ponds. Some of these protozoans can cause more or less pathogenic effects in their fish hosts. This is the case for myxosporidia and microsporidia.

2.3.1 Kudoa spp

The genus *Kudoa* belongs to the phylum *Myxospora*, class *Myxosporea*, order Multivalvulida, and family Kudoidae.

Myxosporean parasites affect many fish families and are common in cichlids, cyprinids, and mugilids [21]. In Africa, more than 135 species of Myxosporea are known to infect freshwater, brackish, and marine fish [22].

Kudoa spp. have a global distribution and infect a wide range of host species. One of the main concerns is that these species are responsible for economic losses in the fishing sector by causing post-mortem myoliquefaction.

K. septempunctata was recently identified as the causative agent of a previously unidentified foodborne illness associated with the consumption of olive flounder (*Paralichthys olivaceus*) in Japan. Since 2003, outbreaks of unidentified foodborne illnesses associated with the consumption of raw fish have increased, and this Myxosporean is implicated as the etiological agent, demonstrating the pathogenic potential of Kudoa spores. Clinical symptoms include severe diarrhea and vomiting 2–20 hours after ingesting raw, parasitized fish. In a study, anti-*Kudoa* spp. IgE antibodies were observed in patients experiencing allergic reactions after consuming fish. In experimental models, oral administration of pseudocysts to mice induced specific IgE antibodies. These IgE responses confirm the possible allergenic nature of certain parasite components [23].

Depending on the site of infestation, two forms of *Myxosporea* have been defined:

Coelozoic forms are free in the lumen of organs such as the gall bladder and urinary bladder.

Hystozoic forms are localized in host tissues where they generally induce cyst formation. Hystozoic species are the most pathogenic. In severe infestations, they can lead to the destruction of parasitized tissues and result in the death of the host. Additionally, Myxosporea infestation can expose fish to secondary contamination by other microorganisms such as viruses or bacteria (**Figure 4**) [24].

2.3.2 Glugea spp

The genus *Glugea* spp. is a microsporidian belonging to the phylum Microsporidia, class Microsporea, order Glugeida, and family Glugeidae [25]. They are strict

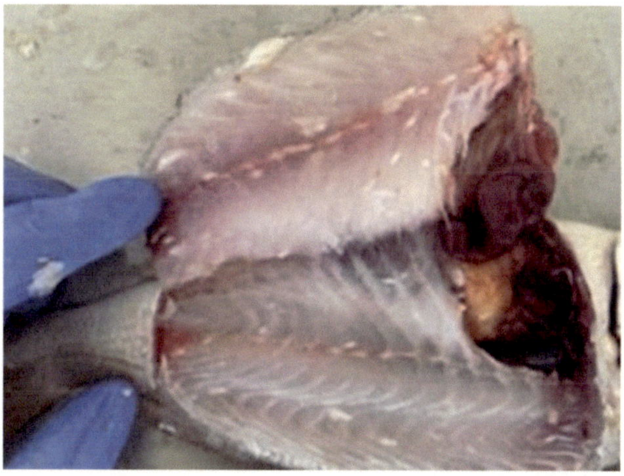

Figure 4.
Xenoparasite formation in Axillary seabream.

intracellular parasites that infect both vertebrates and invertebrates. There are more than 1300 species of microsporidia worldwide. Their classification is primarily based on morpho-anatomical characteristics obtained through light and electron microscopy. All microsporidia exhibit a form of resistance and dissemination, the spore, which is often small (1 to 5 μm long, rarely reaching 20 μm) and usually ovoid or spherical [24].

Fish hosts become infected by ingesting infectious spores from contaminated fish or food. Infected cells generally enlarge (xenomes) to accommodate proliferating parasites, which develop through merogony and sporogony inside the xenomes, leading to spore production. Infected cells hypertrophy and can reach macroscopic sizes, often resulting in characteristic pathological signs, such as multiple whitish nodules in tissues or, in the case of the bladder, significant thickening of the walls. The impact of microsporidia infestation on fish hosts varies. Some fish hosts seem to survive even in the presence of huge xenomes exerting pressure on organs, while in others, microsporidia have a morbid effect. Intranuclear infection of hematopoietic cells is often associated with acute anemia [22].

2.4 Parasitic crustaceans

Crustacean parasites are arthropods characterized by two pairs of antennae and branchial respiration. In higher forms, their chitin is calcified. Their adaptation to parasitism often leads to significant regression of organs and limbs, and they are classified as crustaceans mainly based on their characteristic larval stages [26].

They pose increasingly serious problems in both farmed and wild fish populations. These ectoparasites attach to the gills, body, and fins of fish hosts [22].

2.4.1 Copepods

Copepods are a group of small crustaceans found in almost all freshwater and saltwater habitats. There are planktonic species (living in seawater) and benthic species (living on the ocean floor). Their size varies considerably, but they generally measure 1 to 2 mm in length, with a tear-shaped body and large antennae. Like other crustaceans, they have a tough exoskeleton, but they are so small that in most species, this fine armor and the entire body are almost entirely transparent.

Parasitic copepods are characterized by monoxenous and heteroxenous cycles, going through several larval stages (molts) to reach the adult stage. Nauplius, copepodite, chalimus, and preadult stages are characteristic stages of the copepod development cycle. Parasites with a complex life cycle, using multiple hosts, are generally less specific than those with a direct cycle. Parasites with a direct life cycle often actively search for their host, while the transfer of parasitic stages in species with a complex cycle occurs passively, mainly through predation interactions [27].

Copepods have a pathogenic effect that manifests as tissue destruction during parasite penetration, anemia, extensive damage to the gills, and skin erosion. Generally, the attachment points are marked by a circular red depression, while the peripheral area becomes hemorrhagic and inflamed, sometimes ulcerated with partial loss of the epithelium. Pathogenic copepods include the Pennellidae and Sphyridae families (**Figure 5**) [24].

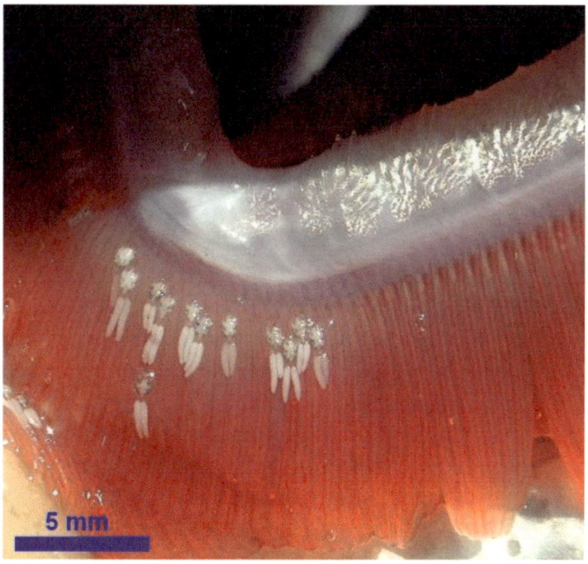

Figure 5.
Ergasilus sp. (a genus of copepod crustaceans) females, each carrying a pair of eggs on the gills.

2.4.2 Isopods

Parasitic isopods measure from 1 to 100 mm in length and are easily distinguished from other crustaceans by their body segmentation (seven thoracic segments and six posterior segments). The most significant ones belong to the family Cymothoidae, the adult forms are found in the mouth or gill cavities. Juveniles are swimming forms looking for a host, on which they attach, transform into males, and later into females [26].

These parasites often cause various pathologies in their hosts, such as epithelial erosions, inflammation, and necrosis of the dermis developing at the attachment point of the parasite to the skin, as well as deformations of gill filaments, and sometimes significant mortality. Infested individuals become unsuitable for consumption [24].

3. Search for parasites in fish

We adopted a fieldwork approach, examining 354 pieces of fish belonging to 29 different species. This examination involves looking by eye, firstly for ectoparasites on the skin, oral cavity and fins, and secondly for internal parasites in the abdominal cavity and flesh. At the end of this research, we found 60 pieces of infested fish containing 657 parasites of different species, thus giving an overall prevalence of 16.94%, an overall abundance of 1.86, and an absolute intensity of 10.95. These infestation parameters vary depending on the species of fish and the type of parasite.

The L3 infesting larva of the *Anisakis* nematode dominates with a prevalence of 11.30%. The plerocercoid larva of the cestode *Gymnorhynchus gigas* was found with a prevalence of 3.11% and appears to exclusively infest the pomfret (*Brama brama*), in which the prevalence is 100%. Xenomas, a whitish nodular formation, were found only in species of the sparid family, with a prevalence of 1.42%. Isopod parasitic crustaceans were found in the pomfret and the Axillary seabream (*Pagellus acarne*) with a prevalence of 1.12%. The pomfret and the Silver scabbardfish (*Lepidopus caudatus*), show a higher level of risk for parasitism with respective prevalences of 100 and 76.92%.

A positive correlation was demonstrated between the total length, the weight of the fish and the intensity of parasitism.

Fish caught off the Moroccan coast as everywhere in the world are infested by nematodes, trematodes and cestodes with varying prevalence depending on the species of fish and therefore constitutes a subject of concern to the consumer and a challenge for the health authorities and professionals in a co-regulatory framework. These parasites are responsible for emerging zoonotic diseases and can be transmissible to humans despite being generally neglected in discussions on the safety of fish products [28]. These zoonosis were considered specific to low-income populations, but tend to evolve due to the diversification of international markets, the development of means of transport and demographic changes [29]. According to the Health Organization World, more than 18 million people are infected with fish-borne parasites; worldwide, more than half a billion people are at risk of being infected [30]. Prioritization of public health systems in countries must give more resources and attention to these parasitic zoonosis of fish and must overcome the lack of data on their health and economic impact. Fish parasites are transmitted to humans following the consumption of raw or undercooked fish, inducing a form of morbidity rather than mortality [31]. Food inspection and control rules vary from country to country and are often inadequate [32]. Indeed, European Union legislation specifies in Commission Regulation No. 1276/2011 of December 8 [33], 2011 amending Annex III to Regulation (EC) No. 853/2004 of the European Parliament and of the Council [34], the axes measures to combat these parasites, namely their removal when they are visible and the application of a sanitizing treatment for products intended to be consumed raw, making it possible to kill any parasites that may have escaped visual inspection. Regulation (EC) No. 2074/2005 defines the visual inspection of fishery products as non-destructive, and specifies the methods of carrying it out in terms of sampling [35]. The visual inspection is carried out with the naked eye, and can be supplemented by the candling technique when the latter is adapted to the products subject to inspection (thin-thickness parts). However, despite the sanitizing treatment, the presence of dead larvae has been associated with allergenicity in sensitive people, due to the thermostability of certain allergens, notably Anisakis [36].

4. Conclusions

The phenomenon of fish parasitism remains a serious health problem (Fish products that are visibly parasitized can transmit parasitic diseases to humans), also leading to significant economic losses since it is considered as main reason for refoulement and seizure. Controlling the hazard of parasites in fish is based on a shared responsibility between professionals in the fishing industry and the competent health authorities. In this regard, the search for parasites in fish should be systematically conducted before their commercialization in markets. Raising consumer awareness about methods to kill parasites, namely: freezing (−20°C for 24 hours or −35°C for 15 hours), cooking, or hot smoking.

Among the perspectives to be considered in future research for parasites, the molecular analysis of larvae collected from the Moroccan coasts to better understand their distribution, their origins and their infectious power. This would help to better assess the risk for sensitized people. Furthermore, training on parasites in fishery products should be considered and carried out to reach the maximum number of professionals within the fish supply chain, in order to avoid the marketing of fishery products containing parasites and to prevent human infection.

Furthermore, it is crucial to observe the "One Health" concept by training students at universities, research centers and cross-sectoral organizations to regulate and prevent zoonoses by integrating all levels to achieve the desired public health outcomes examining the relationships between people, animals and plants and their shared environment.

Conflict of interest

The authors declare no conflict of interest.

Author details

Said Dahani* and Rachid Khatouf
Department of Veterinary Pathology and Public Health, Food Safety Unit, Hassan II Agronomic and Veterinary Institute, Rabat, Morocco

*Address all correspondence to: s.dahani@iav.ac.ma

References

[1] Menghi C, Gatta G, Liliana E, Gabriela S, Federico N, Smayevsky J, et al. Human infection with Pseudoterranova cattani by ingestion of "ceviche" in Buenos Aires, Argentina. Revista Argentina de Microbiología. 2019, 2020;**52**(2):118-120

[2] Seesao Y. Caractérisation des Anisakidae dans les poissons marins: Développement d'une méthode d'identification par séquençage à haut-débit et étude de prévalence Médecine humaine et pathologie. France: Université du Droit et de la Santé—Lille II; 2016

[3] Ángeles-Hernández JC, Gómez-de Anda FR, Reyes-Rodríguez NE, Vega-Sánchez V, García-Reyna PB, Campos-Montiel RG, et al. Genera and species of the Anisakidae Family and their geographical distribution. Animals. 2020;**10**:2374. DOI: 10.3390/ani10122374

[4] Orain M. Apport De L'histologie Dans La Detection D'Anisakis Simplex Et De Kudoa Sp. In: Dans Les Poissons Et Les Matieres Premieres Utilisees Dans L'industrie Ou Dans Les Produits Finis. These de doctorat vétérinaire. France: Université Paul-Sabatier de Toulouse; 2010

[5] Smith J, Wootten R. Pseudoterranova larvae ('Codworm') (Nematoda) in fish. Fiches d'identification des maladies et parasites des poissons, crustaces et mollusques. 1984;7:3-4

[6] Cohen S. Les risques parasitaires liés à la consommation de poisson cru Thèse de doctorat vétérinaire (Thèse vétérinaire). Université Paris-Est Créteil Val de Marne Doukkali, M. R. A. K., 2018. Système marocain de production halieutique et sa dépendance du reste du monde, 117 p. 2004

[7] Falaise P. Les parasites de poisson, agents de zoonoses. Université de Toulouse. Thèse d'exercice, Médecine vétérinaire, Ecole Nationale Vétérinaire de Toulouse—ENVT, 248 p. FAO, 1982. Parasites, infections et maladies du poisson en Afrique. 2017

[8] Gonzales S. Risques d'infection parasitaire par le poisson cru: Cas de l'anisakidose et de la bothriocéphalose. Thèse de doctorat en pharmacie. France: Université de Limoges; 2013. p. 123

[9] Berland B. Hysterothylacium Ad Uncum (nematoda) in Fish. ICES Identification Leaflets for Diseases and Parasites of Fish and Shellfish 2-4, Dk-1261 Copenhague k, Danemark. 1991. DOI: 10.17895/ices.pub.5215

[10] Audicana M, Kennedy M. Anisakis simplex: From obscure infectious worm to inducer of immune hypersensitivity. Clinical Microbiology Reviews. 2008;**21**(2):360-379

[11] Migaki G, Heckmann R, Albert T. Gastric nodules caused by "anisakis type" larvae in the bowhead whale (*Balaena mysticetus*). Journal of Wildlife Diseases. 1982;**18**(3):353-357. DOI: 10.7589/0090-3558-18.3.353

[12] Smith JW, Wootten R. Anisakis and Anisakiasis. In: Advances in Parasitology. Academic Press; 1978. pp. 93-163. DOI: 10.1016/S0065-308X(08)60573-4

[13] Sato H, Suzuki K. Gastrointestinal helminthes of feral raccons (Procyon lotor) in Wakayama prefecture, Japan. The Journal of Veterinary Medical Science. 2006;**68**(4):311-318

[14] Santoro M, Mattiucci S, Paoletti M, Liotta A, Degli UB, Galiero G, et al. Molecular identification and pathology

of Anisakis pegreffii (Nematoda: Anisakidae) infection in the Mediterranean loggerhead sea turtle (Caretta caretta). Veterinary Parasitology. 2010;**174**(1-2):65-71

[15] AFSSA. Avis de l' Agence Française de Sécurité Sanitaire des Aliments relativf à la consommation de la viande de crocodile en France, AFSSA, Saisine n°2006-SA-0229. Maison Alfort, France; 2007;**1**:1-22

[16] Leuckart. Infección pr Anisakis simplex: Anisakiasis parasitación en niño de Groenladia Prevalencia desconocida Epidemiología. 1876. Available from: http://www.alergomurcia.com [consulté le February 20, 2023]

[17] Ibukun EA, Peter MS, Andreas LA. Anisakis nematodes in fish and shellfish-from infection to allergies. International Journal for Parasitology: Parasites and Wildlife. 2019:384-393. DOI: 10.1016/j.ijppaw.2019.04.007

[18] Vázquez-López C, Armas-Serra C, Rodríguez-Caa F. *Gymnorhynchus gigas*: taxonomía, morfología, biología y aspectos sanitarios. Departamento de Microbiología y Parasitología Facultad de Farmacia. España: Universidad de Alcalá; 2001

[19] Rodero M, Cue'llar C. Humoral immune responses induced by Gymnorhynchus gigas extracts in BALB/c mice. Journal of Helminthology. 1999;**73**:239-243

[20] Panebianco F. Biologia caratteri morfologici strutturali metodi di pesca parassitosi linea di condotta nella i.c. Progresso Veterinario. 1952;**8**:65-68

[21] Paperna I. Parasites, infections et maladies du poisson en Afrique. Vol. 7. Rome: Food & Agriculture Organisation; 1982

[22] Iyaji F, Eyo J. Parasites and their freshwater fish host. Bio-Research. 2009;**6**(1):328-338. DOI: 10.4314/br.v6i1.28660

[23] Daschner A. Risks and possible health effects of raw fish intake. In: Fish and Fish Oil in Health and Disease Prevention. Elsevier Inc.; 2016. pp. 341-353. DOI:10.1016/B978-0-12-802844-5.00031-2

[24] Khalifa SO. Contribution A l'etude Des Parasites Et Parasitoses Des Poissons Marins Des Cotes Mauritaniennes, études approfondies de productions animales. (Universite cheikh anta diop de dakar). 2006

[25] Lores B, Rosales MJ, Mascaró C, Osuna A. In vitro culture of Glugea sp. Veterinary Parasitology. 2003;**112**(3):185-196. DOI: 10.1016/S0304-4017(02)00411-9

[26] Alexandre AF. Les Parasites Et Parasitoses Des Poissons D'ornementaux D'eau Douce, Aide Au Diagnostic Et Propositions De Traitements. These pour Le doctorat veterinaire. France: École Nationale Veterinaire D'alfort; 2005

[27] Boualleg C, Seridi M, Kaouachi N, Quiliquini Y, Bensouillah M. Les Copépodes parasites des poissons téléostéens du littoral Est-algérien. Bulletin de l'Institut Scientifique, Rabat, section Sciences de la Vie. 2010;**32**(2):65-72

[28] Shamsi S. Seafood-borne parasitic diseases: A "one-health" approach is needed. Fishes. 2019;**4**(1):9. DOI: 10.3390/fishes4010009

[29] Chai JY, Murrell KD, Lymbery AJ. Fish-borne parasitic zoonoses: Status and issues. International Journal for Parasitology. 2005;**35**(11-12):1233-1254. DOI: 10.1016/j.ijpara.2005.07.013

[30] Ziarati M, Zorriehzahra MJ, Hassantabar F, Mehrabi Z, Dhawan M, Sharun K, et al. Zoonotic diseases of fish and their prevention and control. Veterinary Quarterly. 2022;**42**(1):95-118. DOI: 10.1080/01652176.2022.2080298

[31] Cong W, Elsheikha HM. Biology, epidemiology, clinical features, diagnosis, and treatment of selected fish-borne parasitic zoonoses. Yale Journal of Biology and Medicine. 2021;**94**(2):297-309

[32] Williams M, Hernandez-Jover M, Shamsi S. Parasites of zoonotic interest in selected edible freshwater fish imported to Australia. Food and Waterborne Parasitology. 2022;**26**(November 2021):e00138. DOI: 10.1016/j.fawpar.2021.e00138

[33] Commission Regulation (EC) No. 1276/2011 of 8 December 2011 amending Annex III to Regulation (EC) No. 853/2004 of the European Parliament and of the Council as regards treatments aimed at killing viable parasites in food products. fishing intended for human consumption

[34] Commission Regulation (EC) No. 853/2004 of the European Parliament and of the Council of April 29, 2004 establishing specific hygiene rules applicable to foodstuffs of animal origin. Regulation (EC) No. 854/2004 of the European Parliament and of the Council of April 29, 2004 laying down specific rules for the organization of official controls concerning products of animal origin intended for human consumption

[35] Commission Regulation (EC) No 2074/2005 of 5 December 2005 establishing implementing measures relating to certain products governed by Regulation (EC) No 853/2004 of the European Parliament and of the Council and to the organization of official controls provided for by Regulations (EC) No 854/2004 of the European Parliament and of the Council and (EC) No 882/2004 of the European Parliament and of the Council, derogating from Regulation (EC) No 852/2004 of the European Parliament and of the Council and amending Regulations (EC) No 853/2004 and (EC) No 854/2004

[36] EFSA, Biohaz H. Scientific opinion on risk assessment of parasites in fishery products. EFSA Journal. 2010;**8**(4):1543. DOI: 10.2903/j.efsa.2010.1543

Chapter 12

Advancement in the Identification of Parasites and Obstacles in the Treatment of Intestinal Parasitic Infections: A Brief Overview

Km. Deepika, Amit Baliyan, Anshu Chaudhary and Bindu Sharma

Abstract

Nowadays, intestinal parasite infections (IPIs) continue to be a serious public health issue worldwide. Helminth and protozoa are common examples of infections caused by poverty and inadequate sanitation, which act as two variables linked to IPIs. In response to the growing impact of IPIs, more advanced detection techniques have been researched and developed. To identify these parasites, the diagnostic method's efficacy is paramount. In view of the above, microscopy as a traditional method is now assisted by serology and molecular biological tools. The modern technological tools will help to assess the efficacy of eliminating these parasitic illnesses and future control programs.

Keywords: intestinal parasites, helminths, diseases management, infection, protozoa

1. Introduction

Infectious illnesses have long posed a hazard to the global population throughout history. Nowadays, intestinal parasites account for a significant portion of the world's illness burden. A variety of parasite species are known to be common worldwide, particularly in sub-Saharan Africa, the United States, and Asia [1–3]. The intestinal parasitic infections (IPIs) are widely documented in underdeveloped nations and nowadays also continue to impair human well-being in affluent countries. *Ascaris lumbricoides*, *Trichuris trichiura*, and hookworm are examples of helminths that commonly cause infections, while protozoa such as *Blastocystis hominis*, *Cryptosporidium* sp., *Entamoeba histolytica*, and *Giardia duodenalis* causes infections that are typically due to significant morbidity and mortality, especially in endemic countries [4]. An estimated 2 billion people suffer intestinal parasite infections, and the number is estimated to have increased significantly every year, with an additional 4 billion people at risk of contracting infections [5, 6]. Among the reasons causing these diseases are extreme poverty, inadequate sanitation, social stigma, and a lack of knowledge about the prevention and treatment of these conditions [7]. Moreover, in a study it was

 IntechOpen

	Diagnostic approaches				
	Microscopy-based	**Serology-based**	**Molecular-based**	**Proteomics**	**References**
Helminth					
Schistosoma species	Using Kato-Katz technique	IHA, ELISA, dipstick	PCR, real-time PCR, multiplex PCR	LC-MS/MS	[12–18]
Soil-transmitted helminths	Using sedimentation or concentration techniques	ELISA	Multiplex real-time PCR	—	[19, 20]
Taenia solium	Using sedimentation or concentration techniques	ELISA, Immunoblo	Nested PCR	LC-MS/MS	[21–24]
Protozoa					
C. parvum, C. hominis	Using modified acid-fast staining	DFA, ICT assay kit	PCR, real-time PCR, multiplex real-time PCR, LAMP, Luminex	LC-MS/MS	[21, 25–29]
Giardia lamblia	Using trichrome or ion hematoxylin staining; Using concentration or sedimentation techniques	DFA, ICT assay kit	Multiplex real-time PCR	—	[21, 30–33]
Entamoeba histolytica	Using staining methods	IHA, IIF, ELISA, ICT assay	Multiplex real-time PCR, LAMP	LC-MS/MS	[34–39]

Table 1.
Diagnostic approach for the detection of intestinal parasites.

reported that the host immune system, the afflicted organ, and the type of parasite were all factors that affect IPIs [8]. IPIs seldom result in death, but they can stunt a person's development, especially in young children [9].

As the parasite infections increase, new advanced techniques and methods for the identification of parasite have been used [10]. Modern methods should also take less time to complete without sacrificing the caliber of the output. Many researchers prompt diagnosis is so essential and has remained a top goal to accurately identify the parasites, provide the proper treatment, and ultimately prevent patient deaths [11]. This brief review article will go over the various methodologies that were frequently employed in previous laboratory diagnostics, although each method has its own pros and cons. Here provides an additional summary of the techniques utilized in the diagnosis of many parasites that cause IPIs, the data was tabulated (**Table 1**) [40–42].

2. Advancement in parasite diagnosis

Several assays have been developed during the past few decades to improve the sensitivity and specificity of the test done for parasite identification. The diagnosis of parasitic illnesses has reached a new height because of advances in knowledge and technology. These methods have been used in many research projects around the globe, which has made it possible to combat with disease [41].

2.1 Microscopy-based approach

The only method available at the time for identifying parasites from cerebrospinal fluid, feces, blood smears, and tissue specimens was routine laboratory diagnosis, which includes the conventional microscopy technique. For the morphological identification of parasites, this technique has been widely used as this approach just needs a microscope and cheap reagents or dyes [11]. Nevertheless, over the time, even though microscopy examination has been regarded as the gold standard, it has become increasingly challenging to identify or differentiate the species with the unaided eye. This is because high-quality results require the expertise of a skilled microscopist, and the entire process—from sample collection to the concentration of the parasite's identification—takes time. This condition was further demonstrated by the fact that morphological inspection alone was insufficient to differentiate between the species. Dual procedures such formalin-ether sedimentation, trichrome, and Ziehl-Neelsen staining are typically applied jointly despite the drawback.

Furthermore, other methods like Kato-katz and McMaster counting methods are also widely used nowadays and have been considered as standard techniques for the detection and quantification of IPIs for nearly forty years. Since then, the WHO has recommended them. In the meanwhile, the McMaster counting method is widely used to evaluate STHs or soil-transmitted helminths. The sensitivity of both approaches was shown to vary significantly across trials. The McMaster technique is based on the floating of eggs, whereas the Kato-Katz method covers a larger quantity of feces but has a downside when the infection intensity is relatively low. Additionally, both methods can be used to diagnose IPIs, though, because of its robust factor, the latter is better suited for additional standardization.

2.2 Serology-based approach

If the parasite density is low, for example, as in the case of *Toxoplasma gondii*, it cannot be directly identified because of its life cycle in the host. Therefore, an indirect method of parasite identification employed a serology-based technique needs to be used. Together with the ability to view the parasites under a microscope, the advent of serology-based approaches has made it possible to diagnose IPIs more quickly and effectively. The two subcategories of serology-based diagnosis are antigen detection assays and antibody detection assays. It includes hemagglutination (HA) test, complement fixation (CF) test, immunoblotting, enzyme-linked immunosorbent assay (ELISA), indirect or direct immunofluorescent antibody (IFA or DFA), and rapid diagnostic tests (RDTs) [41]. In the laboratory diagnosis techniques, ELISA test is the most widely used antibody detection test. Although, dipstick assays that are simpler and have a higher sensitivity than microscopy when it comes to identifying intestinal schistosomiasis, have also been thought to be a more sensible option [16].

Because of their sensitivity, two more serology-based tests are also frequently used in laboratories, i.e., indirect hemagglutination (IHA) and indirect immunofluorescence (IIF). However, few researches have been done to examine their repeatability [43]. Moreover, immunoassays have emerged as a primary diagnostic method for parasites [44, 45]. Several commercial kits in the market use an immunoassay-based method to test the parasites using FITC-monoclonal antibodies that target cell wall antigens to detect *Giardia* and *Cryptosporidium* [41]. It took less time to conduct the test and is easier to comprehend the assay's results. But one drawback of the serology-based approach is that, because antibodies are present at different times after infection, the diagnosis is made retrospectively (**Figure 1**) [40, 41].

2.3 Molecular-based approach

Polymerase chain reaction (PCR) technology has grown in importance as a tool for quantifying parasites and assessing the effectiveness of treatment regimens. This method provides higher specificity and sensitivity than the existing diagnostic tests. As technologies have developed, nested, multiplexed, and real-time PCR have replaced classical PCR. By focusing on the 18S rRNA, the PCR technique has effectively identified Cryptosporidium from ambient samples in cases of protozoan illnesses [26]. Furthermore, as noted, the multiplex real-time PCR assay, which was utilized to identify *E. histolytica*, *G. lamblia,* and *C. parvum/C. hominis*, was shown to be similar to microscopy and permit the simultaneous detection of several sequences within a single reaction tube [21]. By using a pentaplex real-time PCR approach, in a previous study four species of soil-transmitted helminths: *Ancylostoma, Necator americanus, Ascaris lumbricoid*es, and *Strongyloides stercoralis* was effectively detected [20]. For the detection of DNA of *Taenia solium* based on the TSO31 gene, nested PCR has demonstrated 100% sensitivity and specificity [48]. Other earlier research has shown the sensitivity of real-time PCR in identifying *Giardia* and *Cryptosporidium* (oo) cysts [49, 50]. The traditional PCR-based approach takes a long time and yields non-quantitative results [51]. Though cost is an issue for both real-time and multiplex PCR, both have produced quick results in comparison to 64 Advances in Parasite Diagnosis and Challenges using the traditional approach [11]. Additionally, one of the most used methods for identifying parasites like *Toxoplasma gondii* is restriction fragment length polymorphism (RFLP) [11, 52]. This method can identify several genotypes from a single sample, based on the digestion of PCR products by restriction enzymes, is appropriate for environmental samples [53].

In addition to the PCR-based methods, numerous alternative amplification techniques also have been developed. Loop-mediated isothermal amplification (LAMP) is

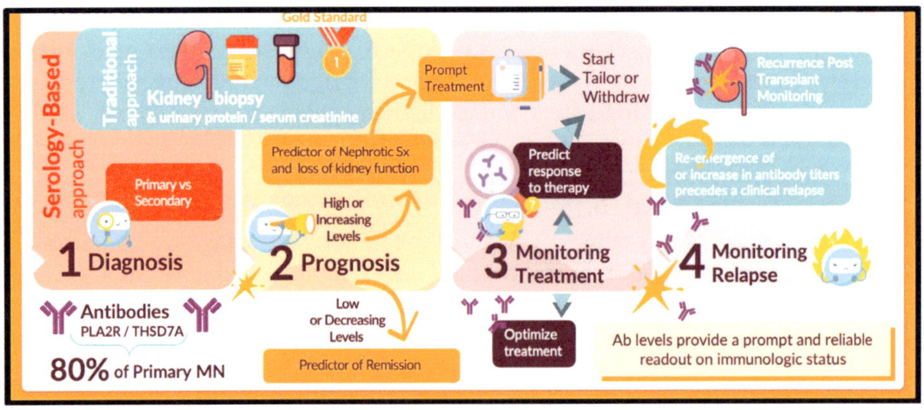

Figure 1.
Representing serology-based approach (figure taken from De Vriese et al. [46], see reference [47]).

a unique gene amplification method that was first employed in several investigations [54]. The advantages of the LAMP approach are its excellent specificity for the target sequence and its capacity to amplify DNA with high efficiency under isothermal condition [54]. This procedure just needs four primers, DNA polymerase, and a standard laboratory water bath or heat block for the reaction; it is also thought to be straightforward and simple to carry out [11]. Additionally, LAMP may amplify RNA sequences very effectively when combined with reverse transcription. Furthermore, as stated reagents can be stored at room temperature without the need for any post-PCR procedures [41]. LAMP has been utilized in the identification of DNA and RNA viruses, including SARS and West Nile viruses, as per earlier research conducted [55, 56]. Additionally, a previous study compared LAMP with multiplex PCR using stool samples from taeniasis patients [57]. In the meantime, a recent work described a unique diagnostic strategy that combines the LAMP and MinION sequencing technology to identify human Plasmodium species [58].

Furthermore, in recent years, the analysis of proteins expressed by parasites has been a fast-expanding field of proteomics research [59]. The demand for sensitivity has since grown as a result of the present interest in proteomics, which helped researchers overcome the obstacles to early diagnosis and therapy [60]. Two methods were used to identify the proteins: top-down and bottom-up. In the top-down approach, two-dimensional polyacrylamide gel electrophoresis was used [40]. Proteomics has been applied to a number of different disorders, including taeniasis, malaria, and Chagas disease [61–63]. A different novel strategy known as microsatellites was based on simple sequence tandem repeats and was also reported in studies on parasites that could rapidly evolve and were taken from both people and animals [64, 65]. Due to the prominent polymorphism shown, microsatellites are regarded as valuable genetic markers [66]. Luminex-based assays, which integrate flow cytometry, fluorescent beads, lasers, and digital signal processing, have also surfaced as a potential method for identifying parasite infections [11, 67]. In a study, Luminex was used to distinguish between the *C. hominis* and *C. parvum* species using just one nucleotide. Other serological testing or antigen detection cannot differentiate between the two species [28]. The assay's research enhances the other PCR procedures' speed, accuracy, and dependability [11, 68, 69].

3. Challenges in the management of parasitic infections

A disease arises from the daily exposure of the human body to parasites from our surroundings. It has been demonstrated that intestinal parasites, which were formerly thought to be benign commensals, may potentially be pathogens [68]. More number of parasites can be discovered at the same time with further improvement of diagnostics procedures as the researchers increasingly try to concentrate on refining existing diagnostic techniques rather than developing new ones. Mass screening and quick diagnostics are helpful features that will increase our knowledge of parasites and lessen the spread of illness [69]. Moreover, to prevent significant delays, the development of field-based diagnosis is also required. Cost is still a problem, as are sensitivity and specificity. Particularly in endemic areas, renewed and sustainable intervention is required. The status of public health, particularly in the area of medical parasitology, can be improved globally in several ways, including by enacting appropriate regulations or policies and by tracking, assessing, and bolstering the surveillance of parasitic diseases [70, 71]. Monitoring the resistance to anti-parasite medications and other options is essential for creating improved patient treatments. Increased awareness is required, especially in targeted areas, and preventive interventions including routine deworming [72]. To improve and eradicate possible diseases, more financing for parasitological research and interventions is also required [73].

4. Conclusion

The utilization of microscopy-based techniques is still beneficial in the diagnosis of patients with parasitic illnesses, even with the rapid advancement of other methods. On the other hand, molecular and serology-based techniques are seen to be superior substitutes, particularly for infections with a narrow spectrum of parasites. The current state of research and methodologies for illness detection offers a better foundation for the development of more effective, dependable, and affordable approaches, thereby enhancing life quality and paving the way for future drops in the global disease burden. Higher authorities, including public health and healthcare organizations, medical experts, and funding suppliers, must fully commit to implementing these recommendations. The efforts to combat IPIs would be strengthened by the support of all stakeholders, and more work needs to be done to fulfill the largest gap in science.

Acknowledgements

Authors are grateful to the facilities provided by the head, department of Zoology, Chaudhary Charan Singh University, Meerut, India.

Conflict of interest

The authors declare no conflict of interest.

Author details

Km. Deepika[1], Amit Baliyan[2], Anshu Chaudhary[3]* and Bindu Sharma[1]

1 Department of Zoology, Molecular Parasitology Laboratory, Chaudhary Charan Singh University, Meerut, Uttar Pradesh, India

2 Maharaj Singh College, Saharanpur, Uttar Pradesh, India

3 Department of Zoology, Molecular Taxonomy Laboratory, Chaudhary Charan Singh University, Meerut, Uttar Pradesh, India

*Address all correspondence to: anshuchaudhary81@gmail.com

References

[1] Del Brutto OH, Santibanez R, Idrovo L, et al. Epilepsy and neurocysticercosis in Atahualpa: A door-to-door survey in rural coastal Ecuador. Epilepsia. 2005;**46**(4):583-587

[2] Medina MT, Duron RM, Martinez L. Prevalence, incidence, and etioloy of epilepsies in rural Honduras: The Salama study. Epilepsia. 2005;**46**:124-131

[3] Montano SM, Villaran MV, Ylquimiche L, et al. Neurocysticercosis: Association between seizures, serology, and brain CT in rural Peru. Neurology. 2005;**65**(2):229-234

[4] White AC Jr. Neurocysticercosis: Updates on epidemiology, pathogenesis, diagnosis, and management. Annual Review of Medicine. 2000;**51**:187-206

[5] Mas-Seśe G, Vives-Pínera I, Ferńandez-Barreiro A, et al. Estudio descriptivo de neurocisticercosis en un hospital terciario. Revista de Neurologia. 2008;**46**(4):194-196

[6] Serpa JA, Graviss EA, Kass JS, White AC. Neurocysticercosis in Houston, Texas: An update. Medicine. 2011;**90**(1):81-86

[7] Sorvillo F, Wilkins P, Shafir S, Eberhard M. Public health implications of cysticercosis acquired in the United States. Emerging Infectious Diseases. 2011;**17**(1):1-6

[8] Del Brutto OH, Sotelo J, Roman G. Neurocysticercosis: A Clinical Handbook. Lisse, The Netherlands: Swets & Zeitlinger; 1988

[9] Gonzalez AE, Lopez-Urbina T, Tsang B, et al. Transmission dynamics of *Taenia solium* and potential for pig-to-pig transmission. Parasitology International. 2006;**55**:S131-S135

[10] Willms K. Morphology and biochemistry of the pork tapeworm, *Taenia solium*. Current Topics in Medicinal Chemistry. 2008;**8**(5):375-382

[11] Escobar A, Weidenheim KM. The pathology of neurocysticercosis. In: Singh G, Prabhakar S, editors. *Taenia Solium* Cysticercosis. From Basic to Clinical Science. Oxon, UK: CAB International; 2002. pp. 289-305

[12] Katz N, Chaves A, Pellegrino J. A simple device for quantitative stool thick-smear technique in *schistosomiasis mansoni*. Revista do Instituto de Medicina Tropical de São Paulo. 1972;**14**(6):397-400

[13] van Gool T, Vetter H, Vervoort T, et al. Serodiagnosis of imported shistosomiasis by a combination of a commercial indirect hemagglutination test with *Schistosoma mansoni* adult worm antigens and an enzyme-linked immunosorbent assay with *S. Mansoni* egg antigens. Journal of Clinical Microbiology. 2002;**40**(9):3432-3437

[14] Ten Hove RJ, Verweij JJ, Vereecken K et al. Multiplex real-time PCR for the detection and quantification of *Schistosoma mansoni* and *S. Haematobium* infection in stool samples collected in northern Senegal. 2008

[15] Cnops L, Soentjens P, Clerinx J, et al. A *Schistosoma haematobium*-specific real-time PCRfor diagnosis of urogenital schistosomiasis in serum samples of international travellers and migrants. PLOS Neglected Tropical Diseases. 2013;7(8):e2413

[16] Lodh N, Naples JM, Bosompem KM, et al. Detection of parasite-specific DNA in urine sediment obtained by filtration differentiates between single and mixed infections of *Schistosoma mansoni* and *S. Haematobium* from endemic areas in Ghana. PLoS One. 2014;**9**(3):e91144

[17] Del Brutto OH, Castillo PR, Mena IX, Freire AX. Neurocysticercosis among patients with cerebral gliomas. Archives of Neurology. 1997;**54**(9):1125-1128

[18] Wang T, Zhao M, Rotgans BA, et al. Proteomic analysis of the *Schistosoma mansoni* miracidium. PLoS One. 2016;**11**(1):e0147247

[19] Bungiro RD Jr, Cappello M. Detection of excretory/secretory coproantigens in experimental hookworm infection. The American Journal of Tropical Medicine and Hygiene. 2005;**73**:915-920

[20] Garćıa HH, Evans CAW, Nash TE, et al. Current consensus guidelines for treatment of neurocysticercosis. Clinical Microbiology Reviews. 2002;**15**(4):747-756

[21] Del Brutto OH, Rajshekar V, White AC Jr, et al. Proposed diagnostic criteria for neurocysticercosis. Neurology. 2001;**57**:177-183

[22] Bueno EC, Scheel CM, Vaz AJ, et al. Application of synthetic 8-kD and recombinant GP50antigens in the diagnosis of neurocysticercosis by enzyme-linked immunosorbent assay. American Journal of Tropical Medicine and Hygiene. 2005;**72**:278-283

[23] Deckers N, Dorny P, Kanobana K, et al. Use of protein Chip technology for identifying biomarkers of parasitic diseases: The example of porcine cysticercosis (Taenia solium). Experimental Parasitology. 2008;**120**(4):320-329

[24] Mayta H, Gilman RH, Prendergast E, et al. Nested PCR for specific diagnosis of Taenia solium Taeniasis. Journal of Clinical Microbiology. 2008;**46**:286-289

[25] Weber R, Bryan RT, Bishop HS, et al. Threshold of detection of *cryptosporidium* oocysts in human stool specimens: Evidence for low sensitivity of current diagnostic methods. Journal of Clinical Microbiology. 1991;**29**:1323-1327

[26] Garcia HH, Del Brutto OH, Nash TE, White AC, Tsang VCW, Gilman RH. New concepts in the diagnosis and management of neurocysticercosis (*Taenia solium*). American Journal of Tropical Medicine and Hygiene. 2005;**72**(1):3-9

[27] Johnston SP, Ballard MM, Beach MJ, et al. Evaluation of three commercial assays for detection of *giardia* and *cryptosporidium* organisms in fecal specimens. Journal of Clinical Microbiology. 2003;**41**:623-626

[28] Bandyopadhyay K, Kellar KL, Moura I et al. Rapid microsphere assay for identification of *Cryptosporidium hominis* and *Cryptosporidium parvum* in stool and environmental samples. Journal of Clinical Microbiology. 2007;**45**:2835-2840

[29] Jothikumar N, da Silva AJ, Moura I, et al. Detection and differentiation of *Cryptosporidium hominis* and *Cryptosporidium parvum* by dual Taq man assays. Journal of Medical Microbiology. 2008;**57**:1099-1105

[30] Danciger M, Lopez M. Numbers of *giardia* in the feces of infected children. The American Journal of Tropical Medicine and Hygiene. 1975;**24**:237-242

[31] Young KH, Bullock SL, Melvin DM, et al. Ethyl acetate as a substitute for diethyl ether in the formalin-ether sedimentation technique. Journal of Clinical Microbiology. 1979;**10**:852-853

[32] Garcia LS, Shimizu RY. Evaluation of nine immunoassay kits (enzyme immunoassay and direct fluorescence) for detection of *Giardia lamblia* and *Cryptosporidium parvum* in human fecal specimens. Journal of Clinical Microbiology. 1997;**35**:1526-1529

[33] Siddiki AZ. Proteome analysis of *Cryptosporidium parvum* and C. Hominis using two-dimensional electrophoresis, image analysis and tandem mass spectrometry. Iran. Journal of Biotechnology. 2012;**10**(3):198-207

[34] Hira PR, Iqbal J, Al-Ali F, et al. Invasive amebiasis: Challenges in diagnosis in a non-endemic country (Kuwait). The American Journal of Tropical Medicine and Hygiene. 2001;**65**:341-345

[35] Gonin P, Trudel L. Detection and differentiation of *Entamoeba histolytica* and *Entamoeba dispar* isolates in clinical samples by PCR and enzyme-linked immunosorbent assay. Journal of Clinical Microbiology. 2003;**41**:237-241

[36] Fotedar R, Stark D, Beebe N, et al. Laboratory diagnostic techniques for *Entamoeba* species. Clinical Microbiology Reviews. 2007;**20**:511-532

[37] Liang SY, Chan YH, Hsia KT, et al. Development of loop-mediated isothermal amplification assay for detection of *Entamoeba histolytica*. Journal of Clinical Microbiology. 2009;**47**:1892-1895

[38] Ali IKM, Haque R, Siddique A, et al. Proteomic analysis of the cyst stage of *Entamoeba histolytica*. PLOS Neglected Tropical Diseases. 2012;**6**(5):e1643

[39] Luna-Nacar M, Navarrete-Perea J, Moguel B, et al. Proteomic study of Entamoeba histolytica trophozoites, cysts, and cyst-like structures. PLoS One. 2016;**11**(5):e0156018

[40] Pittella JEH. Neurocysticercosis. Brain Pathology. 1997;**7**(1):681-693

[41] Del Brutto OH. Stroke and vasculitis in patients with cysticercosis. In: Caplan LR, editor. Uncommon Causes of Stroke. New York, NY, USA: Cambridge University Press; 2008. pp. 53-58

[42] Flisser A, Correa D, Evans CAW. *Taenia solium* Cysticercosis. In: Singh G, Prabhakar S, editors. From Basic to Clinical Science. Oxon, UK: CAB International; 2002

[43] Del Brutto OH, Dolezal M, Castillo PR, Garcıa HH. Neurocysticercosis and oncogenesis. Archives of Medical Research. 2000;**31**(2):151-155

[44] Del Brutto OH, Santibanez R, Noboa CA, Aguirre R, Diaz E, Alarcon TA. Epilepsy due to neurocysticercosis: Analysis of 203 patients. Neurology. 1992;**42**(2):389-392

[45] Garcia HH, Del Brutto OH. Neurocysticercosis: Updated concepts about an old disease. The Lancet Neurology. 2005;**4**(10):653-661

[46] De Vriese AS, Glassock RJ, Nath KA et al. A Proposal for a Serology-Based Approach to Membranous Nephropathy. Journal of the American Society of Nephrology. 2016;**28**:421-430

[47] García HH, Del Brutto OH. Imaging findings in neurocysticercosis. Acta Tropica. 2003;**87**(1):71-78

[48] Nash TE, Singh G, White AC, et al. Treatment of neurocysticercosis: Current status and future research needs. Neurology. 2006;**67**(7):1120-1127

[49] Sotelo J, Diaz-Olavarrieta C. Neurocysticercosis: Changes after 25 years of medical therapy. Archives of Medical Research. 2010;**41**(1):62-63

[50] Sotelo J, Escobedo F, Rodriguez-Carbajal J, et al. Therapy of parenchymal brain cysticercosis with praziquantel. New England Journal of Medicine. 1984;**310**(16):1001-1007

[51] Escobedo F, Penagos P, Rodriguez J, Sotelo J. Albendazole therapy for neurocysticercosis. Archives of Internal Medicine. 1987;**147**(4):738-741

[52] Garcia HH, Pretell EJ, Gilman RH, et al. A trial of antiparasitic treatment to reduce the rate of seizures due to cerebral cysticercosis. New England Journal of Medicine. 2004;**350**(3):249-258

[53] Keilbach NM, De Aluja AS, Sarti-Gutierrez E. A programme to control taeniasis-cysticercosis (*T. Solium*): Experiences in a Mexican village. Acta Leidensia. 1989;**57**(2):181-189

[54] Pawlowski ZS. Role of chemotherapy of taeniasis in prevention of neurocysticercosis. Parasitology International. 2006;**55**:S105-S109

[55] Codd EE, Ng HH, McFarlane C, et al. Preclinical studies on the pharmacokinetics, safety, and toxicology of oxfendazole: Toward first in human studies. International Journal of Toxicology. 2015;**34**:129-137

[56] Siddiqua T, Habeeb A. Neurocysticercosis. Saudi Journal of Kidney Diseases and Transplantation. 2020;**31**:254. DOI: 10.4103/1319-2442.279948,2020

[57] Panic G, Duthaler U, Speich B, Keiser J. Repurposing drugs for the treatment and control of helminth infections. International Journal for Parasitology: Drugs and Drug Resistance. 2014;**4**:185-200

[58] Imai K, Tarumoto N, Misawa K, et al. A novel diagnostic method for malaria using loop-mediated isothermal amplification (LAMP) and MinION nanopore sequencer. BMC Infectious Diseases. 2017;**17**:621

[59] Boersema PJ, Kahraman A, Picotti P. Proteomics beyond large-scale protein expression analysis. Current Opinion in Biotechnology. 2015;**34**:162-170

[60] Petricoin EF, Zoon KC, Kohn EC, et al. Clinical proteomics: Translating benchside promise into bedside reality. Nature Reviews Drug Discovery. 2002;**1**:683-695

[61] Nyunt N, Pisciotta J, Feldman AB, et al. Detection of *plasmodium falciparum* in pregnancy by laser desorption mass spectrometry. The American Journal of Tropical Medicine and Hygiene. 2005;**73**(3):485-490

[62] Santamaria C, Chatelain E, Jackson Y, et al. Serum biomarkers predictive of cure in chagas disease patients after nifurtimox treatment. BMC Infectious Diseases. 2014;**14**:302

[63] Temperley ND, Webster LM, Adam A, et al. Cross-species utility of microsatellite markers in Trichostrongyloid nematodes. The Journal of Parasitology. 2009;**95**(2):487-489

[64] Johnson PC, Webster LM, Adam A, et al. Abundant variation in microsatellites of the parasitic nematode *Trichostrongylus tenuis* and linkage to a tandem repeat. Molecular and Biochemical Parasitology. 2006;**148**(2):210-218

[65] Karanis P, Thekisoe O, Kiouptsi K, et al. Development and preliminary evaluation of a loop-mediated isothermal amplification procedure for sensitive detection of *cryptosporidium* oocysts in fecal and water samples. Applied and Environmental Microbiology. 2007;**73**:5660-5662

[66] Abdul-Muneer PM. Application of microsatellite markers in conservation genetics and fisheries management: Recent advances in population structure analysis and conservation strategies. Genetics Research International. 2014;**691759**:1-12. DOI: 10.1155/2014/691759

[67] Chen T-H, Lee F, Lin Y-L, et al. Development of a multiplex Luminex assay for detecting swine antibodies to structural and non-structural proteins of foot-and-mouth disease virus in Taiwan. J Microbiol Immunol infect. 2016; 13:196-207. Journal of Clinical Microbiology. 2007;**45**:2835-2840

[68] Lukes J, Stensvold CR, Jirku-Pomajbikova K, et al. Are human intestinal eukaryotes beneficial or commensals? PLoS Pathogens. 2015;**11**(8):e1005039

[69] Yansouni CP, Merckx J, Libman MD, et al. Recent advances in clinical parasitology diagnostics. Current Infectious Disease Reports. 2014;**16**:434

[70] Colley DG. Parasitic diseases: Opportunities and challenges in the 21st century. Memórias do Instituto Oswaldo Cruz, Rio de Janeiro. 2000;**95**(1):79-87

[71] CDC. Centers for Disease Control and Prevention Global Health Strategy 2012-2015. Available from: https://www.cdc.gov/globalhealth/strategy/pdf/cdc-globalhealthstrategy.pdf.2012 [Accessed: April 18, 2017]

[72] Traversa D. Pet roundworms and hookworms: A continuing need for global worming. Parasites and Vectors. 2012;**5**:91

[73] Zilungile MK, Musawenkosi M. Status of medical parasitology in South Africa: New challenges and missed opportunities. Trends in Parasitology. 2012;**28**(6):217-219

Chapter 13

New Developments in Diagnosis of Intestinal Parasites

Yohannis Derbew Molla and Hirut Tesfahun Alemu

Abstract

The field of intestinal parasite diagnosis has experienced significant advancements in recent years, propelled by technological innovations and the pursuit of more precise and effective diagnostic methods. A notable development in this area is the widespread adoption of molecular diagnostic techniques, such as polymerase chain reaction and loop-mediated isothermal amplification. These cutting-edge methods provide improved sensitivity and specificity compared to traditional microscopy-based approaches, enabling the detection of intestinal parasites even at low concentrations and in complex clinical samples. Additionally, the creation of multiplex polymerase chain reaction assays allows for the simultaneous identification of multiple parasite species in a single test, streamlining the diagnostic process and reducing turnaround time. Furthermore, the integration of artificial intelligence and machine learning algorithms into diagnostic platforms shows great potential for enhancing the accuracy and efficiency of parasite detection. In conclusion, these recent advancements present unparalleled opportunities to enhance the precision, speed, and accessibility of parasite diagnosis, ultimately leading to better patient outcomes and more effective public health interventions in endemic regions.

Keywords: parasites, intestinal, diagnosis, microscopy, molecular techniques, new developments

1. Introduction

Intestinal parasites continue to present significant health risks on a global scale, particularly in regions where sanitation and hygiene practices are lacking. These parasites, varying in pathogenicity, remain prevalent and continue to cause illness and discomfort in both animals and humans. Despite the advancements made by the pharmaceutical industry in developing treatments for parasitic infections, these infections persist and impose a substantial burden of disease in many parts of the world.

For instance, as indicated by the recent Pan-European Economic Assessment, the economic impact of helminth infections in ruminants is estimated to be comparable to or greater than that of animal diseases, amounting to an estimated €941 million annually [1]. The repercussions of neglected parasitic diseases on human populations, particularly children in low-resource settings, are profound [2]. Furthermore, zoonotic parasites have the ability to move between different hosts, compounding the disease burden for individuals who come into contact with contaminated food, water, soil, or vectors [3, 4].

Parasites, though minuscule and imperceptible to the naked eye, can be observed under a microscope. The community of parasites that pose a threat to human health includes protozoa, helminths, and ectoparasites. It is estimated that 357 million cases of morbidity, predominantly caused by protozoa such as Cryptosporidium, Entamoeba, and Giardia, resulted in 33,900 deaths and the loss of 2.94 million disability-adjusted life years annually [5] Furthermore, over 1.4 billion individuals are afflicted with helminth infections [6]. In addition to their impact on human health, parasites also play a role in causing diseases in plants and other organisms. Notable examples include Giardia, which is transmitted through contaminated water, toxoplasmosis, which is spread by cats, and malaria which is spread by mosquitos [7]. Globally, one species of helminth parasite alone infects over 800 million people [8]. The prevalence and impact of parasitic infections underscore the importance of continued research and intervention efforts to mitigate their detrimental effects on public health.

In developing regions such as East Asia, South America, and Saharan Africa, there exists a plethora of over 100 species of human intestinal parasites that collectively produce an astonishing 200,000 eggs daily. Alarmingly, an estimated 41,500 human fatalities are reported annually as a direct result of parasitic infections [9]. The manifestations of these infections vary widely, encompassing clinical presentations that range from malnutrition to asymptomatic anemia, and in some cases, even leading to the development of cancer [10, 11]. Despite advancements in diagnostic techniques, conventional light microscopic examination continues to serve as the gold standard method for the detection and diagnosis of several parasitic diseases, notably malaria [12].

Timely and accurate diagnosis is paramount for the effective management and control of parasitic infections. Throughout the years, a multitude of diagnostic techniques have been developed and refined to improve sensitivity, specificity, and efficiency. Understanding the composition of parasite communities and their impact on disease risk is crucial for any surveillance program aimed at reducing the parasite burden. Equally important is the utilization of cutting-edge diagnostic tools to optimize resource allocation for parasite control.

For many years, parasitologists have predominantly relied on traditional diagnostic methods involving microscopic examination. Conventional light microscopy remains the preferred method for diagnosing certain parasitic diseases, such as malaria [12]. While these techniques are cost-effective and straightforward, they are often plagued by issues of reproducibility and lack the necessary specificity and sensitivity. Moreover, microscopic methods are labor-intensive and necessitate skilled personnel for accurate interpretation.

As we transition toward a future centered around molecular tools, the reliance on traditional diagnostic techniques may pose challenges [13]. The shortage of trained professionals proficient in identifying parasites through conventional means underscores the importance of embracing advancements in diagnostic technology. By staying abreast of the latest tools and methodologies, we can enhance our ability to combat parasitic infections effectively. In this chapter, we will be exploring the latest advancements in the diagnosis of intestinal parasites. Prior to delving into these new developments, it is imperative to provide a brief overview of the traditional diagnostic methods that have been utilized in the past.

2. Conventional methods

Traditional diagnostic methods for identifying intestinal parasites primarily rely on microscopic analysis of stool samples. These methods include direct smear microscopy, formalin-ether concentration technique, Kato-Katz thick smear technique, and Fecal Floatation Technique. These techniques allow for the visualization of parasite eggs, larvae, or cysts under a microscope, aiding in the detection of various parasitic infections. In addition to these conventional methods, Fecal Immunoassays, specifically enzyme-linked immunosorbent assays (ELISA), are also utilized for diagnosing intestinal parasites. These tests target specific antigens or antibodies produced by parasites in the stool sample, making them particularly effective in identifying certain protozoan infections such as Giardia and Cryptosporidium. Overall, these diagnostic approaches play a crucial role in accurately identifying and treating intestinal parasitic infections, ultimately contributing to improved patient outcomes.

While cost-effective, these methods have limitations in terms of sensitivity, particularly for low-intensity infections, and they may necessitate skilled personnel for accurate interpretation. There are also additional numerous shortcomings associated with these methods, including variable sensitivity, resource, and time consumption, all of which have the potential to significantly impact the results of clinical examinations.

Additionally, the traditional clinical parasitology classification and detection process faces challenges in maintaining staff competency and engagement. The clinical parasitology laboratory is further hindered by the fact that educated technologists are increasingly drawn to technology-driven and automated disciplines within the laboratory, leaving a shortage of adequately trained personnel to manage the traditional methods effectively [14]. Results obtained through the diagnosis of parasites are often reliant on clinical signs and symptoms, which are susceptible to human error. This can result in higher mortality rates, unnecessary drug purchases, and economic burdens [15]. Consequently, there is a pressing need for alternative methods that can provide more accurate and reliable diagnosis results.

3. Point-of-care testing (POCT) devices

Point-of-care testing (POCT) devices are sophisticated medical diagnostic tools engineered to swiftly and conveniently provide diagnostic results directly at the patient's point of care, whether it be in a clinic, doctor's office, or out in the field. These devices are typically compact, user-friendly, and have the ability to produce precise results with minimal sample processing. The advent of POCT devices for diagnosing intestinal parasites has revolutionized decentralized testing and enhanced access to diagnostic services, particularly in areas with limited resources. These portable and intuitive devices employ a variety of detection methods, such as immunochromatographic assays, nucleic acid amplification, and digital microscopy. Examples include rapid diagnostic tests (RDTs) for identifying specific parasite antigens in stool samples and smartphone-based microscopy systems equipped with advanced image analysis algorithms for automated parasite detection.

Some drawbacks of point-of-care testing (POCT) devices include the potential for user error, limited test menu options, and the need for proper training and quality control measures. User error can occur if healthcare providers are not adequately trained on how to use the devices, leading to inaccurate results. Additionally, POCT devices may have a limited test menu, which could restrict the types of tests that can be performed at the point of care. Finally, maintaining quality control measures and ensuring the accuracy of results can be challenging with POCT devices, requiring ongoing monitoring and oversight.

4. Molecular techniques

The introduction of nucleic acid-based detection methods has the potential to not only enhance the accuracy of diagnosis but also improve the efficiency and impartiality of intestinal parasite diagnosis. This is particularly significant given the opportunity to integrate complementary assays into highly automated platforms. Through the refinement of diagnostics, there is a likelihood of better assigning effective antiparasitic treatments, a critical consideration in light of the escalating cases of drug resistance.

In recent years, molecular diagnostic techniques have transformed the field of parasitology by enabling swift and precise detection of parasites. PCR, first described in 1985, is a groundbreaking technique that allows for the in vitro amplification of a specific DNA fragment through a cyclic process involving denaturation, primer hybridization, and DNA strand elongation using a thermostable DNA polymerase [16, 17]. Polymerase chain reaction (PCR)-based assays, such as conventional PCR, real-time PCR, and multiplex PCR, offer exceptional sensitivity and specificity in identifying a broad spectrum of intestinal parasites. These advanced techniques enable the detection of parasite DNA even at minimal concentrations, facilitating early diagnosis and treatment [16, 17]. Following the initial publications on DNA amplification by PCR, it was foreseen that this innovative technology would revolutionize molecular parasitology and the diagnosis of parasitic infections [18, 19]. Prior to this breakthrough, the use of specific DNA probes in research and diagnostics was hindered by the limited sensitivity of direct hybridization assays without amplification. The advent of PCR offered a solution by enabling the specific amplification of minute DNA quantities. In 1995, a comprehensive review by J.B. Weiss highlighted the abundance of research papers on DNA-based methods for detecting and identifying various parasitic infections [20].

During that period, the utilization of polymerase chain reaction (PCR) was still restricted, with most studies focusing on malaria, leishmania, trypanosome, and toxoplasma parasites, all of which are tissue parasites. Furthermore, with the exception of toxoplasmosis, the application of PCR on DNA extracted directly from patient samples was limited. In the past decade or so, numerous clinical microbiology laboratories have been equipped with the necessary tools to conduct molecular diagnostics [21]. Technical advancements, particularly the introduction of real-time PCR, have addressed many of the challenges associated with early PCR methods, such as the risk of contamination from amplified products. Additionally, the ability to incorporate multiple targets in a single multiplex assay has become more straightforward. The implementation of automated DNA/RNA isolation techniques has enabled the use of nucleic acid-based detection methods in a high-throughput manner. Various molecular detection, differentiation, and genotyping techniques for numerous parasites have been developed and integrated into both diagnostic and research environments.

4.1 Techniques of DNA isolation

In the absence of a suitable nucleic acid isolation method, the reliability of DNA amplification techniques is compromised. It is imperative to consider two key factors. Firstly, the isolation method must effectively liberate nucleic acids from the parasitic stage present in the clinical sample, such as cysts, spores, or eggs. Secondly, the isolated nucleic acids should be devoid of any substances that could impede or hinder the amplification reaction. This is particularly crucial when isolating parasite DNA from complex matrices like feces [22].

Various strategies can be employed to prevent inhibition of the amplification reaction, such as heating the stool specimen, incorporating absorbent substances like polyvinyl polypyrrolidone, or utilizing inhibitor-resistant DNA polymerases in the PCR mixture [21, 23–25]. Additionally, the inclusion of an internal inhibition control in each reaction mixture is essential. For instance, the use of phocin herpesvirus (PhHV) as a control allows for monitoring of inhibition within the amplification process [26].

Maintaining consistency in the amplification cycles across samples is also crucial, as any deviation may indicate inhibition. In such instances, repeating the DNA isolation and PCR processes using a diluted sample is recommended. The efficient release of nucleic acids is contingent upon a well-balanced approach in the DNA isolation procedure.

The amplification of a target sequence in PCR relies on the activity of a DNA polymerase enzyme, which catalyzes the synthesis of new DNA molecules by adding free nucleotides to a pre-existing DNA template. Primers play a crucial role in initiating DNA synthesis by providing a starting point for the polymerase. These primers are short, single-stranded nucleic acid sequences typically consisting of 16–30 base pairs that are designed to be complementary to the specific target sequence being amplified.

During PCR, the polymerase enzyme initiates replication at the 3′-end of the primer and proceeds to synthesize a new DNA strand that is complementary to the target sequence. This process allows for the selective amplification of the desired DNA target, enabling the detection and analysis of specific genetic sequences [27].

4.2 Conventional PCR

Conventional PCR, also known as traditional PCR, is a widely used molecular biology technique that amplifies a specific segment of DNA through a series of temperature cycles. This method involves the use of a DNA template, primers, DNA polymerase, and nucleotides to generate multiple copies of the target DNA sequence. The conventional polymerase chain reaction (PCR) plays a crucial role in the accurate diagnosis of intestinal parasites. By targeting specific DNA sequences of the parasites, conventional PCR can detect even low levels of infection with high sensitivity and specificity. This method is particularly valuable in cases where traditional diagnostic techniques may yield false-negative results. The precision and reliability of conventional PCR make it an indispensable tool in the identification and management of intestinal parasite infections. Conventional PCR offers a sensitive and specific method for the diagnosis of intestinal parasites like *Giardia lamblia*. It allows for rapid detection of parasite DNA in clinical samples, aiding in accurate diagnosis and appropriate management of patients with parasitic infections.

However, there are several limitations associated with conventional PCR in the diagnosis of intestinal parasites. One major drawback is the potential for false-negative results due to the presence of PCR inhibitors in the sample. Additionally, conventional PCR may not be able to detect all species of intestinal parasites, leading to incomplete or inaccurate diagnoses. Furthermore, the sensitivity and specificity of conventional PCR can be affected by variations in sample collection, storage, and processing techniques.

4.3 Reverse transcriptase PCR

To enhance the capabilities of PCR amplification to the transcriptome level, the initial step involves the reverse transcription of RNA into complementary DNA (cDNA). Reverse transcriptase PCR (RT-PCR) emerges as a superior method for scrutinizing RNA transcripts, particularly when dealing with limited quantities of starting material. In contrast, traditional blotting hybridization assays necessitate a larger amount of RNA for analysis and lack the efficiency and convenience provided by PCR-based techniques. RT-PCR boasts numerous advantages, including its adaptability, sensitivity, swift processing time, and the ability to concurrently compare multiple samples. Within the realm of reverse transcriptase PCR (RT-PCR), cDNA replicas are generated from RNA, followed by the standard PCR amplification of the desired target.

Reverse transcriptase PCR (RT-PCR) plays a crucial role in the diagnosis of intestinal parasites. This molecular technique allows for the detection of parasite genetic material in clinical samples, providing a highly sensitive and specific method for identifying infections. By targeting specific RNA sequences of the parasite, RT-PCR can accurately differentiate between different parasite species and strains. This precision is essential for guiding appropriate treatment strategies and monitoring the effectiveness of interventions. In addition, RT-PCR can detect low levels of parasite DNA, making it particularly useful in cases of low parasite burden or chronic infections. Overall, the use of RT-PCR in the diagnosis of intestinal parasites represents a valuable tool in the clinical management of these infections.

4.4 Real-time PCR

Real-time PCR, or quantitative PCR, is a powerful molecular biology technique used to quantify and monitor the amplification of specific DNA sequences in real time. This technique allows researchers to accurately measure the amount of DNA present in a sample at each cycle of the PCR reaction, providing precise and quantitative results. Real-time PCR is widely used in research, clinical diagnostics, and forensic analysis due to its sensitivity, specificity, and speed. It has revolutionized the field of molecular biology by enabling rapid and accurate detection of genetic material in a wide range of applications.

In the realm of real-time PCR, the quantification of amplicons occurs in "real time" as the amplification process unfolds. Various techniques have been developed, ranging from the utilization of non-specific staining of double-stranded DNA with intercalating dyes to the incorporation of fluorescence-labeled DNA probes.

A significant advancement in the field of diagnostic applications of PCR was the emergence of real-time or quantitative PCR (qPCR) assays. This development led to the rapid introduction of various detection chemistries for real-time PCR, resulting in the gradual disappearance of older detection methods such as gel electrophoresis and allele-specific oligonucleotide blots from laboratory practices. qPCR integrates the amplification steps of traditional PCR with simultaneous detection steps that eliminate the need for post-PCR manipulation, as the PCR process is directly monitored within the reaction vessel.

In qPCR, the exponential phase of PCR is closely monitored in real time using fluorescently labeled molecules, allowing for the direct correlation between the amount of PCR product present in the reaction vessel and the emitted fluorescence, as well as the initial target quantity. This quantitative aspect of qPCR makes it a valuable tool in molecular diagnostics.

There are two primary types of detection chemistries utilized in qPCR: those employing intercalating DNA binding dyes like SYBR Green I, and those utilizing various fluorescently labeled probes such as TaqMan. The key advantages of qPCR include the rapid analysis of samples without the need for post-PCR processing steps, the closed-tube design that minimizes the risk of contamination, and its quantitative capabilities.

Following qPCR, two main post-analysis methods are commonly employed: amplification curve analysis for quantifying the amount of amplicon by comparison to a known standard, and melt curve analysis based on the denaturation property of double-stranded DNA with heat. This denaturation process is monitored using fluorescent dyes that emit fluorescence when bound to double-stranded DNA.

As the temperature is increased, the double strand begins to dissociate, releasing the dye and causing a decrease in fluorescence intensity. The resulting fluorescence data is depicted as a curve of fluorescence intensity plotted against temperature. The melting temperature (Tm) is the point at which 50% of the DNA is in the double-stranded state, and it is indicated by the peak of the melting curve derivative. When DNA binding dyes are present in saturating concentrations, a specific amplicon sequence will exhibit a distinct Tm and melting curve shape. This unique melting curve can be utilized to identify DNA sequence variations within the amplicon without the need for post-PCR processing.

The streamlined nature of probe-based real-time PCR chemistry, such as scorpion probes, reduces the risk of contamination, minimizes labor time, and optimizes reagent costs, making it a valuable tool in molecular biology research [28, 29]. The individual quantification of probes utilizing distinct fluorophores that emit fluorescence at varying wavelengths facilitates the execution of multiplex polymerase chain reactions (PCRs) involving DNA fragments of comparable sizes with uniform efficacy.

The advancement of high-resolution qPCR instruments and novel saturating DNA dyes has enabled a more accurate assessment of sequence variations through melting analysis. High-resolution melting analysis (HRMA) can differentiate DNA sequences based on factors such as composition, length, GC content, and strand complementarity. It is valuable for mutation scanning, methylation studies, and genotyping. The method's ease of use, high sensitivity and specificity, cost-effectiveness, and rapid turnaround time make it well-suited for routine diagnostic applications. However, the accuracy of HRMA is contingent upon the quality of the instrumentation, saturation dyes, and analysis software employed, potentially leading to variability in different clinical diagnostic settings [30, 31].

Real-time PCR plays a crucial role in the diagnosis of intestinal parasites by providing a rapid and accurate method for detecting the presence of these pathogens in clinical samples. This advanced molecular technique allows for the amplification and quantification of specific DNA sequences from parasites, enabling healthcare professionals to identify the exact species causing the infection. Real-time PCR is particularly beneficial in cases where traditional microscopy techniques may yield false-negative results or fail to differentiate between similar parasite species. By offering high sensitivity and specificity, real-time PCR aids in the timely and precise diagnosis of intestinal parasites, ultimately guiding appropriate treatment strategies for patients.

4.5 Multiplex PCR

Another significant advancement in the progression of PCR technology is the enhancement of assay multiplexing capabilities. Multiplex PCR is a highly effective technique that enables the amplification of two or more products simultaneously within a single reaction tube. This method typically involves the utilization of different primer or probe pairs in the same reaction to amplify multiple targets concurrently.

Multiplex PCR is extensively utilized in various genotyping applications and across multiple areas of DNA testing within research, forensic, and diagnostic laboratories. Its applications range from gene expression and deletion analysis to SNP genotyping, forensic identity testing such as STR typing, and pathogen detection. The ability to quantify multiple genes within a single reaction not only reduces reagent costs and conserves sample material but also enhances throughput capabilities [27].

Multiplex PCR plays a crucial role in the diagnosis of intestinal parasites by allowing for the simultaneous detection of multiple parasite species in a single test. This advanced molecular technique offers increased sensitivity and specificity compared to traditional methods, enabling healthcare providers to accurately identify a wide range of parasites in a timely manner. By detecting multiple parasites at once, multiplex PCR streamlines the diagnostic process and helps guide appropriate treatment decisions for patients with suspected intestinal parasitic infections. Its ability to identify a diverse array of parasites makes it an invaluable tool in the field of diagnostic medicine, providing healthcare professionals with a comprehensive and efficient approach to diagnosing intestinal parasites.

4.6 Random amplified polymorphic DNA

Random amplification of polymorphic DNA (RAPD) is conducted using single primers with arbitrarily selected short nucleotide sequences to amplify products from genomic DNA. Following optimization, distinct banding patterns specific to genus, species, or strain can be observed, representing various DNA regions across the entire genome. The utilization of these non-specific primers necessitates DNA from a pure isolate free from contamination by DNA from other organisms, rendering this method unsuitable for genomic DNA extracted from clinical samples. Specific DNA products can be isolated, sequenced, and utilized for the development of targeted assays [32].

Random amplified polymorphic DNA (RAPD) analysis plays a crucial role in the diagnosis of intestinal parasites by providing a highly sensitive and specific method for detecting genetic variations within parasite populations. This technique allows for the identification of unique DNA markers that can differentiate between different parasite species, strains, or isolates. By analyzing the RAPD profiles of parasite samples, healthcare professionals can accurately diagnose and monitor infections, track the spread of parasites, and assess the effectiveness of treatment strategies.

Addressing the limitations of current molecular techniques, Next-generation sequencing (NGS) was introduced. NGS is a cutting-edge technology that allows for rapid and high-throughput sequencing of DNA or RNA. This advanced method has revolutionized the field of genomics by enabling researchers to efficiently analyze large amounts of genetic information in a shorter amount of time. Next-generation sequencing has opened up new possibilities for studying complex biological processes, identifying genetic variations associated with diseases, and advancing personalized medicine.

NGS has revolutionized the rapid generation of extensive data from parasitic species in a single individual, population, or environmental sample within a single sequencing run. NGS technologies have emerged as robust tools for comprehensive parasite detection and genomic analysis [33, 34]. NGS offers numerous advantages over traditional Sanger sequencing, including high throughput, cost-effectiveness, rapid processing, enhanced sensitivity (detecting as low as ~10 ng DNA), and decreased labor to mitigate cloning bias. Platforms like Illumina and Oxford Nanopore can sequence complete parasite genomes from clinical samples, yielding crucial insights into parasite diversity, drug resistance, and transmission dynamics. Furthermore, metagenomic strategies enable the concurrent detection of multiple pathogens in complex clinical specimens, improving diagnostic accuracy in cases of polyparasitism.

5. Imaging studies

Imaging plays a pivotal role in the diagnosis of intestinal parasites, providing a range of techniques to visualize the gastrointestinal tract and identify parasitic infections. Radiographic imaging methods, including X-rays, barium studies, and computed tomography (CT) scans, can unveil structural abnormalities in the gastrointestinal tract resulting from parasitic infections. Specific parasites, such as Ascaris lumbricoides (roundworm), may be discernible on abdominal X-rays due to their distinctive appearance, aiding in the diagnostic process. Barium studies, encompassing barium swallow and barium enema, can pinpoint irregularities like strictures or obstructions caused by large parasites or their associated complications [35].

Ultrasonography proves particularly valuable in detecting liver and biliary tract involvement in parasitic infections, such as liver flukes (e.g., *Fasciola hepatica*) or echinococcosis (caused by Echinococcus spp.). It can also pinpoint intestinal wall thickening, fluid collections, or abscesses stemming from parasitic infections. Endoscopic procedures, such as esophagogastroduodenoscopy (EGD) and colonoscopy, enable direct visualization of the gastrointestinal mucosa and the sampling of suspicious lesions. Endoscopy may unveil characteristic mucosal alterations linked to specific parasitic infections, such as ulceration, nodularity, or inflammation. In certain instances, parasites may be directly observed during endoscopy, facilitating the diagnostic process. For instance, adult worms of Strongyloides stercoralis or *Enterobius vermicularis* (pinworm) may be identified in the gastrointestinal lumen.

Recently, Capsule endoscopy involves the ingestion of a pill-sized camera that captures images as it traverses the digestive tract, providing a comprehensive view of the small intestine. This non-invasive procedure is particularly valuable for diagnosing small bowel parasitic infections, such as hookworms (e.g., *Ancylostoma duodenale*, *Necator americanus*) or *Giardia lamblia*, which may not be easily identified through traditional endoscopy or stool analysis. Wireless video capsule endoscopy, which operates similarly to capsule endoscopy, enables real-time visualization of the small intestine, facilitating the detection of mucosal irregularities and parasitic infections. This advanced technology is instrumental in diagnosing conditions like giardiasis, as it allows for the direct observation of characteristic changes in the small bowel mucosa, such as mucosal inflammation or villous atrophy.

Furthermore, the integration of various imaging modalities or contrast agents for the simultaneous detection of multiple parasites or gastrointestinal abnormalities, along with the utilization of nanoparticles that are specifically tailored to bind to parasite antigens, holds promise for enhancing the sensitivity of parasite detection in imaging techniques.

6. Nanoparticles in the diagnosis of intestinal parasites

Nanoparticles are minuscule particles with dimensions on the nanometer scale, typically ranging from 1 to 100 nanometers in size. These particles exhibit unique physical and chemical properties due to their small size, high surface area-to-volume ratio, and quantum effects. Nanoparticles, owing to their distinctive physical and chemical attributes, have generated considerable interest in the realm of biomedical applications, particularly in disease diagnosis. In the domain of intestinal parasites, nanoparticles present a plethora of benefits, including high sensitivity, specificity, and adaptability. Various diagnostic methodologies for detecting intestinal parasites have leveraged the advantages offered by nanoparticles, encompassing:

Immunoassays: nanoparticles adorned with antibodies or antigens tailored to parasite biomarkers facilitate the highly sensitive detection of parasite antigens in clinical specimens. Immunoassays such as enzyme-linked immunosorbent assays (ELISA) and lateral flow assays (LFAs) expedite the specific identification of parasite proteins or antigens in stool samples, thereby expediting early diagnosis.

Nucleic acid detection: nanoparticles coupled with nucleic acid probes, such as DNA or RNA aptamers, enable the precise detection of parasite DNA or RNA sequences with exceptional sensitivity and specificity. This approach, often integrated with polymerase chain reaction (PCR) or loop-mediated isothermal amplification (LAMP), enables the swift and accurate identification of parasite genetic material in clinical samples.

Imaging and contrast agents: nanoparticles possessing imaging capabilities, such as quantum dots, gold nanoparticles, and magnetic nanoparticles, function as contrast agents for imaging modalities like fluorescence microscopy, computed tomography (CT), and magnetic resonance imaging (MRI). These nanoparticles can be customized with targeting ligands to specifically target and visualize parasites in the gastrointestinal tract, thereby facilitating diagnostic imaging and localization.

Recent research efforts have been devoted to the development of innovative nanoparticle-based diagnostic platforms for intestinal parasites. Nanostructured biosensors, which incorporate nanoparticles into biosensor platforms, enable label-free and real-time detection of parasite biomarkers in clinical samples. Biosensors utilizing surface plasmon resonance (SPR), impedance spectroscopy, and electrochemical techniques offer rapid and sensitive detection of parasite antigens or nucleic acids, with potential applications in point-of-care diagnostics.

Theranostic nanoparticles, capable of both diagnosis and therapy, show promise for targeted treatment of intestinal parasitic infections. These multifunctional nanoparticles can deliver therapeutic agents, such as antiparasitic drugs or immunomodulators while facilitating non-invasive imaging for disease monitoring and assessment of treatment response.

The utilization of nanotechnology presents numerous unique opportunities for enhanced diagnostics of parasitic diseases in the future. Current diagnostic tools for detecting parasitic diseases include light and fluorescence microscopy, rapid diagnostic tests (RDT) like immunochromatographic lateral flow tests, serology, quantitative Buffy-coat (QBC) techniques, and nucleic acid amplification techniques such as polymerase chain reaction (PCR) [36–39]. Various types of nanoparticles, including fluorescent, magnetic, and metal nanoparticles, are being investigated for their diagnostic potential. Among these, gold and silver nanoparticles are the most extensively studied, as they exhibit intense absorption when stimulated by electromagnetic radiation [40]. Molecules like antibodies, antigens, and enzymes can be attached to nanoparticles as electrochemical markers, optical probes, and signal enhancers. For instance, magnetic nanoparticles with an iron oxide core and silver coating are being explored for early detection of malaria [41, 42].

7. Artificial intelligence and machine

Deep technology, also known as deep tech, currently lacks a universally accepted formal definition. However, it can be understood as a fusion of science, engineering, and design, aimed at providing societal benefits that surpass those of individual technologies [43]. This interdisciplinary approach is geared toward generating innovative solutions in various sectors such as healthcare, agriculture, space, and energy [44–46]. Deep tech projects are rooted in problem-focused research, with a focus on creating unique and complex products that are challenging to replicate. Cutting-edge technologies like machine learning, artificial intelligence, robotics, and quantum computing play a pivotal role in the design, development, and testing of these advanced solutions [47].

The integration of artificial intelligence (AI) and machine learning algorithms into diagnostic platforms is becoming increasingly prevalent, aimed at enhancing accuracy and efficiency. AI-based image analysis software is now capable of swiftly analyzing microscopic images of stool samples, accurately detecting and quantifying parasite eggs, cysts, and larvae. Furthermore, AI algorithms, trained on extensive datasets, can assist healthcare providers in interpreting intricate diagnostic results, offering diagnostic recommendations and treatment guidelines tailored to individual patient parameters. The field of medical diagnostics is undergoing a profound transformation with the advent of artificial intelligence (AI).

A study titled "Detection of Intestinal Protozoa in Trichrome-Stained Stool Specimens by Use of a Deep Convolutional Neural Network" sheds light on this paradigm shift, focusing on the pivotal role of convolutional neural networks (CNN) in parasitology. The findings of the study are unequivocal: the CNN model exhibited remarkable accuracy, successfully identifying parasites in specimens that had previously eluded detection through manual methods. This underscores the immense potential of AI in significantly enhancing diagnostic precision [48].

A significant increase in literature has been observed regarding the research, development, and utilization of deep tech innovations in the identification of parasites (both single and multispecies in a sample), detection of life cycle stages, and classification of eggs from human intestinal parasites [49–51]. There has been a particular focus on the application of deep learning for the analysis of protozoan images, leading to highly sensitive parasite detection. This has facilitated the creation of extensive public datasets for various parasites such as plasmodium, toxoplasma, leishmania, and trypanosome [52–54].

Within the framework of the Department of Biotechnology (DBT), advanced machine learning modules, both supervised and unsupervised, have been established and trained with vast amounts of data using artificial intelligence algorithms and neural network models. These modules have been seamlessly integrated into user-friendly interfaces, including mobile applications, resulting in unparalleled performance with no interpretation bias [55]. A groundbreaking approach utilizing computer vision screening and visualization algorithms analyzed over 19.6 billion floating point operations (flops) of digitized blood smears, achieving an impressive 99.52% accuracy in detecting malarial parasites [56].

Furthermore, a more computationally efficient model requiring only 4600 flops demonstrated a 99.23% accuracy rate, highlighting its enhanced commercial viability [56]. Deep technologies are also delving into the assessment of parasitic motility as a biomarker for precise parasite detection [57]. Zhang et al. developed a platform utilizing lensless holographic speckle analysis and deep learning to automatically detect and count motile parasites in body fluids by analyzing holographic time-lapse speckle patterns [58].

Despite the significant research and development progress in the field of deep technologies, the commercial utilization of these advancements remains relatively constrained, with minimal indications of widespread market adoption. An example of a cutting-edge commercial tool within this realm is the VETSCAN IMAGYST scanning and analyzing systems. When utilized in conjunction with the VETSCAN IMAGYST fecal preparation techniques, this innovative system enables the swift and accurate detection of Ancylostoma, Toxocara, Trichuris vulpis, and taeniid eggs in the fecal matter of both dogs and cats, all within a mere 15-minute timeframe and without the necessity for highly specialized personnel [59].

8. Challenges and future directions

Despite the considerable advancements in diagnostic methodologies, obstacles persist in the integration of these technologies into everyday clinical practice, especially in resource-limited environments. Challenges such as financial constraints, infrastructure demands, and the necessity for skilled personnel may impede widespread utilization. Furthermore, continued endeavors are essential to authenticate and establish standardized novel diagnostic assays, guaranteeing their dependability and consistency across various contexts.

9. Conclusion

Recent advancements in diagnostic techniques present promising opportunities for the precise and timely detection of intestinal parasites. Molecular methods, point-of-care testing (POCT) devices, nanoparticles, and artificial intelligence-driven approaches hold the potential to transform parasite diagnosis, ultimately enhancing patient outcomes and bolstering the efficacy of parasitic infection control measures. Nevertheless, overcoming current obstacles and ensuring equal access to these innovations are imperative for their effective deployment across a range of healthcare environments. Continued research and collaboration are necessary to refine and incorporate these diagnostic tools into standard clinical protocols, thereby playing a pivotal role in the worldwide campaign against intestinal parasitic diseases.

Acknowledgements

The author acknowledges the use of Grammarly software for language polishing of the manuscript.

Abbreviations

AI	artificial intelligence
CNN	convolutional neural networks
CT	computed tomography
DBT	department of biotechnology
EGD	esophagogastroduodenoscopy
ELISA	enzyme-linked immunosorbent assay
LFA	lateral flow assays
MRI	magnetic resonance imaging
NGS	next-generation sequencing
PCR	polymerase chain reaction
POCT	point-of-care testing
RDT	rapid diagnostic tests

Author details

Yohannis Derbew Molla* and Hirut Tesfahun Alemu
College of Medicine and Health Sciences, University of Gondar, Gondar, Ethiopia

*Address all correspondence to: yderbew73@gmail.com

References

[1] Charlier J, Rinaldi L, Musella V, Ploeger HW, Chartier C, Vineer HR, et al. Initial assessment of the economic burden of major parasitic helminth infections to the ruminant livestock industry in Europe. Preventive Veterinary Medicine. 2020;**182**:105103

[2] Pullan R, Brooker S. The health impact of polyparasitism in humans: Are we under-estimating the burden of parasitic diseases? Parasitology. 2008;**135**(7):783-794

[3] van der Giessen J, Deksne G, Gómez-Morales MA, Troell K, Gomes J, Sotiraki S, et al. Surveillance of foodborne parasitic diseases in Europe in a one health approach. Parasite Epidemiology and Control. 2021;**13**:e00205

[4] Torgerson PR, Macpherson CNL. The socioeconomic burden of parasitic zoonoses: Global trends. Veterinary Parasitology. 2011;**182**(1):79-95

[5] Torgerson PR, Devleesschauwer B, Praet N, Speybroeck N, Willingham AL, Kasuga F, et al. World Health Organization estimates of the global and regional disease burden of 11 foodborne parasitic diseases, 2010: A data synthesis. PLoS Medicine. 2015;**12**(12):e1001920

[6] Hotez PJ, Brown AS. Neglected tropical disease vaccines. Biologicals. 2009;**37**(3):160-164

[7] CDC – DPDx – Parasites A-Z Index. Google Search. 2021. Available from: https://www.cdc.gov/dpdx/az.html [Accessed: November 20, 2021]

[8] Schistosomiasis and soil-transmitted helminthiases: Numbers of people treated in 2017. Available from: https://www.who.int/publications/i/item/who-wer9350essed [Accessed: Novenber 20, 2021]

[9] Pullan RL, Smith JL, Jasrasaria R, Brooker SJ. Global numbers of infection and disease burden of soil transmitted helminth infections in 2010. Parasites & Vectors. 2014;**7**(1):37

[10] Dematei A, Fernandes R, Soares R, Alves H, Richter J, Botelho MC. Angiogenesis in *Schistosoma haematobium*-associated urinary bladder cancer. APMIS. 2017;**125**(12):1056-1062

[11] Marcilla A, Trelis M, Cortés A, Sotillo J, Cantalapiedra F, Minguez MT, et al. Extracellular vesicles from parasitic helminths contain specific excretory/secretory proteins and are internalized in intestinal host cells. PLoS One. 2012;**7**(9):e45974

[12] Hart BL, Hart LA. How mammals stay healthy in nature: The evolution of behaviours to avoid parasites and pathogens. Philosophical Transactions of the Royal Society B: Biological Sciences. 2018;**373**(1751):20170205

[13] Baltrušis P, Höglund J. Digital PCR: Modern solution to parasite diagnostics and population trait genetics. Parasites & Vectors. 2023;**16**(1):143

[14] Bennett A, Garcia E, Schulze M, Bailey M, Doyle K, Finn W, et al. Building a laboratory workforce to meet the future: ASCP task force on the laboratory professionals workforce. American Journal of Clinical Pathology. 2014;**141**(2):154-167

[15] Petti CA, Polage CR, Quinn TC, Ronald AR, Sande MA. Laboratory medicine in Africa: A barrier to effective

health care. Clinical Infectious Diseases. 2006;**42**(3):377-382

[16] Saiki RK, Gelfand DH, Stoffel S, Scharf SJ, Higuchi R, Horn GT, et al. Primer-directed enzymatic amplification of DNA with a thermostable DNA polymerase. Science. 1988;**239**(4839): 487-491

[17] Saiki RK, Scharf S, Faloona F, Mullis KB, Horn GT, Erlich HA, et al. Enzymatic amplification of β-globin genomic sequences and restriction site analysis for diagnosis of sickle cell anemia. Science. 1985;**230**(4732):1350-1354

[18] Barker RH. DNA probe diagnosis of parasitic infections. Experimental Parasitology. 1990;**70**(4):494-499

[19] de Bruijn MHL. Diagnostic DNA amplification no respite for the elusive parasite. Parasitology Today. 1988;**4**(10):293-295

[20] Weiss JB. DNA probes and PCR for diagnosis of parasitic infections. Clinical Microbiology Reviews. 1995;**8**(1):113-130

[21] Verweij JJ, Stensvold CR. Molecular testing for clinical diagnosis and epidemiological investigations of intestinal parasitic infections. Clinical Microbiology Reviews. 2014;**27**(2):371-418

[22] Monteiro L, Bonnemaison D, Vekris A, Petry KG, Bonnet J, Vidal R, et al. Complex polysaccharides as PCR inhibitors in feces: *Helicobacter pylori* model. Journal of Clinical Microbiology. 1997;**35**(4):995-998

[23] Demeler J, Ramünke S, Wolken S, Ianiello D, Rinaldi L, Gahutu JB, et al. Discrimination of gastrointestinal nematode eggs from crude fecal egg preparations by inhibitor-resistant conventional and real-time PCR. PLoS One. 2013;**8**(4):e61285

[24] Morgan UM, Pallant L, Dwyer BW, Forbes DA, Rich G, Thompson RCA. Comparison of PCR and microscopy for detection of *Cryptosporidium parvum* in human fecal specimens: Clinical trial. Journal of Clinical Microbiology. 1998;**36**(4):995-998

[25] Kreader CA. Relief of amplification inhibition in PCR with bovine serum albumin or T4 gene 32 protein. Applied and Environmental Microbiology. 1996;**62**(3):1102-1106

[26] Niesters HGM. Clinical virology in real time. Journal of Clinical Virology. 2002;**25**:3-12

[27] Al-Turkmani MR, Deharvengt SJ, Lefferts JA. Chapter 31 – Molecular assessment of human diseases in the clinical laboratory. In: Coleman WB, Tsongalis GJ, editors. Essential Concepts in Molecular Pathology. 2nd ed. Lebanon, NH, United States: Dartmouth Hitchcock Medical Center; 2020. pp. 563-578. Available from: https://www.sciencedirect.com/science/article/pii/B9780128132579000310

[28] Espy MJ, Uhl JR, Sloan LM, Buckwalter SP, Jones MF, Vetter EA, et al. Real-time PCR in clinical microbiology: Applications for routine laboratory testing. Clinical Microbiology Reviews. 2006;**19**(1):165-256

[29] Klein D. Quantification using real-time PCR technology: Applications and limitations. Trends in Molecular Medicine. 2002;**8**(6):257-260

[30] Schaaf CP, Wiszniewska J, Beaudet al. Copy number and SNP arrays in clinical diagnostics. Annual Review of Genomics and Human Genetics. 2011;**12**(1):25-51

[31] Whale AS, Huggett JF, Cowen S, Speirs V, Shaw J, Ellison S, et al. Comparison of microfluidic digital PCR and conventional quantitative PCR for measuring copy number variation. Nucleic Acids Research. 2012;**40**(11):e82

[32] Williams JGK, Kubelik AR, Livak KJ, Rafalski JA, Tingey SV. DNA polymorphisms amplified by arbitrary primers are useful as genetic markers. Nucleic Acids Research. 1990;**18**(22):6531-6535

[33] Hutchison CA III. DNA sequencing: Bench to bedside and beyond †. Nucleic Acids Research. 2007;**35**(18):6227-6237

[34] Ekblom R, Galindo J. Applications of next generation sequencing in molecular ecology of non-model organisms. Heredity. 2011;**107**(1):1-15

[35] Palmer PES. Diagnostic imaging in parasitic infections. Pediatric Clinics of North America. 1985;**32**(4):1019-1040

[36] Tangpukdee N, Duangdee C, Wilairatana P, Krudsood S. Malaria diagnosis: A brief review. The Korean Journal of Parasitology. 2009;**47**(2):93-102

[37] Yetisgin AA, Cetinel S, Zuvin M, Kosar A, Kutlu O. Therapeutic nanoparticles and their targeted delivery applications. Molecules. 2020;**25**(9):2193

[38] Moyano A, Serrano-Pertierra E, Salvador M, Martínez-García JC, Rivas M, Blanco-López MC. Magnetic lateral flow immunoassays. Diagnostics. 2020;**10**(5):288

[39] Thakur S, Joshi J, Kaur S. Leishmaniasis diagnosis: An update on the use of parasitological, immunological and molecular methods. Journal of Parasitic Diseases. 2020;**44**(2):253-272

[40] Tallury P, Malhotra A, Byrne LM, Santra S. Nanobioimaging and sensing of infectious diseases. Advanced Drug Delivery Reviews. 2010;**62**(4):424-437

[41] Nash MA, Waitumbi JN, Hoffman AS, Yager P, Stayton PS. Multiplexed enrichment and detection of malarial biomarkers using a stimuli-responsive iron oxide and gold nanoparticle reagent system. ACS Nano. 2012;**6**(8):6776-6785

[42] Baptista V, Peng WK, Minas G, Veiga MI, Catarino SO. Review of microdevices for hemozoin-based malaria detection. Biosensors. 2022;**12**(2):110

[43] Lee K. Philosophy and Revolutions in Genetics: Deep Science and Deep Technology. London, UK: Palgrave Macmillan; 2003

[44] Verma J. Deep Technologies using big data in: Energy and waste management. In: Kadyan V, Singh TP, Ugwu C, editors. Deep Learning Technologies for the Sustainable Development Goals: Issues and Solutions in the Post-COVID Era. Singapore: Springer Nature; 2023. pp. 21-39. (Advanced Technologies and Societal Change). DOI: 10.1007/978-981-19-5723-9_2

[45] Hinton G. Deep learning—A technology with the potential to transform health care. Journal of the American Medical Association. 2018;**320**(11):1101-1102

[46] Lee K. The Natural and the Artefactual: The Implications of Deep Science and Deep Technology for Environmental Philosophy. United States: Lexington Books; 1999. 310 p

[47] Patil T, Pandey S, Visrani K. A review on basic deep learning technologies and

applications. In: Kotecha K, Piuri V, Shah HN, Patel R, editors. Data Science and Intelligent Applications. Singapore: Springer Singapore; 2021. pp. 565-573. (Lecture Notes on Data Engineering and Communications Technologies; vol. 52). Available from: http://link.springer.com/10.1007/978-981-15-4474-3_61

[48] Mathison BA, Kohan JL, Walker JF, Smith RB, Ardon O, Couturier MR. Detection of intestinal protozoa in trichrome-stained stool specimens by use of a deep convolutional neural network. Journal of Clinical Microbiology. 26 May 2020;**58**(6):e02053-19

[49] Zhang Y, Jiang H, Ye T, Juhas M. Deep learning for imaging and detection of microorganisms. Trends in Microbiology. 2021;**29**(7):569-572

[50] Butploy N, Kanarkard W, Maleewong IP. Deep learning approach for Ascaris lumbricoides parasite egg classification. Magalhães LG, editor. Journal of Parasitology Research. 2021;**2021**:1-8

[51] Routledge & CRC Press [Internet]. Computational Vision and Medical Image Processing V: Proceedings of the 5th Eccomas Thematic Conference on Computational Vision and Medical Image Processing (VipIMAGE 2015, Tenerife, Spain, October 19-21, 2015). Available from: https://www.routledge.com/Computational-Vision-and-Medical-Image-Processing-V-Proceedings-of-the/Tavares-Natal-Jorge/p/book/9781138029262

[52] Quinn JA, Nakasi R, Mugagga PKB, Byanyima P, Lubega W, Andama A. Deep convolutional neural networks for microscopy-based point of care diagnostics. In: Proceedings of the 1st Machine Learning for Healthcare Conference. Los Angeles, CA: PMLR; 2016. pp. 271-281. Available from: https://proceedings.mlr.press/v56/Quinn16.html

[53] Ljosa V, Sokolnicki KL, Carpenter AE. Annotated high-throughput microscopy image sets for validation. Nature Methods. 2012;**9**(7):637-637

[54] Anantrasirichai N, Chalidabhongse TH, Palasuwan D, Naruenatthanaset K, Kobchaisawat T, Nunthanasup N, et al. ICIP 2022 challenge on parasitic egg detection and classification in microscopic images: Dataset, methods and results. In: 2022 IEEE International Conference on Image Processing (ICIP). Bordeaux, France: IEEE; 2022. pp. 4306-4310. Available from: https://ieeexplore.ieee.org/document/9897267/

[55] Jo T. Machine Learning Foundations: Supervised, Unsupervised, and Advanced Learning [Internet]. Cham: Springer International Publishing; 2021 [cited 2024 Oct 10]. Available from: http://link.springer.com/10.1007/978-3-030-65900-4

[56] Fuhad KMF, Tuba JF, Sarker MRA, Momen S, Mohammed N, Rahman T. Deep learning based automatic malaria parasite detection from blood smear and its smartphone based application. Diagnostics. 2020;**10**(5):329

[57] Zhang Y, Koydemir HC, Shimogawa MM, Yalcin S, Guziak A, Liu T, et al. High-throughput and label-free detection of motile parasites in bodily fluids using lensless time-resolved speckle imaging. In: Conference on Lasers and Electro-Optics (2019), Paper ATu4K2. Optica Publishing Group; 2019. p. ATu4K.2. Available from: https://opg.optica.org/abstract.cfm?uri=CLEO_AT-2019-ATu4K.2

[58] Zhang Y, Ceylan Koydemir H, Shimogawa MM, Yalcin S, Guziak A,

Liu T, et al. Motility-based label-free detection of parasites in bodily fluids using holographic speckle analysis and deep learning. Light: Science & Applications. 2018;**7**(1):108

[59] Nagamori Y, Hall Sedlak R, DeRosa A, Pullins A, Cree T, Loenser M, et al. Evaluation of the VETSCAN IMAGYST: An in-clinic canine and feline fecal parasite detection system integrated with a deep learning algorithm. Parasites & Vectors. 2020;**13**(1):346

Chapter 14

The Immunodominant Determinants of the Host-Protective Recombinant Oncosphere Antigens of Cestode Parasites are Conformational Epitopes

Emmanuel Assana and André Pagnah Zoli

Abstract

Host-protective antigens isolated from the oncosphere of taeniid cestodes are highly effective vaccine antigens against cysticercosis and hydatid diseases in mammals, achieving 99 to 100% of protection in vaccinated intermediate hosts against an experimental challenge infection and in field trials. The principal immune mechanism induced by recombinant oncosphere antigens is believed to be complement-fixing antibodies that kill the oncosphere or early developing parasites. Knowledge of the nature of antigenic sites recognized by antibodies is an important component in understanding the characteristics of a vaccine antigen and the development of associated immunological assays. Efforts to identify and characterize protective epitopes have been made for two recombinant oncosphere antigens: EG95 and TSOL18 vaccines against *Echinococcus granulosus* in sheep and *Taenia solium* in pigs, respectively. The objective of this paper is to give a short review of the investigations that were undertaken to characterize whether the principal antibody specificities raised by these oncospheral antigens are against linear or conformational determinants.

Keywords: antigen, antibody, conformational epitopes, cestodes, oncosphere

1. Introduction

Cysticercosis and hydatid diseases are parasitic diseases of humans and several mammals with important public health and economic impacts in low- and middle-income countries. These diseases are caused by the larvae stage of cestode parasites. An attractive strategy to control cysticercosis and hydatid diseases is the use of vaccines to prevent infections in the animal intermediate hosts, thereby breaking the parasite's life cycle and removing the source of infections for definitive hosts [1]. The first effective recombinant oncosphere vaccine was developed against *Taenia ovis* [2, 3]. This vaccine has been recognized as a milestone in the history of parasitology [4]. The success in the development of the vaccine against *Taenia ovis* was the basis of the research on vaccines against other cestode parasites. Recombinant oncosphere vaccine antigens have been developed against *Taenia saginata* in cattle [5], *Echinococcus granulosus* [6] and *Taenia multiceps* in sheep [7], and *Taenia solium* in pigs [8, 9]. Oncosphere vaccine antigens seem to target the parasites at the early stage of their development [10]. The principal immune mechanism is believed to be complement-fixing antibodies that kill activated oncosphere or early developing parasites [10, 11]. Evidence of the implication of complement in antibody-mediated protection against cestode infection was provided in an early investigation on *Taenia taeniaeformis* infection (reviewed by Lightowlers et al. [12]). Cobra venom factor blocks the classical and alternative pathways of the complement cascade system on the parasite surface and abrogates the protective effect of antibodies against *Taenia taeniaeformis* in mice and rats. However, high level of immune protection induced by a single recombinant oncosphere remains a mystery in parasitology. Helminths are known as efficient immune manipulators able to modulate and modify the innate and adaptive immune responses of mammals through specific molecules [13]. Why are antigens from oncospheres of cestodes highly protective in intermediated hosts? Part of the answer may be linked to the fibronectin type III domain (FN-III) found in all oncosphere vaccines [14, 15]. FN-III domains are folded modules found in a variety of multidomain proteins of eukaryotic organisms [16]. It is believed that FN-III is associated to the host-protective and conformational epitopes of oncosphere antigens of cestodes parasites [9, 14]. The objective of this paper is to give a short review of the investigations that were undertaken to characterize whether the principal antibody specificities raised by the oncospheral antigens are against linear or conformational determinants.

2. Antibody specificities raised by the oncosphere antigens in sheep and pig models

The EG95 and TSOL18 recombinant oncosphere vaccine antigens against *Echinococcus granulosus* in sheep and *Taenia solium* in pigs, respectively, have provided models for investigations to characterize whether the principal antibody specificities raised by the oncosphere antigens in animals are against linear or conformational determinants. *Echinococcus granulosus* oncosphere protein EG95 is a 16.5 kDa antigen as a fusion protein with glutathione S-tranferase (GST). Linear antibody-binding epitopes on EG95 were mapped using 25 overlapping synthetic peptides [17]. Four immunodominant regions of EG95 were found. Sheep were immunized with these four synthetic peptides corresponding to these immunodominant epitope peptides and challenged with *E. granulosus* eggs. All of the peptides induced specific antibodies, but these antibodies did not kill the parasite in *in vitro* culture assays and the challenged sheep were not protected [18, 19]. Three overlapping truncated regions of EG95 were also expressed in *E. coli*. In vaccination trials, none of the truncated regions provided any significant protection of sheep against challenge infection [20]. Since linear epitopes did not protect against infection, it was concluded that the protective epitopes of EG95 are conformational and the full length of the EG95 molecule is required to produce immunity.

The investigations that were undertaken to characterize linear or conformational determinants of *T. solium* oncosphere protein TSOL18 were similar to those undertaken with EG95 antigen, with slight differences in immunoassays based on inhibition enzyme-linked immunosorbent assay (i-ELISA) as described by Assana et al. [9]. The TSOL18 antigen used in these investigation was identical to the vaccine protein used in the successful vaccine trials described by Assana et al. [21]. The protein was expressed as a C-terminal fusion to glutathione *S*-transferase (TSOL18-GST) and to maltose-binding protein (TSOL18-MBP) [9]. TSOL18 was also expressed in two truncated forms fused to GST (TSOL18-1-GST and TSOL18-2-GST) representing either the amino terminal portion or the carboxy-terminal portion of the antigen. TSOL18-1 contained 71 amino acids starting from the amino terminus of TSOL18. TSOL18-2 consisted of the carboxy-terminal 66 amino acids of TSOL18. The two truncated proteins overlapped each other by 25 amino acids. The whole protein (TSOL18) and the two truncations (TSOL18-1 and TSOL18-2) were used in i-ELISA to determine their ability to inhibit the binding of pig antibodies to TSOL18. TSOL18 was shown to be capable of completely inhibiting the binding of pig anti-TSOL18 antibodies to TSOL18 in i-ELISA [9]. However, neither TSOL18-1 nor TSOL18-2, either alone or combined, was capable of inhibiting any detectable amount of reactivity of pig anti-TSOL18 antibodies (**Figure 1**). Taking in account these results described by Assana et al. [9] and also the results from the investigations on EG95 [20], it was concluded that the dominant antibody

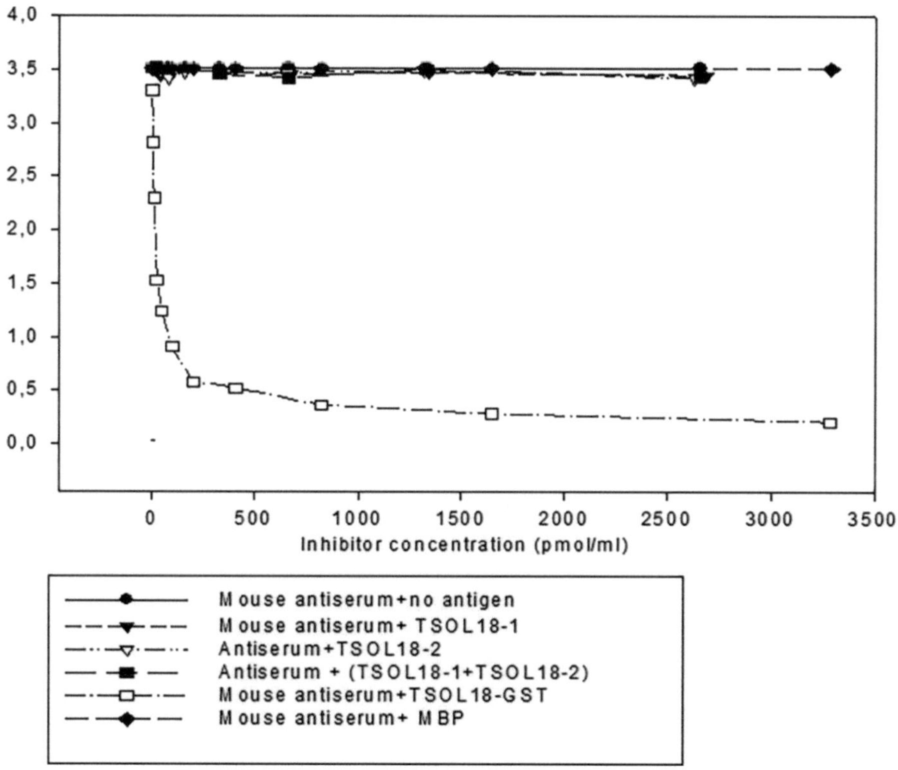

Figure 1.
Inhibition enzyme-linked immunosorbent assay (i-ELISA) using a serial dilution of antiserum from mouse immunized with TSOL18-GST.

specificities, and probably the host-protective specificities, of recombinant onco-sphere vaccines developed against cysticercosis and hydatid diseases are conformational epitopes [9, 20].

3. Similarity of pig and mouse antibody responses to *Taenia solium* oncosphere protein TSOL18

Studies were undertaken to compare antibody responses of pig and mouse to TSOL18 for further monoclonal antibody production in mouse against the antigenic epitopes of oncospheres antigens [22]. Two hypotheses have directed this part of investigations: (1) Antibody responses to TSOL18 pigs and mice are not similar; therefore, it would not be relevant to produce mouse monoclonal antibodies for further characterization and identification of conformational epitopes on the recombinant oncosphere proteins [23, 24] and (2) the structure of recombinant oncosphere proteins fused with GST or MBP causes interference with the binding of antibodies to some epitopes.

Inhibition ELISA (i-ELISA) and competition ELISA (c-ELISA) were used as described by Assana et al. [9] and Assana [22], respectively, to provide the evidence of the similarity of pig and mouse antibody responses to TSOL18 antigen. As demonstrated previously in pigs, the i-ELISA indicated that the entire TSOL18 inhibited completely mouse anti-TSOL18 antibodies, but the truncated forms (TSOL-18-1 and TSOL18-2) caused no inhibition in i-ELISA, suggesting that mice also recognized predominantly conformational epitopes of TSOL18 (**Figures 1** and **2**).

Antibody responses in pigs and mice for the same epitopes on TSOL18 were evaluated with the c-ELISA [22]. Briefly, serum samples collected from 10 pigs immunized

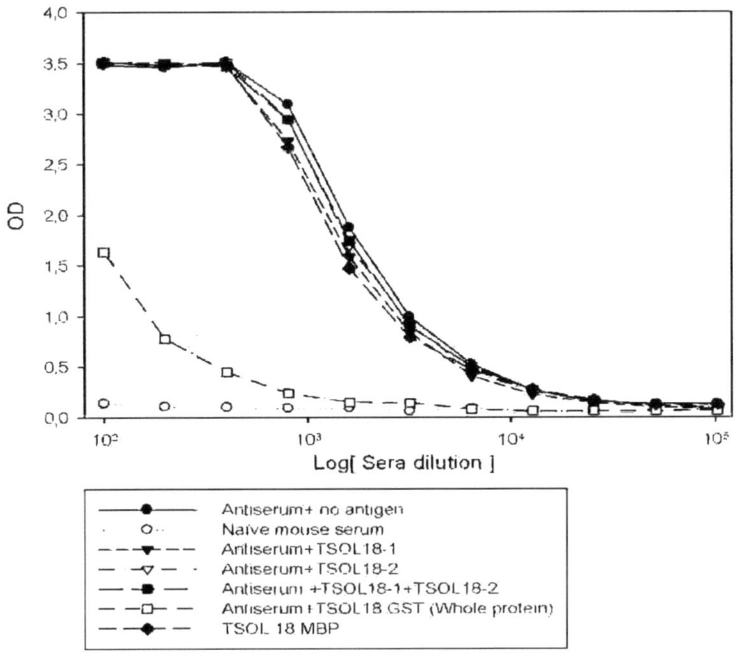

Figure 2.
Inhibition enzyme-linked immunosorbent assay (i-ELISA) using constant dilution of antigen.

with TSOL18 antigen were serially diluted in phosphate buffered saline-bovine serum albumin (PBS-BSA) and distributed on the plates coated with TSOL18-MBP antigen. Constant dilution (1/50) in PBS-BSA of pooled mouse serums immunized with TSOL18 was added to serial diluted pig serums. Pre-immune serum was used as control (no competition). Goat anti-mouse IgG conjugated to horseradish peroxidase was used to reveal the competition between pig and mouse anti-TSOL18 antibodies for the same epitopes on TSO18 antigen. The results indicated that pig serums exhibited strong and different inhibition profiles of the binding of pooled mouse serums from optical density (OD) approaching 0 to approximately 1, suggesting the majority of pig and mouse antibodies raised to TSOL18 recognized by the same epitopes on TSOL18 (**Figure 3**).

Phage display mimotope technology has been used to identify the conformational epitopes EG95 [23, 24]. Only one momotope was identified representing a minor component of the protective antibody produced by the EG95 vaccine [24]. An alternative technology that may be applied to identify and characterize the antigenic epitopes of the recombinant oncosphere antigens is the use of monoclonal antibodies. From the results demonstrating the similarity of pig and mouse antibody responses to TSOL18 protein, monoclonal antibody technology may provide a suitable method to further characterization and identification of the conformational epitopes of

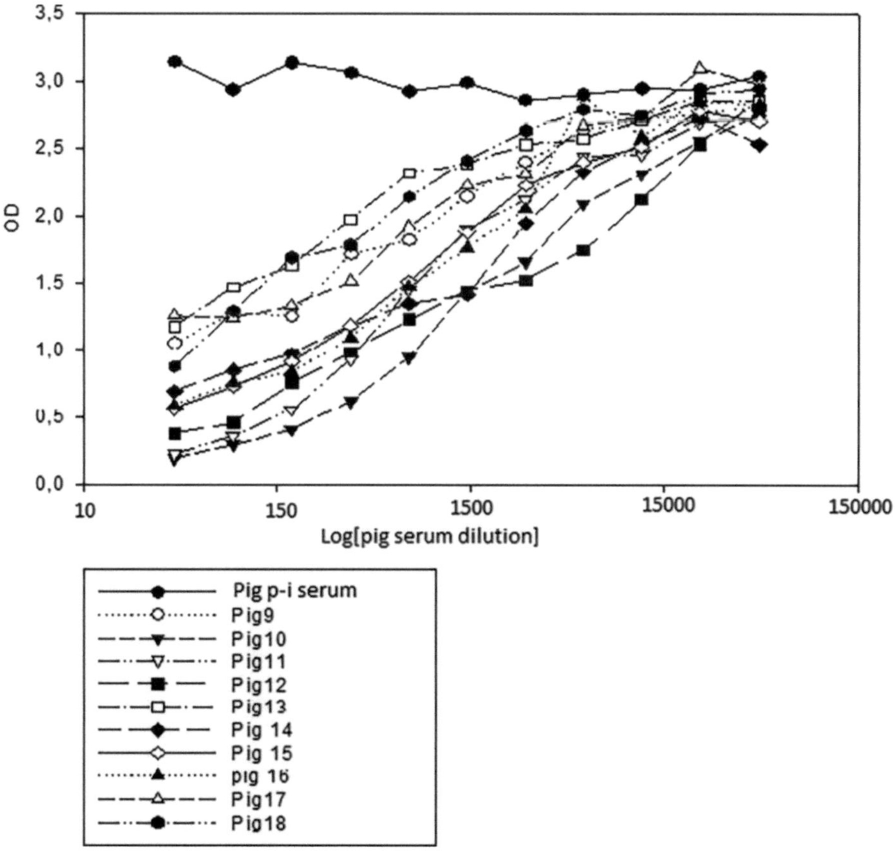

Figure 3.
Competition ELISA for pig and mouse anti-TSOL18 antibodies reacting with the same epitopes.

host-protective recombinant oncosphere antigens of cestode parasites developed to date. Consequently, investigations were undertaken for the generation of mouse monoclonal antibodies against TSOL18 [25].

4. Generation and characterization of mouse monoclonal antibodies against TSOL18 protein

Monoclonal antibodies were generated against TSOL18 protein as described by Assana et al. [22, 25]. The production procedure resulted in 20 cell clones producing MoAb (**Table 1**). An i-ELISA was carried out as described above [9] for the selection of MoAb directed against conformational epitopes of TSOL18. The isotypes of the MoAb were determined by an immunoassay kit [20]. Subsequently, 18 IgG1 and 2 IgM monoclonal antibodies were identified (**Table 2**). All IgG1 (18), representing 90% of generated MoAb to TSOL18, reacted only with full-length TSOL18 protein and not with the two linear forms of TSOL18 (TSOL18-1 and ISOL18-2) suggesting that the great majority of the specific antibodies induced in pigs and mice following

Plate N°	Line	Column	ELISA optical density	Cryopreserved cell lines
2	F	4	0,836	2F4 Assana
4	A	9	0,73	4A9 Assana
4	D	6	0,73	4D6 Assana
9	B	8	1316	9B8 Assana
10	D	8	0,187	10D8 Assana
10	D	9	0,144	10D9 Assana
10	H	1	1209	10H1 Assana
12	C	8	0,282	12C8 Assana
13	A	3	0,965	13A3 Assana
13	H	8	0,439	13H8 Assana
15	F	1	1177	15F1 Assana
17	G	9	0,37	17G9 Assana
19	A	2	0,289	19A2 Assana
21	C	2	0,191	21C2 Assana
21	H	7	0,219	21H7Assana
22	A	12	0,7	22A12 Assana
22	B	7	0,246	22B7 Assana
25	D	12	0,593	25D12 Assana
25	E	9	0,389	25E9 Assana
25	H	7	1005	25H7 Assana

Table 1.
Cell lines producing monoclonal antibodies to TSOL18 protein [22].

MoAB	MoAbs isotypes reacting in immunoassay kit (Southern Biotechnology, Associates, USA)						Reactivity of MoAbs with full length and the two truncated TSOL18 proteins in i-ELISA		
	IgM	IgG1	IgG2a	IgG2b	IgG3	IgA	TSOL18	TSOL18-1	TSOL18-2
4A9	—	+	—	—	—	—	+	—	—
21C2	—	+	—	—	—	—	+	—	—
25D12	—	+	—	—	—	—	+	—	—
10H1	—	+	—	—	—	—	+	—	—
19A2	+	—	—	—	—	—	+	—	—
22A12	—	+	—	—	—	—	+	—	—
2F4	—	+	—	—	—	—	+	—	—
15F1	+	—	—	—	—	—	+	—	+
13H8	+	—	—	—	—	—	+	—	+
21H7	+	—	—	—	—	—	+	—	—
25H7	—	+	—	—	—	—	+	—	—
13A3	—	+	—	—	—		+	—	—
4D6	—	+	—	—	—		+	—	—
9B8	—	+	—	—	—		+	—	—
10D8	—	+	—	—	—		+	—	—
10D9	—	—	—	—	—		+	—	—
17G9	—	+	—	—	—		+	—	—
12C8	—	+	—	—	—		+	—	—
22B7	—	+	—	—	—		+	—	—
25E9	—	+	—	—	—		+	—	—

Table 2.
Characterization of anti-TSOL18 monoclonal antibodies (MoAbs) [25].

immunization with TSOL18-GST are IgG1 subtypes directed against conformational determinants rather than linear determinants of TSOL18. Predominant IgG1 isotypes induced by TSOL18-GST in pigs were previously reported by Kyngdon et al. [11]. This may suggest the IgG1 isotypes are implicated in the protection against cestode parasites in intermediate hosts. The IgM isotype MoAb against TSOL18 reacted only with the Tsol18-2 [25], suggesting that the linear epitopes of TSOL18 are located within the amino acid sequence AKTIYRVDVDGYRNEIMVFGSQRFATTLPKKQIKHKKVRRS. Surprisingly, linear epitope(s) of TSOL18 recognized by 93% of pig antisera reacting with linear overlapped peptides 13 and 14 described by Kyngdon et al. [11] are located within amino acid sequence FATTLPKKQIKHKKVRRS, which is the terminal portion of TSOL18-2. Taking into account the results of overlapped linear synthetic peptides reacting with pig antisera to TSOL18 protein [11] and the mouse monoclonal antibodies against TSOL18 [22, 25], it could be concluded that the immunodominant linear epitopes of TSOL18 are located within the carboxy-terminal 41 amino acids of TSOL18 (**Table 3**).

Proteins	Sequence of amino acids	Number of amino acids
TSOL18 (full length)	DRTFGDDIFVPYLRCFALSATEIGVF WDAGEMVGHGVEEIK VKVEKAIHPYKIWNATVSANNGKVIIRDLKAKTIYRVDVDGYR NEIMVFGS QRFATTLPKKQIKHKKVRRS	112
TSOL18-1 (front half of TSOL18)	DRTFGDDIFVPYLRCFALSATEIGVFWDAGEMVGHGVEEIKV KVEKAIHPYKI WNATVSANNGKVIIRDLK	71
TSOL18-2 (back half of TSOL18)	AIHPYKIWNATVSANNGKVIIRDLKAKTIYR VDVDGYRNEIMVFGSQRF ATTLPKKQIKHKKVRRS	66
Overlapped portion of TSOL18-1 and TSOL18-2	AIHPYKIWNATVSANNGKVIIRDLK	25
The carboxy-terminal 41 amino acids of TSOL18 containing linear epitopes reacting with mouse MoAb and pig antisera [11, 22, 25]	AKTIYRVDVDGYRNEIMVFGSQ RFATTLPKKQIKHKKVRRS	41

Table 3.
Sequence of amino acids in TSOL18, TSOL18-2, and TSOL18-2 proteins [9].

5. Concluding remarks

Investigations that were undertaken to characterize linear and conformational determinants of EG95 and TSOL18 recombinant oncosphere antigens [9, 17–20] and the generation of monoclonal antibodies against conformational and linear epitopes of *Taenia solium* oncosphere protein TSOL18 [22, 25] provide a foundation for the understanding of the antibody responses to host-protective recombinant oncosphere antigens of cestode parasites in intermediate hosts. To this time, definitive studies have not been undertaken for all oncosphere antigen vaccines; however, it can be concluded from the data and studies described above that the dominant antibody specificities, and likely the host-protective specificities of the various oncosphere vaccine antigens developed to date, are conformational epitopes. These antigens comprise predicted FN-III domains, which may be responsible for their tertiary structure [14, 15]. The similarity of pig and mouse antibody responses to conformational epitopes of TSOL18 [22, 25] and homology between recombinant oncosphere antigens developed to date [14, 15] would suggest that monoclonal antibodies generated against these oncosphere antigens are suitable tools for the identification of the conformational antigenic epitopes and the development of synthetic peptide-based vaccines [23, 24] and associated immunological assays [25].

Acknowledgements

The authors are grateful to the Wellcome Trust, Animal Health in the Developing World Grant 075818 for the funding. Marshall Lightowlers (Department of Biosciences, Melbourne Veterinary School, Faculty of Veterinary and Agricultural Sciences, the University of Melbourne) provided the antigens TSOL18-GST and TSOL18-MBP and the two truncated forms of TSOL18 (TSOL18-1-GST and TSOL18-2-GST). Lea Brys (Free University of Brussels, Belgium) provided methodical and procedural assistance for the generation of mouse monoclonal antibodies against TSOL18 protein.

Conflict of interest

None.

Author details

Emmanuel Assana* and André Pagnah Zoli
School of Veterinary Medicine and Sciences, University of Ngaoundéré, Ngaoundéré, Cameroon

*Address all correspondence to: assana_e@yahoo.fr

References

[1] Lightowlers MW, Gasser RB, Hemphill A, Romig T, Tamarozzi F, Deplazes P, et al. Advances in the treatment, diagnosis, control and scientific understanding of taeniid cestode parasite infections over the past 50 years. International Journal for Parasitology. 2021;**51**:1167-1192. DOI: 10.1016/j.ijpara.2021.10.003

[2] Johnson KS, Harrison GB, Lightowlers MW, O'Hoy KL, Cougle WG, Dempster RP, et al. Vaccination against ovine cysticercosis using a defined recombinant antigen. Nature. 1989;**338**:585-587

[3] Lightowlers MW. Vaccination against animal parasites. Veterinary Parassitology. 1994;**54**:177-204

[4] Cox FEG. Milestones in parasitology. Parasitology Today. 1993;**9**:347-348

[5] Lightowlers MW, Rolfe R, Gauci CG. *Taenia saginata*: Vaccination against cysticercosis in cattle with recombinant oncosphere antigens. Experimental Parasitology. 1996;**84**:330-338

[6] Lightowlers MW, Jensen O, Fernandez E, Iriarte JA, Woollard DJ, Gauci CG, et al. Vaccination trials in Australia and Argentina confirm the effectiveness of the EG95 hydatid vaccine in sheep. International Journal for Parasitology. 1999;**29**:531-534

[7] Gauci C, Vural G, Öncel T, Damia V, Kyndon CT, Craig PS, et al. Vaccination with recombinant oncosphere antigens reduces the susceptibility of sheep to infection with *Taenia multiceps*. International Journal for Parasitology. 2008;**38**:1041-1050

[8] Flisser A, Gauci CG, Zoli A, Martinez-Ocaña J, Garza-Rodriguez A, Dominguez-Alpizar JL, et al. Induction of protection against porcine cysticercosis by vaccination with recombinant oncosphere antigens. Infection and Immunity. 2004;**72**:5292-5297. DOI: 10.1128/iai.72.9.5292-5297.2004

[9] Assana E, Gauci CG, Kyngdon C, Geerts S, Dorny P, Zoli AP, et al. Antibody responses to the host-protective *Taenia solium* oncosphere protein TSOL18 in pigs are directed against conformational epitopes. Parasite Immunology. 2010a;**32**:399-405. DOI: 10.1111/j.1365-3024.2009.01197.x

[10] Kyngdon CT, Gauci CG, Rick A, Rolfe RA, Velásquez Guzmán JC, Farfán Salazar MJ, et al. In vitro oncosphere-killing assays to determine immunity to the larvae of *Taenia pisiformis*, *Taenia ovis*, *Taenia saginata*, and *Taenia solium*. The Journal of Parasitology. 2006;**92**:273-281

[11] Kyngdon CT, Gauci CG, Gonzalez AE, Flisser A, Zoli A, Read AJ, et al. Antibody responses and epitope specificities to the *Taenia solium* cysticercosis vaccines TSOL18 and TSOL45-1A. Parasite Immunology. 2006;**28**:191-199. DOI: 10.1111/j.1365-3024.2006.00820.x

[12] Lightowlers MW, Colebrook AL, Gauci CG, Gauci SM, Kyngdon CT, Monkhouse JL, et al. Vaccination against cestode parasites: Anti-helminth vaccines that work and why. Veterinary Parasitology. 2003;**115**:83-123. DOI: 10.1016/S0304-4017(03)00202-4

[13] Chakraborty P, Aravindhan V, Mukherjee S. Helminth-derived biomacromolecules as therapeutic agents for treating inflammatory and

infectious diseases: What lessons do we get from recent findings? International Journal of Biological Macromolecules. 2023:124649. DOI: 10.1016/j.ijbiomac.2023.124649

[14] Gauci C, Lightowlers MW. Molecular cloning of genes encoding oncosphere proteins reveals conservation of modular protein structure in cestode antigens. Molecular & Biochemical Parasitology. 2003;**127**:193-198

[15] Lightowlers MW, Flisser A, Gauci CG, Heath DD, Jensen O, Rolfe R. Vaccination against Cysticercosis and hydatid disease. Parasitology Today. 2000;**16**:191-196

[16] Siggers K, Soto C, Palmer AG III. Conformational dynamics in loop swap mutants of homologous fibronectin type III domains. Biophysical Journal. 2007;**93**:2447-2456. DOI: 10.1529/biophysj.106.100578

[17] Woollard DJ, Gauci CG, Heath DD, Lightowlers MW. Epitope specificities and antibody responses to the EG95 hydatid vaccine. Parasite Immunology. 1998;**20**:535-540

[18] Woollard DJ, Gauci CG, Lightowlers MW. Synthetic peptides induce antibody against a host-protective antigen of *Echinococcus granulosus*. Vaccine. 2000;**18**:785-794

[19] Woollard DD, Gauci CG, Heath DD, Lightowlers MW. Assessment of protective immune response against hydatid disease in sheep by immunization with synthetic peptide antigens. Parasitology. 2000;**121**:145-153

[20] Woollard DD, Gauci CG, Heath DD, Lightowlers MW. Protection against hydatid disease induced with the EG 95 vaccine is associated with conformational epitopes. Vaccine. 2001;**19**:498-507

[21] Assana E, Kyngdon CT, Gauci CG, Geerts S, Dorny P, De Deken R, et al. Elimination of *Taenia solium* transmission to pigs in a field trial of the TSOL18 vaccine in Cameroon. International Journal for Parasitology. 2010b;**40**:515-519. DOI: 10.1016/j.ijpara.2010.01.006

[22] Assana E. TSOL18 vaccine antigen of *Taenia solium*: Development of monoclonal antibodies and field testing of the vaccine in Cameroon [thesis]. Ghent: Ghent University; 2010

[23] Read AJ, Gauci CG, Lightowlers MW. Purification of polyclonal anti-conformational antibodies for use in affinity selection from random peptide phage display libraries: A study using the hydatid vaccine EG95. Journal of Chromatography. B, Analytical Technologies in the Biomedical and Life Sciences. 2009;**877**:1516-1522

[24] Read AJ, Casey JL, Coley AM, Gauci CG, Jackson DC, Lightowlers MW. Isolation of antibodies specific to a single conformation-dependant antigenic determinant on the EG95 hydatid vaccine. Vaccine. 2009;**27**:1024-1031. DOI: 10.1016/j.vaccine.2008.11.096

[25] Assana E, Zoli AP, Gauci CG, Lightowlers MW, Dorny P. Immunodiagnostic usefulness of monoclonal antibodies specific to conformational epitopes of *Taenia solium* oncosphere protein TSOL18. Journal of Immunological Methods. 2021;**197**:113121. DOI: 10.1016/j.jim.2021.113121

Chapter 15

Antiparasitic Efficacy of the Root Bark Powder of *Oldfieldia Dactylophylla* (Welw. Ex Oliv.) J. Léonard on the Digestive Strongyles of Grazing Goats in Lubumbashi (DR Congo)

Victor Okombe Embeya, Gaël Nzuzi Mavungu, Welcome Muyumba Nonga, Célestin Pongombo Shongo, Amandine Nachtergael and Pierre Duez

Abstract

In order to evaluate the efficacy of the root bark powder of *Oldfieldia dactylophylla* (Welw. ex Oliv.) J. Léonard (a Picrodendraceae), 32 locally breed grazing goats naturally infested with various gastrointestinal helminths were randomly assigned to four groups of eight animals: one untreated control, one positive control group treated with a reference anthelmintic (albendazole, 5 mg/kg), and two groups treated *per os* with *O. dactylophylla* root bark powder (100 and 200 mg/kg body weight, respectively). Four doses of these respective treatments were administered monthly. To evaluate parasitological, blood and zootechnical parameters, samples were taken on day 0, just before administration of the first treatment and on 14, 31, 45, 62, 76, 92 and day 126. *O. dactylophylla* was effective on day 14 after treatment with 69% strongle egg fecal excretion (both doses) versus 90% albendazole. However, efficacy was stabilized at 85, 86 and 89% for *O. dactylophylla* (100 and 200 mg/kg) and albendazole, respectively. These data support the ethnoveterinary use of this plant in the control of digestive parasitism in goat breeding. However, phytochemical studies support that the plant should make contributions to human studies in the future.

Keywords: gastrointestinal parasite, *Oldfieldia dactylophylla*, *Haemonchus contortus*, goat, Haut-Katanga

1. Introduction

In Lubumbashi (Haut-Katanga Province, southeastern DR Congo) and in its green belt, as in most tropical areas, goat husbandry has low productivity because of inadequate management and poor animal health [1]. Parasite infections by gastro-intestinal helminths remain among the main causes of this weak production [2–4]. *Haemonchus contortus* is one of the nematode species that dominate the parasite spectrum of goats in sub-Saharan Africa [5–7].

It is therefore of great importance, because of its prevalence and pathogenicity [8].

Control of these infections is generally based on the strategic use of anthelmintics [9, 10]. However, these anthelmintics are not always available or, when they are, their costs are so high that they are not readily available to farmers and breeders [11]. And so, in developing countries, that are heavily affected by these parasitic infections, the traditional methods of control used by herders remain largely dependent on medicinal plants [12–14]. It is therefore essential to find means of control that would be inexpensive and accessible to breeders.

In a survey we conducted in the regions of Kamina and Kaniama (Haut-Katanga province, DR Congo), *Vitex thomasii* De Wild (Verbenaceae) was the most cited traditional plant-based remedy applied to the control of gastrointestinal disorders in livestock [13, 15]. We have however recently determined that this species name is incorrect, the plant being locally confused with *Oldfieldia dactylophylla* (Welw. ex Oliv.) J.Léonard (Picrodendraceae); all the "*Vitex thomasii* " samples we could examine so far are in fact *Oldfieldia dactylophylla* [15].

O. dactylophylla is found in Africa, south of the Sahara (DR Congo, Tanzania, Angola, Zambia, Malawi), at altitudes from 1000 to 1800 m [16]. Our survey among breeders showed that root bark powder is used in animals on wounds or given, *per os*, against gastrointestinal parasitosis [13]. In humans, it is administered, always *per os*, against gastrointestinal parasitosis, back pain, hip or various joint pain. Its decoction is also administered orally in case of threats of miscarriage, asthenia, rheumatism, gonorrhea and diarrhea [17].

The aim of the present work was to evaluate the purported antiparasitic efficacy of the root bark powder of *O. dactylophylla* in grazing goats raised under natural conditions in DR Congo.

2. Material and methods

2.1 Plant material

The root barks of *O. dactylophylla* (vernacular name, kikoto muchi); previously wrongly identified as were harvested in Kelambwe (8°35′335 S; 24°414′422 E), Kankundwe (8°45′636 S; 24°50′491 E) and Kiabukwa (8°44′270 S; 24°54′253 E). A voucher sample was deposited in the Kipopo herbarium (Botanic Laboratory of the University of Lubumbashi; specimen N°9-OKOMBE). The plant was identified by Nsenga Nkulu (Université de Lubumbashi, UNILU) and confirmed by P. Meerts (Université Libre de Bruxelles, ULB). The material was dried in the shade and powdered. The powder was cohesive enough to be compressed "*as is*" into 500 mg tablets that were administered *per os* to the animals.

2.2 Chromatographic profiling of *Oldfieldia dactylophylla* root bark

O. dactylophylla root bark powder (1.0 g) was extracted with 10 mL of n-heptane; after vortexing, ultrasonication and centrifugation, the supernatant was evaporated

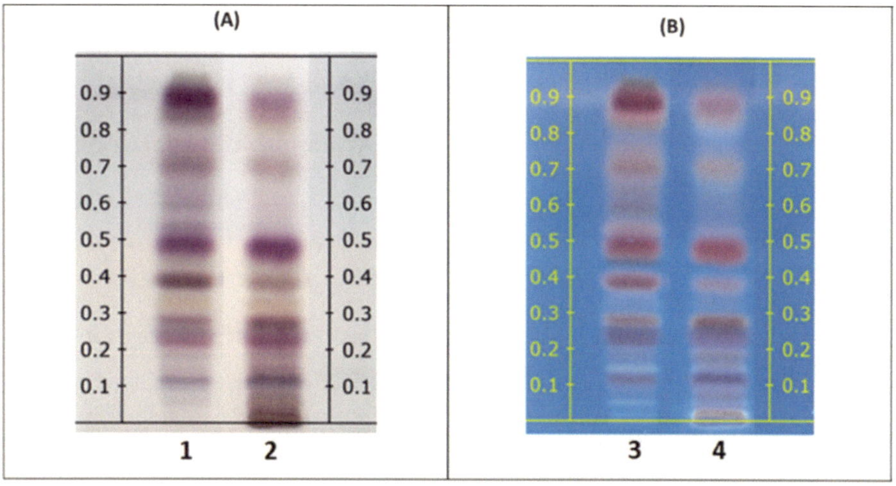

Figure 1.
Chromatographic profiles of Oldfieldia dactylophylla *root bark. HPTLC plate (20 × 10 cm), silica gel 60 F254. Mobile phase, petroleum ether (40–60°C)—acetone—ethyl acetate (85: 15: 5, v/v/v); derivatization with vanillin reagent and visualization (A) under white light; (B) under UV light (365 nm). Tracks 1 and 3,* O. dactylophylla *root bark n-heptane extract; Tracks 2 and 4,* O. dactylophylla *root bark dichloromethane extract.*

to dryness and dissolved in 1 mL of methanol. The plant residue was then similarly extracted with 10 mL of dichloromethane and the extract was dissolved in 1 mL of methanol. The high-performance thin-layer chromatography (HPTLC) of extracts was performed according to the procedure of the European Pharmacopoeia 10 [18] using Camag Automatic TLC Sampler (ATS 4), Automatic Developing Chamber 2 (ADC 2), Derivatizer and TLC Visualizer 2. The Camag systems were driven by the software visionCATS version 2.5. The HPTLC was performed on silica gel 60 F254 HPTLC plates (Merck, Germany); 5 μL of samples were applied in 8-mm wide bands, the plates were activated on MgCl2 (~33% RH) and the tank saturated for 20 min; the solvent system was petroleum ether (40–60°C)—acetone—ethyl acetate (85: 15: 5, v/v/v). The plate development was performed at 70 mm from the lower edge of the plate. 5 mL of a vanillin reagent (2 mL of sulfuric acid added to 100 mL of a 10 g/L solution of vanillin in 96% ethanol) was applied on the plate that was then heated at 110°C for 3 min. The plate was examined under visible light and UV_{366nm} (**Figure 1**).

2.3 Experimental setup and treatment

The applied sampling protocols met the Unified Ethical Principles and an Animal Research 'Helsinki' declaration [19]. The study was conducted at the Naviundu Farm of the University of Lubumbashi (RD Congo). It included 32 locally breed goats, at least 2 months old, naturally infected with various gastrointestinal helminths and randomly assigned to four groups of eight homogeneous animals. All animals graze together on the same pastures and the groups were not physically separated throughout the study period. No anthelmintics were received in the 4 months prior to the experiment.

Four consecutive treatments (excluding the control group) were administered once a month to the different groups for four consecutive months according to the scheme described below:

- group 1 was the untreated control group (control);
- group 2 was treated with albendazole orally (Vermitan®, Laprovet) at a dose of 5 mg/kg body weight (positive control); albendazole is a broad-spectrum benzimidazole anthelminthic, effective against most nematodes, but at these doses would have little efficacy against cestodes [20];
- group 3 was treated with a tablet containing bark powder from the root of *O. dactylophylla per os*, 100 mg/kg body weight;
- group 4 was treated with a tablet containing bark powder from the root of *O. dactylophylla per os*, 200 mg/kg body weight.

The treatments were administered on the same day by two experimenters used to handling animals, one of whom assisted with the restraint by raising the neck of the animal and the other by inserting the drug into the pocket of the animal's cheek with a small amount of water to facilitate the administration of the treatment. Our ethnopharmacological study indicated that, in traditional veterinary treatments, the doses of kikoto muchi (vernacular name of *O. dactylophylla* root bark) are not standardized and depend on the experience of individuals [13]; we determined the doses to be tested by considering the dosages indicated by interviewed farmers. All procedures performed were in accordance with the ethical standards committee of the University of Lubumbashi (license N° UNILU/CEM/167/2011). Fecal, blood samples and weight measurements were taken on day 0 (before administration of the first treatment) and on days 14, 31, 45, 62, 76, 92 and 126 post-treatment (**Figure 2**).

2.4 Stool specimens and coprological analyzes

Individual fecal samples were taken directly from the rectum of animals early in the morning and immediately placed in separate plastic bags, clearly identified with the animal identification number. When the stool examination did not directly follow the collection, samples were temporarily placed at a temperature of 4°C for not longer than 24 h.

For qualitative coprological analyzes, the Willis flotation method [21] was applied. The eggs per gram of fecal matter (EPG) were quantified by the Mc Master technique with a solution of NaCl of density 1.2 (sensitivity: 1 egg observed = 50 EPG, i.e. 50 EPG).

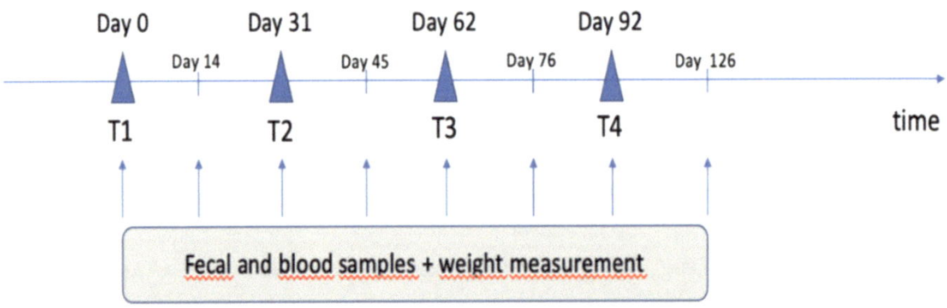

Figure 2.
Time scale of the experiment.

2.5 Blood sampling and analyzing

The blood was collected from the jugular vein using a syringe and transferred in test tubes with or without anticoagulant. The blood collected on tubes with anticoagulant (sodium citrate) was used for the establishment of the hematocrit and the count of total leukocytes. Blood collected on dry tubes was used to obtain serum after centrifugation at 3000 rpm for 10 min for biochemical assays. The hematocrit was determined by a microhematocrit method [22]. The biochemical parameters (total proteins, albumin, creatinine and transaminases) were measured using standard kits from Biomérieux.

2.6 Measure of efficacy of treatments

The efficacy of the treatment was calculated according to the method of Presidente [23], that considers the average EPG before and after the treatments:

$$E\% = \left\{1 - \left(\frac{T1}{T2} \times \frac{C2}{C1}\right)\right\} \times 100 \quad (1)$$

With E% = rate of effectiveness;
T1 = EPG on the day after treatment;
T2 = initial EPG of the treated lot;
C1 = EPG on the day after treatment of control batch.
C2 = initial EPG of the control batch.

2.7 Statistical analysis

For each of the four groups, we performed Multiple Factor Variance Analysis (ANOVA) to compare the various parameters. The EPG values did not follow a Gaussian distribution and were therefore transformed according to the log (x + 10) function. These different statistics were calculated using the software R. For each of the tests, the standard criterion of $p < 0.05$ was used to check whether the measured differences were statistically significant. The effects were noted as very highly significant ($p < 0.001$), highly significant ($p < 0.01$), significant ($p < 0.05$) and not significant ($p > 0.05$).

3. Results

3.1 Chromatographic profiling of *Oldfieldia dactylophylla* root bark

Figure 1 presents HPTLC profiles of the n-heptane and dichloromethane sequential extracts of *O. dactylophylla* root bark. These profiles are quite characteristic, yielding bands probably attributable to terpenoids; a phytochemical study is on-going to identify the compounds of interest.

3.2 Animals

Table 1 shows that all four groups were equilibrated at baseline, regarding sexes, weights and EPG.

Groups	Sex	Body weight (kg)	Fecal worm egg count (EPG)
Control	Female (n = 4)	18.9 ± 3.8[a]	500.0 ± 20.5[a]
	Male (n = 4)	17.9 ± 2.3[a]	497.0 ± 19.9[a]
Albendazole (5 mg/kg)	Female (n = 4)	18.6 ± 4.7[a]	491.3 ± 16.5[a]
	Male (n = 4)	18.2 ± 3.6[a]	498.6 ± 17.1[a]
O. dactylophylla (100 mg/kg)	Female (n = 4)	19.3 ± 4.5[a]	496.0 ± 15.9[a]
	Male (n = 4)	19.0 ± 4.6[a]	500.2 ± 13.4[a]
O. dactylophylla (200 mg/kg)	Female (n = 4)	20.2 ± 5.2[a]	487.1 ± 17.5[a]
	Male (n = 4)	19.9 ± 4.3[a]	498.9 ± 17.2[a]

Values expressed as mean ± sd of body weight and EPG for all groups before the experiment. Means with the same letters are not significantly different through ANOVA and the Tukey test (p < 0.05).

Table 1.
Baseline characteristics of study animals.

3.3 Effects of *Oldfieldia dactylophylla* root bark powder on the gastrointestinal strongyles and evaluation of efficacy

From the 2nd week after the first treatment (day 14), the EPG study indicated a decrease of more than half for the fecal excretion of strongyle eggs in goats receiving *O. dactylophylla* root bark powder ($p < 0.001$ vs. negative control). There was no dose-effect relationship as the two doses of *O. dactylophylla* root bark powder showed non-significant differences in eggs counts. Although a 90% EPG decrease was obtained in the control group treated with albendazole, the within-group variabilities were such that the differences between all treated groups were non-significant. The effectiveness of treatments was also evaluated using the method of Presidente (**Table 2**) [23]. On day 126, the decrease in EPG stabilized at 85, 86 and 89% compared to the initial infestation in *O. dactylophylla* 100 mg/kg, *O. dactylophylla* 200 mg/kg and albendazole-treated groups, respectively.

3.4 Effects of *Oldfieldia dactylophylla* root bark powder on serum total proteins and albumin

The total proteins and albumin of the control group showed non-significant differences throughout the study and remained significantly lower ($p < 0.001$)

Groups	Day of treatment							
	T1		T2		T3		T4	
	0	14	31	45	62	76	92	126
	Effectiveness (%)							
Control	0	0	0	0	0	0	0	0
Albendazole (5 mg/kg)	0	90	89	89	90	87	90	89
O. dactylophylla (100 mg/kg)	0	69	78	80	82	83	83	85
O. dactylophylla (200 mg/kg)	0	69	78	77	79	83	84	86

Table 2.
Effectiveness rate of Oldfieldia dactylophylla *root bark powder treatment.*

compared to those of the groups treated either with albendazole or *O. dactylophylla* root bark powder. The total proteins and albumin in the treated groups significantly increased ($p < 0.001$) from day 14 of treatment and remained steady over the study, with no differences between the two dosages of *O. dactylophylla* and albendazole.

3.5 Effects of *Oldfieldia dactylophylla* root bark powder on total leucocytes count

Total leucocytes of the treated animals and control group showed a marked and significant ($p < 0.05$) decrease in all treated groups throughout the study. Comparison of data at different dates revealed non-significant differences between the two dosages of *O. dactylophylla* root bark powder and albendazole.

3.6 Effects of *Oldfieldia dactylophylla* root bark powder on the hematocrit

The mean values of hematocrit of the control group compared to those of the batches treated with *O. dactylophylla* root bark powder or albendazole showed significant differences ($p < 0.001$) throughout the study.

3.7 Effects of *Oldfieldia dactylophylla* root bark powder on transaminases

The base levels of alanine aminotransferase (ALT) slightly differ ($p < 0.001$) in the groups treated with *O. dactylophylla* (100 mg and 200 mg/kg) compared to the other groups whereas the aspartate aminotransferase (AST) levels slightly differ from group to group ($p < 0.001$). The levels of these enzymes in all groups remained stable throughout the study.

3.8 Effects of *Oldfieldia dactylophylla* root bark powder treatments on serum creatinine

There was no difference in serum creatinine levels between the different groups throughout the experimentation.

3.9 Effects of *Oldfieldia dactylophylla* root bark powder on animal weight

Mean weight values compared at different dates between the four groups of animals involved in our study showed no significant difference throughout the experiment.

4. Discussion

This study indicates that the levels of parasitic eggs fecal excretion were similar in the four groups of goats before onset ($p > 0.05$). After 2 weeks of treatment, there was a significative decrease in the fecal excretion of strongyle eggs in goats receiving *O. dactylophylla* root bark powder at either 100 or 200 mg/kg or albendazole. From the 14th day to the 126th day, we observed in the animals treated monthly with *O. dactylophylla* a significant decrease of infestation in comparison to the untreated group ($p < 0.001$). Compared to the group treated monthly with albendazole, the fecal excretion of eggs in animals treated with *O. dactylophylla* monthly at dosages of 100 and 200 mg/kg showed non-significant differences 14th day after the first treatment and the levels of infestation remained similar until the end of the study. There was no statistical difference between the two doses of *O. dactylophylla* tested ($p > 0.05$), indicating that the lower dosage is sufficient; dose-finding trials are worth conducting to determine the lowest efficient dosage. These results are comparable to those found in several studies using bioactive plants against digestive strongyles: *Eucalyptus staigeriana* leaves [24], *Eucalyptus citriodora* leaves [25] and *Moringa oleifera* leaves [26].

Indeed, several families of molecules present in the root bark of *O. dactylophylla* (tannins, flavonoids, iridoids and triterpenoids) have been evoked in previous works as possessing anthelminthic properties. The action of these molecules, alone or in combination, may explain this decrease of infestation. Similar activities have been demonstrated for sesquiterpenes and lactones in sheep [27], triterpenes and alkaloids in sheep [28–30], anthraquinones in goat [25] saponins [14] and condensed tannins in sheep and goats [14, 31, 32]. In these studies, the use of bioactive plants containing these substances (condensed tannins, triterpenes, alkaloids, anthraquinones or saponins) has been shown to be an alternative to the use of synthetic anthelmintics. As to the efficacy of *O. dactylophylla* monthly administration in our work, we observed a considerable reduction in EPG in the three treated groups (up to 86%). These results are comparable to those obtained by Kommuru et al. [33] with condensed tannins. These molecules have also been identified as effective on some parasites in humans [34]. Thus, to some extent, the use of *O. dactylophylla* may well be extrapolated in the treatment of parasitic nematodes in humans.

Compared to the control group, the serum levels of total proteins and albumin, measured 1 month after the administration of the four monthly treatments, are markedly higher in the treated groups compared to measurements taken 14 days after the first treatment ($p < 0.001$), and similar for the 2 *O. dactylophylla* dosages and albendazole. This suggests that the different treatments have improved the availability of amino acids from dietary proteins. These results are in line with those of Hassan et al. [35] who observed a remarkable increase in serum proteins during treatment with ivermectin; it is likely that the reduction of intestinal parasites burden reduces the diversion of proteins, improving their bioavailability. On the other hand, condensed tannins have been proposed to explain such an increase by an indirect mechanism, the precipitation of food proteins; this would prevent protein degradation in the rumen, improving their intestinal bioavailability [36]. However, certain types of condensed tannins are known for a high toxicity on the digestive mucosa with a consequent reduction of nutrient absorption [37]. But, in goats, physiological adaptations allow them to consume large quantities of plants rich in secondary metabolites, notably tannins [38]; these adaptations include an increase of salivary glands size with the secretion of salivary proteins and three amino acids (glutamine, glycine and proline) with high affinity for tannins [39, 40]. Goats also possess a particular rumen flora that secretes enzymes, such as tannases, active in the rumen [41]. These enzymes specifically break the ester linkages of hydrolyzable tannins, reducing their molecular weight and thus their ability to bind proteins, probably increasing the bioavailability of proteins farther in the digestive tract; such enzymes were notably isolated from the ruminal enterobacteria of goat [42].

From day 14th onwards after the first treatment, the hematocrit of groups treated with albendazole and *O. dactylophylla* show a statistically significant increase compared to the control group. This increase probably corresponds to an anthelmintic activity of tested treatments toward hematophagous parasites [43], including *Haemonchus contortus* that was diagnosed in our study animals. The values of the transaminases (ALT and AST) remained stable in all groups along the study, indicating no hepatotoxicity of tested treatments. There was no difference in serum creatinine levels between the different groups throughout the experimentation, indicating a probable absence of renal toxicity.

Despite the effectiveness of albendazole and *O. dactylophylla* treatments, indicated by a marked decrease in *Haemonchus contortus* bioburden (as seen from EPG data), the evolution of corporeal weights was similar in the treated and control groups throughout the experiment. In a previous study on goats' anthelminthic treatment in Tanzania, during a long dry season, goats were orally dosed with 7.5 mg/kg albendazole and the weight gains were quite limited [20]. At that dosage, albendazole is effective against nematodes but may not be effective against trematodes. The authors explained that their animals may have been infected either with a low level of nematodes, so clearing these would have a small effect, or with a mix of different worms, some of the infections not being cleared by albendazole. In our study, goats are grazing and so are also likely co-infected with different worms, which may explain the non-effectiveness of albendazole on weights. For *O. dactylophylla* treatments, an anti-nutritive effect of tannins on energy production by the rumen flora could yield an additional explanation.

5. Conclusion

The significant decrease, in field conditions, in fecal excretion of parasite eggs after administration of *O. dactylophylla* root bark powder as observed in this study is in line with data obtained in many other earlier works on secondary plant metabolites possessing anthelmintics activities. Moreover, this decrease in fecal excretion underlines the interest that can be gained using *O. dactylophylla* in the control of the digestive parasitism in goat breeding. The goat is an animal particularly well adapted by its physiological and digestive particularities. In view of these initial results, the plant seems to present an ability to be chosen among the alternatives to the control of parasites in agriculture, but it is necessary to complete the analytical approach and to better specify the optimal conditions of its use in farming. The present study has currently highlighted the antiparasitic properties of *O. dactylophylla* on animals; however, phytochemical studies support that the plant should make contributions to human studies in the future.

Acknowledgements

This study was supported by the project "Appui Institutionnel P3-Université de Lubumbashi" of the ARES-CCD (Académie de Recherche et d'Enseignement Supérieur-Commission Coopération au Développement, Belgium).

The authors thank professor Bertrand Losson of the University of Liège for his scientific contribution to the preparation of the project and this present study.

Conflict of interest

The authors declare no conflict of interest regarding the publication of this chapter.

Author details

Victor Okombe Embeya[1,2], Gaël Nzuzi Mavungu[1,2*], Welcome Muyumba Nonga[2,3], Célestin Pongombo Shongo[1], Amandine Nachtergael[2] and Pierre Duez[2]

1 Faculty of Veterinary Medicine, Pharmacology and Toxicology Department, University of Lubumbashi (UNILU), Lubumbashi, Democratic Republic of the Congo

2 Unit of Therapeutic Chemistry and Pharmacognosy, Maistriau, University of Mons (UMONS), Mons, Belgium

3 Department of Chemistry-Physics, High College Training Teachers of Lubumbashi, Lubumbashi, Democratic Republic of the Congo

*Address all correspondence to: mavungug@unilu.ac.cd

References

[1] Armson B, Ekiri AB, Alafiatayo R, Cook AJ. Small ruminant production in Tanzania, Uganda, and Ethiopia: A systematic review of constraints and potential solutions. Veterinary Sciences. 2021;**8**:5. DOI: 10.3390/vetsci8010005

[2] Burke JM, Wells A, Casey P, Miller JE. Garlic and papaya lack control over gastrointestinal nematodes in goats and lambs. Veterinary Parasitology. 2009;**159**:171-174

[3] Abebe R, Gebreyohannes M, Mekuria S, Abunna F, Regassa A. Gastrointestinal nematode infections in small ruminants under the traditional husbandry system during the dry season in southern Ethiopia. Tropical Animal Health and Production. 2010;**42**:1111-1117

[4] Rupa APM, Portugaliza HP. Prevalence and risk factors associated with gastrointestinal nematode infection in goats raised in Baybay city, Leyte, Philippines. Veterinary World. 2016;**9**:728-734

[5] Besier RB, Kahn LP, Sargison ND, Van Wyk JA. Diagnosis, treatment and management of *Haemonchus contortus* in small ruminants. In: Gasser RB, Samson-Himmelstjerna GV, editors. Advances in Parasitology. Amsterdam: Elsevier Ltd; 2016. pp. 181-238

[6] Zvinorova PI, Halimani TE, Muchadeyi FC, Matika O, Riggio V, Dzama K. Prevalence and risk factors of gastrointestinal parasitic infections in goats in low-input low-output farming systems in Zimbabwe. Small Ruminant Research. 2016;**143**:75-83

[7] Arsenopoulos KV, Fthenakis GC, Katsarou EI, Papadopoulos E. Haemonchosis: A challenging parasitic infection of sheep and goats. Animals. 2021;**11**:363. DOI: 10.3390/ani11020363

[8] Mpofu TJ, Nephawe KA, Mtileni B. Prevalence of gastrointestinal parasites in communal goats from different agro-ecological zones of South Africa. Veterinary World. 2020;**13**(1):26-32

[9] Gnoula C, Guissou P, Duez P, Frederich M, Dubois J. Nematocidal compounds from seed of *Balanites aegyptiaca*-isolation and structural elucidation. International Journal of Pharmacology. 2007;**3**:280-284

[10] Selzer PM, Epe C. Antiparasitics in animal health: Quo vadis? Trends in Parasitology. 2021;**37**:77-89

[11] Knox MR, Besier RB, Le Jambre LF, Kaplan RM, Torres-Acosta JFJ, Miller J, et al. Novel approaches for the control of helminth parasites of livestock VI: Summary of discussions and conclusions. Veterinary Parasitology. 2012;**186**:143-149

[12] Hoste H, Torres-Acosta JFJ. Non chemical control of helminths in ruminants: Adapting solutions for changing worms in a changing world. Veterinary Parasitology. 2011;**180**:144-154

[13] Okombe EV, Lumbu Simbi J-B, Stévigny C, Vandenput S, Pongombo Shongo C, Duez P. Traditional plant-based remedies to control gastrointestinal disorders in livestock in the regions of Kamina and Kaniama (Katanga province, Democratic Republic of Congo). Journal of Ethnopharmacology. 2014;**153**:686-693

[14] Oliveira Santos F, Ponce Morais Cerqueira A, Branco A, José Moreira Batatinha M, Borges BM. Anthelmintic

activity of plants against gastrointestinal nematodes of goats: A review. Parasitology. 2019;**146**:1233-1246

[15] Mavungu GN, Mutombo CS, Numbi DM, Nsenga SN, Muyumba WN, Pongombo CS, et al. Smallholders' knowledge about healing goat gastrointestinal parasite infections with wild plants in southern DR Congo. Frontiers in Pharmacology. 2023;**14**. DOI: 10.3389/fphar.2023.1124267

[16] Ruffo C, Birnie A, Tengnäs B. Edible wild plants of Tanzania. Vol. 27. Nairobi: Technical Handbook; 2002. p. 766

[17] Kasonia K, Ansay M, Basegere N, Gustin P, Kaba S, Katsongeri M, et al. Note d'ethnopharmacologie vétérinaire en cas de verminoses, diarrhée, coprostase et météorisme au Kivu et Kibali-Ituri (Zaïre). Tropicultura. 1991;**9**:169-172

[18] Council of Europe. High-performance thin-layer chromatography of herbal drugs and herbal drug preparations (2.8.25). In: European Pharmacopoeia. 10th ed. Strasbourg: Council of Europe; 2019

[19] Petkov CI, Flecknell P, Murphy K, Basso MA, Mitchell AS, Hartig R, et al. Unified ethical principles and an animal research 'Helsinki' declaration as foundations for international collaboration. Current Research in Neurobiology. 2022;**3**:100060. DOI: 10.1016/j.crneur.2022.100060

[20] Bessell PR, Sargison ND, Mirende K, Dash R, Prasad S, Al-Riyami L, et al. The impact of anthelmintic drugs on weight gain of smallholder goats in subtropical regions. Preventive Veterinary Medicine. 2018;**159**:72-81

[21] Thienpont D, Rochette F, Vanparijs OFJ. Diagnosing Helminthiasis through Coprological Examination. Belgium: Jansen Ani Antwerp; 2003

[22] Bamberg R, Gwyn T, Miller J, Thompson M, Transou P. The effects of over-anticoagulated blood on hematocrit values by the microcentrifuge method. Clinical Laboratory Science. 2008;**21**:146-150

[23] Presidente P. Methods for detection of resistance to anthelmintics. In: Anderson N, Waller PJ, editors. Resistance in Nematodes to Anthelmintic Drugs. Melbourne, New South Wales, CISRO: Division of Animal Health and Australian Wool Corporation; 1985. pp. 13-27

[24] Macedo ITF, Bevilaqua CML, de Oliveira LMB, Camurça-Vasconcelos ALF, Vieira L d S, Oliveira FR, et al. Anthelmintic effect of *eucalyptus staigeriana* essential oil against goat gastrointestinal nematodes. Veterinary Parasitology. 2010;**173**:93-98

[25] Sastya S, Kumar RR, Vatsya S. *In vitro* and *in-vivo* efficacy of *Eucalyptus citriodora* leaf in gastrointestinal nematodes of goats. Journal of Entomology and Zoology Studies. 2018;**6**:25-30

[26] Pedraza-Hernández J, Elghandour MMMY, Khusro A, Salem MZM, Camacho-Diaz LM, Barbabosa-Pliego A, et al. Assessment on bioactive role of *Moringa oleifera* leaves as anthelmintic agent and improved growth performance in goats. Tropical Animal Health and Production. 2021;**53**:318. DOI: 10.1007/s11250-021-02745-9

[27] Mendonça-Lima FW, RB dos S, Santos LC, Zacharias F, David JM, David JP, et al. Anthelmintic activity of *Cratylia mollis* leaves against gastrointestinal nematodes in goats.

Revista Brasileira de Saúde e Produção Animal. 2016;**17**:753-762

[28] Githiori JB, Athanasiadou S, Thamsborg SM. Use of plants in novel approaches for control of gastrointestinal helminths in livestock with emphasis on small ruminants. Veterinary Parasitology. 2006;**139**:308-320

[29] Zuorro A, Iannone A, Lavecchia R. Water-organic solvent extraction of phenolic antioxidants from brewers' spent grain. PRO. 2019;**7**:126. DOI: 10.3390/pr7030126

[30] Antonio AP, Perera MLS, García JA, Rehmana MU, Choudhary MI. Anthelminthic activity against sheep gastrointestinal nematodes in chemical compounds from *Tephrosia vogelii* leaves. Journal of Veterinary and Animal Sciences. 2019;**6**:8-17

[31] Quijada J, Fryganas C, Ropiak HM, Ramsay A, Mueller-Harvey I, Hoste H. Anthelmintic activities against *Haemonchus contortus* or *Trichostrongylus colubriformis* from small ruminants are influenced by structural features of condensed tannins. Journal of Agricultural and Food Chemistry. 2015;**63**:6346-6354

[32] Chan-Pérez JI, Torres-Acosta JFJ, Sandoval-Castro CA, Castañeda-Ramírez GS, Vilarem G, Mathieu C, et al. Susceptibility of ten *Haemonchus contortus* isolates from different geographical origins towards acetone: Water extracts of polyphenol-rich plants. Part 2: Infective L3 larvae. Veterinary Parasitology. 2017;**240**:11-16

[33] Kommuru DS, Whitley NC, Miller JE, Mosjidis JA, Burke JM, Gujja S, et al. Effect of *Sericea lespedeza* leaf meal pellets on adult female *Haemonchus contortus* in goats. Veterinary Parasitology. 2015;**207**:170-175

[34] Adak M, Kumar P. Herbal anthelmintic agents: A narrative review. Journal of Traditional Chinese Medicine. 2022;**42**(4):641-651

[35] Hassan MM, Hoque MA, Islam SKMA, Khan SA, Hossain MB, Banu Q. Efficacy of anthelmintics against parasitic infections and their treatment effect on the production and blood indices in black Bengal goats in Bangladesh. Turkish Journal of Veterinary & Animal Sciences. 2012;**36**:400-408

[36] Hassanpour S, Sadaghian M, MaheriSis N, Eshratkhah B, ChaichiSemsari M. Effect of condensed tannin on controlling faecal protein excretion in nematode-infected sheep. The Journal of American Science. 2011;**7**:896-900

[37] Frutos P, Hervás G, Giráldez FJ, Mantecón AR. Review: Tannins and ruminant nutrition. Spanish Journal of Agricultural Research. 2004;**2**:191-202

[38] Silanikove N. The physiological basis of adaptation in goats to harsh environments. Small Ruminant Research. 2000;**35**:181-193

[39] Alonso-Díaz MA, Torres-Acosta JFJ, Sandoval-Castro CA, Hoste H. Tannins in tropical tree fodders fed to small ruminants: A friendly foe? Small Ruminant Research. 2010;**89**:164-173

[40] Torres-AcostaJFJ,Sandoval-CastroCA, Hoste H, Aguilar-Caballero AJ, Camara-Sarmiento R, Alonso-Díaz MA. Nutritional manipulation of sheep and goats for the control of gastrointestinal nematodes under hot humid and subhumid tropical conditions. Small Ruminant Research. 2012;**103**:28-40

[41] Sharma D, Mal G, Kannan A, Bhar R, Sharma R, Singh B. Degradation

of euptox a by tannase-producing rumen bacteria from migratory goats. Journal of Applied Microbiology. 2017;**123**:1194-1202

[42] Singh B, Bhat TK, Sharma OP, Kanwar SS, Rahi P, Gulati A. Isolation of tannase-producing *Enterobacter ludwigii* GRT-1 from the rumen of migratory goats. Small Ruminant Research. 2012;**102**:172-176

[43] Bizimenyera ES, Meyer S, Naidoo V, Eloff JN, Swan GE. Efficacy of *Peltophorum africanum* Sond. (Fabaceae) extracts on *Haemonchus contortus* and *Trichostrongylus colubriformis* in sheep. Journal of Animal and Veterinary Advances. 2008;7:364-371

Chapter 16

Perspectives on the Drug Discovery of Intestinal Protozoan Parasites

Sarika Thakur, Alka Sharma, Reena Negi, Ram Gopal Nitharwal and Inderjeet Kaur

Abstract

The intestinal protozoan parasites pose serious health concerns, infecting more than one billion individuals every year and mainly causing diarrhea in infants and adults. Main pathogens include *Giardia intestinalis, Entamoeba histolytica, Cyclospora cayetanensis*, and *Cryptosporidium* spp. causing giardiasis, amoebiasis, cyclosporiasis, and cryptosporidiosis, respectively. The drug arsenal to treat these diseases is limited (<25 drugs are in clinical use) for the treatment of all protozoal infections. The existing treatment options are decades of years old (discovered in 1930–1980s) and have limitations such as low therapeutic index, toxic side effects during long-term treatment, and drug resistance. Therefore, urgent renewed drug discovery efforts are needed to tackle these neglected protozoal diseases. This chapter discusses the current status of treatment options and their limitations, along with current drug discovery efforts. We conclude that the knowledge gained in the genomic and post-genomic era should be appropriately harnessed to accelerate the futuristic drug discovery process in this field.

Keywords: protozoan parasites, intestinal diseases, drug resistance, drug discovery, therapeutics

1. Introduction

Worldwide, around 1.7 billion incidents of diarrheal illness are recorded annually [1]. According to the WHO report 2024, every year, diarrheal disease kills approximately 443,832 children and is the third leading cause of death among children aged below 5 years. A diverse group of pathogenic microbes, including bacteria, viruses, and parasitic organisms, can cause diarrheal disease. Of these pathogens, protozoan parasites are the major contributors [2]. These intestinal protozoans are a divergent group of unicellular organisms that reaches the intestine through ingestion of contaminated food or drinking water [3], particularly in the tropics and subtropics, causing millions of cases of diarrhea annually.

The intestinal infections are caused by different protozoan parasites such as *Dientamoeba fragilis, Giardia lamblia, Isospora belli, Microsporidia* (*Septata intestinalis, Enterocytozoon bieneusi*), *Entamoeba histolytica, Balantidium coli, Blastocystis hominis, Cyclospora cayetanensis, Cryptosporidium* spp., etc. [4]. However, this manuscript focuses primarily on *Giardia intestinalis, Entamoeba histolytica, Cyclospora cayetanensis*, and *Cryptosporidium* spp. causing giardiasis, amoebiasis, cyclosporiasis, and cryptosporidiosis, respectively [5]. *C. cayetanensis, G. intestinalis*, and *C. pavrum* are the small intestinal parasites that affect children and elderly persons, whereas *Entamoeba*, the large bowel parasite, infects all age groups but mainly adults [6]. They are transmitted through the oral-fecal route *via* indirect or direct contact with the transmittable phase, leading to cases of mortality and morbidity [7].

These intestinal infections can be managed by both preventive measures as well as by appropriate drug treatment. For treating different protozoan parasites, only 25 drugs are used in clinical settings [8]. However, even after the latest advancements in the field, such as the availability of the complete genomes and a comprehensive understanding of the life cycles of these pathogens, there are limited translational breakthroughs from the lab to the clinic, and no major new classes of antiprotozoal drugs have been developed. Moreover, the efficacy of currently available drugs is insufficient, and the emergence of drug resistance is another challenge resulting in clinical treatment failures [9]. Therefore, due to the lack of effective, safe, and reasonable drugs, the impact of protozoan infections on humans has been amplified. Understanding the molecular basis of resistance facilitates the identification of novel drug targets and helps in the advancement of therapeutic agents, thereby necessitating further research to ensure a sustainable discovery of effective compounds. Moreover, the lack of vaccines against these parasites further demands renewed efforts toward the development of novel drugs, especially in the post-genomics era.

This chapter discusses current treatment options for different human intestinal protozoa to understand the scenario of drug-resistant strains, available alternatives, and future therapeutic strategies for the effective management and cure of these infections.

2. Giardiasis

Giardiasis is a small intestinal disease caused by *Giardia intestinalis*, known as *G. lamblia* or *G. duodenalis.* Giardiasis is a global public health concern, with approximately 280 million cases per annum [10]. A huge number of cases of parasitic infections (2-30%) while in developed countries the infection frequency is in the range of 2-7% [11].

G. intestinalis is a human intestinal parasite, that also affects domestic and wildlife animals, particularly mammals. The latest study has revealed the existence of trophozoites similar to *Giardia* in the gut of invertebrate *Heterotermes tenuis* [12]. It was initially elucidated by Antonie van Leeuwenhoek while examining his own diarrheal stool in 1681. Subsequently, Vilém Dušan Lambl discovered *Giardia* in 1859 and explained it in detail, and therefore, the protozoan was named after him. The parasite is transmitted through contaminated water, either freshwater or public water supply. *G. intestinalis* exists in two forms: trophozoite and cyst. It is transmitted in cyst form either through contaminated water or direct oral-fecal route [13]. After consumption, excystation takes place, followed by the release of trophozoites. The trophozoites infect the duodenum and upper intestine, taking advantage of the favorable alkaline pH, resulting in the development of the disease [14].

2.1 Current drug regimen for giardiasis

The therapy administered for giardiasis includes nitroimidazole compounds, which are potent against various bacterial as well as parasitic infections, especially a synthetic 5-nitroimidazole derivative called metronidazole primarily used for the treatment of trichomoniasis [15]. Eventually, Darbon et al. proclaimed that metronidazole can be used against *Giardia* infections [16]. Since the 1960s, it remains the predominant drug used worldwide for the treatment of giardiasis [17]. Its success rate varies from 60 to 100%, and thus is the first-line drug used for the treatment [17, 18]. Metronidazole is a pro-drug that, after entering the trophozoite, is reduced by the parasite's electron transport proteins (ferredoxins) that donate the electrons to the nitro group [19]. This drug builds oxidative stress through binding with thiol groups, resulting in the cysteine adducts and distorting the DNA by developing a double-strand rupture [20]. The activation of metronidazole is intervened by the enzyme nitroreductase-1 (NRT-1) as well as by the reduction pathway mediated by ferredoxin. Other enzymes that result in the reduction of metronidazole are pyruvate: ferredoxin oxidoreductase (PFOR) and thioredoxin reductase (TrxR) [21]. The reduction of the drug creates a gradient that helps in the intracellular transport of the drug, which primarily destructs the replication phase of *G. intestinalis* cell cycle and further results in the DNA fragmentation and failure of its functions, leading to the death of trophozoite (**Figure 1**) [20]. Even though metronidazole is the first-line drug used against various parasites, it has been pointed out to be carcinogenic by the US Department of Health, stating that it created tumors in mice at higher doses, but no cancer-related symptoms have been found in humans (**Table 1**) [34]. Another compound that is extensively used for the treatment of giardiasis is albendazole, a benzimidazole class drug. This compound has been utilized as an anthelmintic for humans since the 1960s in veterinary medicine and as an antifungal in agriculture. Their inhibitory efficiency as anti-protozoan compounds was discovered in the 1980s as they inhibited the growth of *Trichomonas vaginalis*. Its efficiency against *G. intestinalis* was also discovered afterwards [35]. Due to the low cure rate of this drug, it is observed

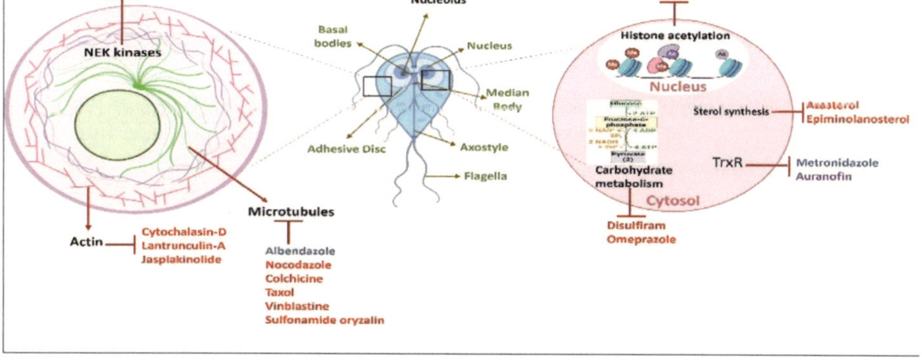

Figure 1.
Schematic representation of the existing and novel drug targets in G. intestinalis. The figure also illustrates the anti-giardia drugs in the current therapy (mentioned in blue) as well as the drugs under various phases of research (mentioned in red). Moreover, auranofin (mentioned in violet) is the only novel drug undertaken for clinical trial. Created with BioRender.com.

S. No.	Drug	Parasite	Mechanism	References
1	Metronidazole	*Entamoeba histolytica* *Giardia intestinalis*	Reduction of nitro groups; DNA fragmentation and cell cycle arrest.	[22, 23]
2	Albendazole	*Giardia intestinalis*	Binds to β-tubulin; cell cycle arrest.	[24]
3	Nitazoxanide	*Giardia intestinalis* *Entamoeba histolytica* *Cyclospora cayetanensis* *Cryptospordium parvum*	Inhibits PFOR, nitroreductase, disrupts plasma membrane	[25–27]
4	Furazolidone	*Giardia intestinalis*	Depletes cytoplasm, produces toxic intermediates	[22]
5	Paromomycin	*Giardia intestinalis* *Entamoeba histolytica* *Cryptospordium parvum*	Inhibits protein synthesis	[28]
6	Quinacrine	*Giardia intestinalis*	Inhibits DNA production	[29]
7	Trimethoprim-Sulfamethoxazole	*Cyclospora cayetanensis*	—	[30–32]
8	Ciprofloxacin	*Cyclospora cayetanensis*	—	[33]
9.	Roxithromycin	*Cryptospordium parvum*	Disrupt bacterial protein synthesis	[26]
10.	Rifabutin and rifaximin	*Cryptospordium parvum*	Inhibits RNA synthesis	[26]

Table 1.
Currently used drugs for the intestinal parasites and their mode of action.

as a secondary option for the treatment. Also, this drug is not recommended during pregnancy due to teratogenic effects in animals and may be in humans as well [17]. Trophozoites metabolize albendazole and result in the formation of toxic intermediates: albendazole sulfone and albendazole sulfoxide with the help of flavohemoglobin, a NADH oxidase (gNADHox) present inside the parasite (**Figure 1**) [36]. It has been established that the albendazole binds to the beta-tubulin of the parasite, and the presence of two amino acids (Glu-198 and Phe-200) in the beta-tubulin sequence renders this protozoan susceptible to benzimidazoles (**Table 1**). However, *E. histolytica* displays resistance due to the presence of different amino acids in this particular region [37]. Other drugs that are employed include furazolidone [38], acridine (quinacrine) [39], aminoglycoside (paromomycin) [40], and nitazoxanide (**Table 1**) [25]. Nitazoxanide, a nitrothiazolide derivative, shows inhibitory activity against bacteria, protozoa, and helminths. It was approved for giardiasis treatment in 2004. It is hypothesized that this drug inhibits enzymes such as PFOR and nitroreductases [41]. Moreover, nitazoxanide destroys the cyst by disrupting the protozoan's cyst wall [42]. Furazolidone is another drug used for the treatment of giardiasis, particularly for pediatric cases [29]. However, due to evident genotoxicity and activation of neoplastic processes, the use of this drug is prohibited in the United States [17]. Even though the mechanism of action of this drug is similar to metronidazole, it is reduced by NADH oxidase instead of PFOR [43]. Quinacrine, another drug used for the treatment of giardiasis, is an acridine derivative with broad-spectrum activity. The usage of this drug is limited due to side effects like vomiting and psychosis, while in some countries, it is used when patients do not respond to metronidazole.

Resistance to the drugs metronidazole and albendazole used for the treatment of giardiasis is a major emerging clinical concern with unspecified consequences. Human giardiasis has been primarily treated with metronidazole for the past 60 years, but the efficiency of this antibiotic has been weakened due to an increase in resistance against metronidazole, a first-line drug. This treatment failure has turned into a major health concern in the last 15 years [44]. Moreover, a large number of giardiasis cases refractory to metronidazole have been documented in low *Giardia* frequency settings. A study conducted in 2010 revealed that the regimen containing one or more nitroimidazoles did not succeed in curing 5.8% of patients out of a group of 170 [45]. Other data from 2008 to 2013 from the Hospital for Tropical Diseases in London reported a sharp rise in metronidazole-refractory cases from 15% to >40% of all the cases [46]. Moreover, it has also been discovered that metronidazole-refractory patients are difficult to treat with other antibiotics, such as nitazoxanide and albendazole. Furthermore, a sharp rise in refractory patients has also been documented in India [47]. *In vitro* studies have illustrated that the induction of resistance to benzimidazole is correlated with β-tubulin mutation, degradation of enzymes involed in glycolysis and arginine metabolism, and reduced mRNA expression of flavohemoglobin [36]. The detailed molecular mechanisms of resistance that lead to 5-nitroimidazole refractory *Giardia* infection as well as other types of resistance is not completely understood despite substantial efforts with laboratory as well as clinical strains. Therefore, it warrants the search for new compounds through screening of libraries or drug repositioning. The drugs commonly used to treat giardiasis are listed in **Table 1**.

2.2 Recent drug discovery efforts against giardiasis

Giardiasis has been overlooked for years, typically in underdeveloped countries. The search and development of novel drugs have been poorly researched, mainly due to economic reasons. The genome sequencing demonstrated that *G. intestinalis* comprises a compact genome of approximately 12 Mb with around 4800 expressed genes [48]. The completion of the *Giardia* genome project and advanced molecular tools helped in the identification of new inhibitors for almost one-tenth of the total potent drug targets in the parasite. High-throughput technologies have also benefited in screening the repurposed drugs as well as new pharmacophores, escalating the depository of anti-giardia compounds, mostly exhibiting activity against metronidazole or albendazole-resistant *Giardia* [49]. The drugs under investigation against giardiasis are highlighted in **Figure 1**.

Auranofin, a gold (Au) containing anti-rheumatic compound, was repurposed against the parasite in 2013. The clinical phase trial IIa (NCT02736968) revealed that it decreases the load of *Giardia* trophozoites and is also safe to use at a dose of 6 mg/day. Even though auranofin has been described as a TrxR activity inhibitor, the mode of action is not fully understood and requires further research [39]. Orlistat, an anti-obesity drug, also exhibited anti-giardia activity *in vitro* both against susceptible and metronidazole-resistant *Giardia,* at lower concentrations than metronidazole (4.3 μM and 11.0 μM) [50]. Robenidine, an anticoccidial drug classified as a guanidine derivative, showed better and faster activity than metronidazole against *G. intestinalis* with minimum lethal concentration (MLC) as low as 2.8 μM. Several analogs of this drug are developed, researched, and patented [51].

Azidothymidine (AZT), an anti-retroviral drug, also exhibits inhibitory activity *in-vivo* against *Giardia,* even against the metronidazole-resistant strains [52]. Disulfiram, a thiuram disulfide drug used to treat alcohol abuse disorder, also exhibited *in vitro* anti-giardia activity with a minimum lethal concentration of 1.23 μM and modest activity *in vivo* with a 21% cure rate in mice against *Giardia* [53]. In addition, mavelertinib, an EFGR-TKI (tyrosine-kinase inhibitor), has also displayed effective activity in mice infected with *G. intestinalis* [54]. Several anticancer drugs have also been suggested to be repurposed against protozoa including *G. intestinalis*. Trichostatin A, tubastatine A, and nicotinamide have inhibitory effects on the growth of trophozoites [55]. Moreover, a new compound, KH-TFMDI, a 3-arylideneindolin-2-one derivative, and KV-46, a 4-[(10H-phenothiazin-10-yl) methyl]-N-hydroxy benzamide, displayed growth inhibitory activity, with IC_{50} less than 1 μM. While these compounds primarily inhibit histone acetylase, there is a possibility that they affect other pathways as well (**Figure 1**) [56].

The cytoskeleton of *G. intestinalis* serves as a potent target for novel drug discovery as existing as well as proposed drugs affect the components of the parasitic cytoskeleton. *Giardia* depends on substrate-level phosphorylation due to the lack of typical mitochondria. Therefore, targeting the enzymes of carbohydrate metabolism is a potential strategy. Various compounds that target metabolic pathways associated with sterol synthesis have been examined *in vitro*. For example, azasterol and epiminolanosterol that suppress the activity of Δ24(25) sterol methyltransferase (24-SMT) have exhibited activity against trophozoites of *Giardia*, although the parasite does not produce 24-alkyl sterols or ergosterol [57]. The enzymes involved in this process can be different from mammalian cells and thus can be potential targets in drug discovery (**Figure 1**) [58]. Few kinase inhibitors against *Giardial* NEK kinases are under investigation. The screening of kinase inhibitors provided five compounds that hinder the growth of *G. intestinalis*. One compound (BKI1213) particularly impacted cytokinesis [59], whereas another notable compound (GW843682X) hinders flagellar length and thus alters cytokinesis [60]. Moreover, a recently discovered nucleolus has also emerged as a potential target [61]. This structure would constitute several transcription initiation features that are unique to the parasite [62], making it a strong candidate for drug discovery (**Figure 1**). Natural compounds such as curcumin, berberine, garlic extract, and grapefruit seed extract have been investigated to demonstrate anti-Giardia activity [63]. Curcumin inhibits *Giardia lamblia* trophozoite adhesion and growth by altering the microtubule cytoskeleton and preventing parasite multiplication [64]. These chemicals have the potential as alternative therapeutics and represent a viable avenue for the development of novel anti-giardia medicines.

3. Amoebiasis

Amoebiasis, also known as amebiasis or amoebic dysentery, is a condition caused by the infection of *Entamoeba* spp., which are protozoan parasites that typically reside in the intestine. Most of the infections are asymptomatic. However, the invasive disease may develop, showing symptoms of abdominal cramps, acute diarrhea, dysentery, and amoebic colitis (bloody diarrhea with mucus). Amoebic liver abscesses (ALA) develop if the parasite reaches the liver through the bloodstream. The symptomatic manifestation of amoebiasis has been attributed mainly to *Entamoeba histolytica,* but other species such as *E. dispar, E. moshkovskii, E. hartmanni, E. polecki,* and *E. bangladeshi* are also implicated [65]. However, further research is required to establish the pathogenicity of *E. dispar* and *E. bangladeshi*. Amoebiasis has been responsible for more than 100,000 annual deaths worldwide [66] and ranks third in the category of parasitic diseases (after malaria and schistosomiasis) responsible for mortality across the globle [67]. The disease is more prevalent in developing countries of Asia, Africa, and Central and South America. It represents the highest disease burden in Asia under the category of neglected tropical diseases. South Africa has a disease prevalence of 12.4% in 2006 [68] while in 2011, India reported the prevalence of intestinal amoebiasis to be ~11.7% [69]. The most affected countries include Bangladesh, China, India, Mexico, Columbia, and Brazil [70]. Although it is considered a tropical disease, it is also being reported in developed countries, especially among travelers returning from endemic places.

The life cycle of *E. histolytica* is a simple two-stage cycle compared to the other protozoan parasites. It consists of an infectious cyst that can survive outside its host for sufficient time to be able to cause transmission [71]. The transmission of the disease occurs by ingestion of the cysts from contaminated food and water [71]. Once the cysts reach the small intestine, the process of excystation starts with the action of intestinal trypsin enzymes, resulting in the formation of eight vegetative trophozoites per cyst that colonize the caecum and colon. The motile trophozoites are responsible for invasive disease as they divide and multiply by binary fission, and can migrate to other tissues. It may cause extraintestinal amoebiasis and also convert back to cysts in a process called encystation to be excreted out in feces. Hence, a new cycle of fecal-oral transmission starts [72]. *E. histolytica* remains in the human intestine, causing asymptomatic disease in about 90% of the cases, and only a minority of cases develop invasive disease. However, the reasons behind this selectivity are poorly understood. It is now established that the pathogenesis of *E. histolytica* is multifactorial, involving interactions of parasitic virulent factors, host cells, and components of the immune system and microbiota of the intestine [72]. The trophozoites adhere to the intestinal epithelium and interact with the TJ junctions, resulting in paracellular permeability and destroying the membrane integrity. The parasite ingests the host target cells and degrades them, leading to the development of ulcers [73].

3.1 Current drug regimen for amoebiasis

Feder Losch, in 1875, first detected amoebae in fecal samples. In 1903, Fritz Schaudinn was the first to distinguish between *E. coli* and *E. histolytica* and named the latter because of its tissue lysing ability. Maintaining basic hygiene practices can easily control the spread of the disease. Prohibiting open defecation, access to toilets, effective sewage water treatment, and improved water purification systems could be crucial measures in the prevention of amoebiasis [74].

Amoebiasis, despite being a significant global public health concern, currently lacks vaccinations or prophylactic drugs for prevention. The WHO recommends that all cases of amoebiasis including asymptomatic patients should be treated [75]. The treatment of asymptomatic cases is necessary not only to stop the invasive disease but also to inhibit the spread and further transmission through excreted cysts. The current lines of drugs that are used in the treatment of this infection have been categorized into two types. Drugs that are used to treat non-invasive colitis are referred to as luminal agents (paromomycin, diloxanide furoate, iodoquinol, and nitazoxanide) that kill the intraluminal cysts. Invasive amoebiasis and extraintestinal disease have been treated with chloroquine, emetine, tinidazole, and metronidazole, which are the elected treatment in patients with symptomatic intestinal amoebiasis

(**Table 1**) [72]. These organic compounds have been the mainstay therapy for this disease since the 1960s and are active only against trophozoites [76]. In particular, metronidazole is used widely as a first line of treatment for amoebic colitis for at least 5 days. The other nitroimidazoles with longer half-lives have also been successfully used for shorter durations such as ornidazole, tinidazole, and secnidazole [77]. Another relatively newer drug, nitazoxanide, successfully cures 80–90% of patients with intestinal amoebiasis in 3 days [78]. The nitroimidazoles are not effective against luminal stages. Therefore, an effective therapy should include a course of luminal agents such as paromomycin following metronidazole treatment [28]. Despite its side effects, metronidazole still remains the chief drug being used in the treatment of amoebiasis, and so far, there is no clear evidence for the clinically resistant strains of *E. histolytica* [72]. However, cases of treatment failure, especially with ALA patients, have been reported [79]. Other studies have described the increase in MIC values by *E. histolytica* when exposed to increased metronidazole concentrations *in vitro* [80]. The drugs commonly used to treat amoebiosis are listed in **Table 1**.

3.2 Recent drug discovery efforts against amoebiasis

Auranofin is the latest drug with potential against *E. histolytica,* even for metronidazole-resistant parasites, and is currently in clinical phase II trials (NCT02736968). In the era of drug repurposing, several compounds have been suggested to be explored against this parasite. Disulfiram or antabuse, used to treat alcohol dependence, has been explored against *E. histolytica* but showed negligible impact on parasite viability [81]; however, its metabolite, ZnDTC, showed efficient antiparasitic effects in a mice model at low nanomolar concentration by inhibiting the ubiquitin-proteasome pathway (**Figure 2A**) [82]. A recent study has identified 26 potential compounds after screening ~12,000 compounds in cell culture, which could be further developed into anti-amoebiasis drugs [83]. Out of them, ponatinib, a multikinase inhibitor, can be the most effective for repurposing strategy. It was found to be 30X more potent than metronidazole *in vitro* [83]. Beloranib and TNP470 (analogs of fumagillin), are a class of MetAP2 inhibitors that can prevent encystation, block reoccurrence, and are most effective against metronidazole-resistant *E. histolytica* parasites. However, the use of beloranib is associated with thromboembolism. This warrants further research and development

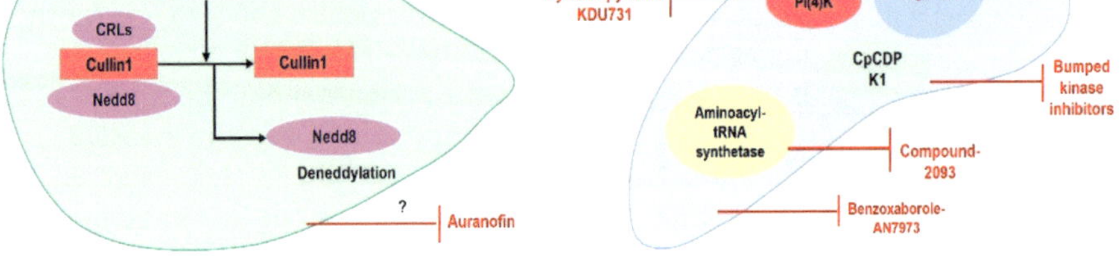

Figure 2.
Schematic representation of recent drug discovery efforts for Entamoeba histolytica and Cryptosporidium parvum. A. Potential drug disulfiram's metabolite, ZnDTC inhibits COP9 signalosome subunit 5 (CSN5) activity in Entamoeba histolytica. The mode of action of auranofin is not completely understood. B. Illustration of putative drugs and their targets within Cryptosporidium parvum.

of newer and safer derivatives of MetAP2 inhibitors [84]. Another class of mTOR/PI3K inhibitors, including dactolisib, sapanisertib, omipalisib, and a few others, have shown inhibitory potential against metronidazole-resistant parasites *in vitro*. The drugs under investigation against amoebiasis are highlighted in **Figure 2A**.

In addition, exploring the molecular pathways and cellular components of *E. histolytica* for developing novel therapeutics holds an enormous potential that necessitates rigorous efforts in the research and development in the field. The update and information on promising drug targets for amoebiasis have been compiled and summarized elsewhere [85].

4. Cyclosporiasis

Cyclosporiasis is an intestinal parasitic disease caused by the coccidian parasite *Cyclospora cayetanensis* [86], first described in 1870. It is the only species known to infect humans, with the first recorded instance in Papua New Guinea in 1979 [87]. The attention toward the parasite has increased due to its capacity to induce gastrointestinal distress among human populations, transcending geographical boundaries and socioeconomic disparities and surge in clinical cases globally [88]. Despite efforts to curtail its proliferation, *C. cayetanensis* infections persist as a significant concern, underscoring the complexity of managing this pathogen in contemporary society [89]. Endemic hotspots for *C. cayetanensis* include tropical and subtropical regions, where poor sanitation results in environmental contamination with human feces [90]. Contaminated food and water sources play a pivotal role in *Cyclospora* transmission, necessitating stringent sanitation measures and enhanced surveillance efforts.

The clinical outcomes of cyclosporiasis are multifactorial and influenced by various factors, including the age and immune status of the host [91]. It is a significant challenge, especially for vulnerable populations such as immunosuppressed individuals, children, and the elderly that are more susceptible to severe forms of the disease, including extraintestinal complications like biliary disease, Guillain-Barré syndrome, reactive arthritis syndrome, and ocular inflammation [92]. *C. cayetanensis* has a complex life cycle involving both sexual and asexual stages. It begins when an individual ingests food or water contaminated with oocysts, which develop into merozoites that invade new epithelial cells [93]. The merozoites then undergo sexual reproduction in the gastrointestinal tract, developing into microgametocytes and macrogametocytes, which are released into the environment through feces [90]. The fertilization occurs in outside environment. The zygote forms sporulated oocysts, capable of infecting new hosts (**Figure 3**). The transmission of *C. cayetanensis* is facilitated by factors like globalization of food supply chains and increasing international travel [90]. Public health interventions should focus on improving food safety standards, enhancing water sanitation infrastructure, promoting hygiene practices, and strengthening surveillance and outbreak response systems [94].

4.1 Current drug regimen for cyclosporiasis

Cyclosporiasis, is a highly prevalent disease, particularly among vulnerable population like those with HIV/AIDS, organ transplant recipients, and those undergoing immunosuppressive or anticancer regimens [6]. The primary treatment option for cyclosporiasis is trimethoprim-sulfamethoxazole (TMP-SMX), also known as co-trimoxazole, which is a combination antibiotic that inhibits Dihydrofolate reductase

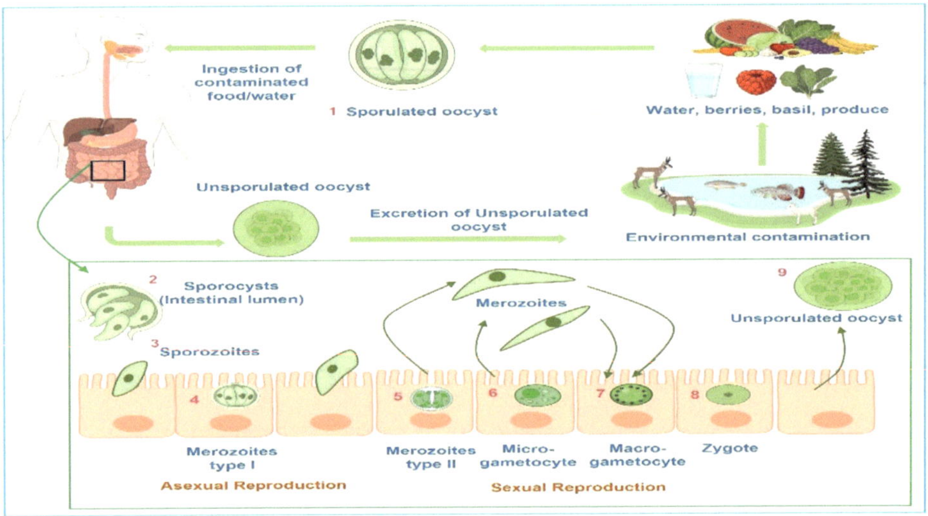

Figure 3.
Life cycle and transmission of Cyclospora cayetanensis. The infection starts with the ingestion of the sporulated oocysts. It shows both the asexual and sexual reproduction. Fertilization occurs in the intestine. Unsporulated oocysts are excreted out in the environment where they sporulate and start the cycle again. It was noted that no drugs for cyclosporidiosis are in the clinical trials. Created with BioRender.com.

(DHFR) in *C. cayetanensis* (**Table 1**). This combination therapy disrupts folate metabolism, hindering DNA synthesis and thereby leading to parasite death. TMP-SMX has shown efficacy in both immunocompetent and immunocompromised patients (HIV/AIDS), with cure rates exceeding 90% in some studies [95]. However, prolonged use can result in antibiotic resistance, hence resulting in drug-resistant strains [96]. The extended use of TMP-SMX has been associated with a wide range of harmful effects on organs, including hematologic problems, liver damage, and skin responses [97].

For patients who cannot tolerate TMP-SMX due to sulpha allergy or treatment failure, alternative antibiotics like ciprofloxacin may be considered. Ciprofloxacin, although less effective than TMP-SMX, can be used as an alternative [33]. However, there have been situations where ciprofloxacin has been reported to be ineffective in treating certain condition, although it is generally acknowledged to be therapeutic in specific cases. Nitazoxanide is another drug with promise in treating cyclosporiasis [98], especially in patients with sulpha allergy (**Table 1**) [99]. Although the drug's exact mode of action is yet unknown, it is believed to function by inhibiting their energy metabolism, damaging cell membranes, and compromising mitochondrial function. It interferes with the pyruvate: ferredoxin/flavodoxin oxidoreductase (PFOR) cycle, essential for energy production, and induces lesions in cell membranes. Additionally, it disrupts mitochondrial membrane potential and inhibits key enzymes, leading to parasite death [100]. Furthermore, it has been observed that nitazoxanide exhibits a direct inhibitory effect on coccidian oocysts, resulting in a reduction in their viability, as evidenced by the ultrastructural analysis [101]. Studies have reported cure rates ranging from 71 to 87% with nitazoxanide treatment, and the drug has been well-tolerated with no serious adverse effects [99]. The drugs commonly used to treat cyclosporiasis are listed in **Table 1**.

However, it is important to note that some antibiotics, such as norfloxacin, metronidazole, tinidazole, and quinacrine, have been shown to be ineffective against *C. cayetanensis* infections, rendering the treatment of *C. cayetanensis* infections highly challenging [90]. The research efforts are underway to explore novel drug targets and therapeutic strategies for *C. cayetanensis* infections using high-throughput screening assays, structure-based drug design, and drug-repurposing approaches. Advances in molecular biology and genomics have provided insights into the molecular mechanisms of *Cyclospora* pathogenesis, paving the way for the development of targeted therapies [1].

4.2 Recent drug discovery efforts against cyclosporiasis

The occurrence of adverse effects linked to trimethoprim-sulfamethoxazole (TMP-SMX) and ciprofloxacin drugs, coupled with the increase in Cyclospora resistance, hinders the efficiency of treatment [96]. This emphasizes the urgent requirement for innovative therapeutic approaches to tackle the issue of multidrug-resistant phenotypes. Recent research has highlighted the promising efficacy of curcumin and curcumin nanoemulsion (CR-NE) as novel therapeutic agents [102]. Studies conducted on mice models have demonstrated that CR-NE exhibits increased efficacy compared to the standard treatment of trimethoprim-sulfamethoxazole (TMP-SMX). It is believed that the anti-protozoal activity of CR is due to its ability to regulate transcription pathways and induce cellular death. They can also trigger apoptosis in injected cells by the activation of intracellular calcium release and mitochondrial membrane depolarization. It also affects cellular signaling pathways by targeting growth factors, receptors, transcription factors, cytokines, enzymes, and genes that are involved in the regulation of apoptosis. Its interference with the ability of *Cyclospora* to survive and proliferate within host cells could potentially lead to new treatments for cyclosporiasis [102].

These findings underscore the potential of curcumin and curcumin nanoemulsion as promising therapeutic options for cyclosporiasis. The enhanced efficacy of CR-NE, as demonstrated by decreased oocyst burden and improved antioxidant biomarkers, suggests its potential superiority over conventional therapies such as TMP-SMX. Further research and clinical studies are warranted to validate these findings and explore the clinical utility of CR-NE in treating cyclosporiasis in humans [102].

Modulating the host immune response represents a novel approach to combat *Cyclospora* infections. Recent research has focused on elucidating the immunopathogenesis of *C. cayetanensis* and identifying host immune factors associated with protection or susceptibility. Immunomodulatory agents, such as cytokine inhibitors or immune checkpoint inhibitors, hold promise for enhancing host defenses against the parasite [95]. Nanoparticle-based drug delivery systems hold promise for targeted drug delivery to the site of infection, minimizing systemic toxicity and enhancing therapeutic outcomes. Another study on magnesium oxide (MgO) nanoparticles reveals their effectiveness against *C. cayetanensis* oocysts, suggesting their potential as a new treatment approach. MgO nanoparticles show promise in inhibiting the viability and infectivity of *C. cayetanensis*, offering a novel strategy for combating this parasitic infection [103]. Further investigation into parasitic-specific research is required in order to acquire a more comprehensive understanding of the molecular pathways, with the aim of identifying novel therapeutic targets (**Figure 3**).

The apicoplast of *C. cayetanensis*, a non-photosynthetic plastid with its own genome, presents a potential focal point for developing novel therapeutic agents to combat the disease [104]. The ferredoxin-NADP+ reductase/ferredoxin redox system, also a key metabolic agent in apicomplexan human parasites, has potential as a therapeutic target due to its involvement in electron transfer reactions. Targeting this system could interfere with crucial metabolic processes essential for parasite survival, offering a promising opportunity for developing new antiparasitic medications [105]. *C. cayetanensis* also harbors a diverse array of proteases from distinct families such as cysteine, serine, and metalloproteases. Understanding the involvement of proteases in the biological processes of *C. cayetanensis* could provide valuable knowledge about its pathogenesis and aid in identifying potential therapeutic targets [106].

5. Cryptosporidiosis

Cryptosporidiosis is a gastrointestinal, watery diarrheal disease of humans, affecting children younger than 2 years and immunocompromised individuals more severely [107]. Cryptosporidiosis is caused by *Cryptosporidium spp.* which is an intracellular, intestinal protozoan parasite. It was first identified by Ernest Tyzzer in 1907 in a common mouse's gastric glands [108]. *Cryptosporidium hominins* and *Cryptosporidium parvum* are the main species responsible for 90% of the cases in humans, causing the largest known outbreak of waterborne disease in the United States in 1993, affecting ~403,000 people [109]. The parasite is transmitted through the fecal-oral route via contaminated food and water [110]. Cryptosporidium, a Coccidia parasite, has a distinctive life cycle consisting of asexual and sexual stages within a single host [111]. It begins with the ingestion of infective oocysts containing four sporozoites, which then invade intestinal epithelial cells, transforming into trophozoites [112]. Trophozoites undergo multiple rounds of asexual replication, which amplifies the infection [113]. The sporozoites are excreted in feces, contributing to environment contamination and transmission to new hosts [114]. The adaptation of Cryptosporidium to a monoxenous life cycle and persistence in the environment pose significant public health challenges.

5.1 Current drug regimen for cryptosporidiosis

Nitazoxanide (NTZ), a nitrothiazole benzamide derivative, is the only FDA-approved drug used for the treatment of cryptosporidiosis [115]. NTZ treats and reduces diarrhea and oocyst shedding in children and adults [116] but does not show efficient results against HIV-infected or immunocompromised patients [117]. Paromomycin, an aminoglycoside, is another drug used against cryptosporidiosis [103]. Roxithromycin, a macrolide, has been found effective in patients having cryptosporidium infections along with AIDS, but only 50% of the medicated individuals had full clearance of parasites [118].

Rifamycin derivatives are the class of drugs that mainly affect mycobacterial infections by binding to DNA-dependent RNA polymerase and inhibiting RNA synthesis [119]. Its derivatives such as rifabutin and rifaximin are shown to be effective in treating cryptosporidiosis in individuals infected with HIV. Additionally, rifabutin was found to be more effective than other derivatives [120]. Letrazuril, a benzene acetonitrile derivative, has shown modest efficacy against advanced AIDS-related cryptosporidial diarrhea (**Table 1**) [121].

Additionally, different combinational therapies have also been used that show promising effectiveness for the treatment of cryptosporidiosis. When azithromycin/paromomycin combination therapy is used to treat cryptosporidial infections, there is a significant reduction in the amount of cryptosporidial oocysts excreted in feces [122]. A combination of azithromycin and nitazoxanide has been found to effectively treat cryptosporidiosis resulting in the total eradication of both diarrhea and parasites [123]. A combination of azithromycin, nitazoxanide, paromomycin, or rifaximin used in triple treatment resulted in a complete clinical parasitological recovery in kidney transplant recipients, with no instances of the recurrence [124]. The drugs commonly used to treat cryptosporidiosis are listed in **Table 1**.

5.2 Recent drug discovery efforts against cryptosporidiosis

Till now there has been no permanent treatment against cryptosporidium in humans as well as in animals. Due to the limited genetic tractability of Cryptosporidium, the absence of conventional targets, unique host cell location, and insufficient cell culture platforms, the progress in understanding host-parasite interactions is hampered [107], and subsequent drug discovery or development efforts are affected. However, recently, there have been advancements in drug discovery for the treatment of cryptosporidial infections due to improvements in the methods of its culture and genetic manipulation [125]. Currently, certain drugs such as bump kinase inhibitors (BKIs), pyrazolopyrimidine-based KDU731, triazolopyradizine MMV665917, benzoxaborole AN7973, and compound 2093 have demonstrated potential in treating cryptosporidiosis in animals (**Figure 2B**) [126]. Several studies have reported that BKI-1294 significantly reduces the shedding of oocysts and improves clinical symptoms by inhibiting *C. parvum* calcium-dependent protein kinase 1 (CpCDPK1) [127]. This enzyme is necessary for invading host cells [126]. However, BKI-1294 does not completely eliminate diarrhea and dehydration in infected bovines and neonatal calves [127]. Alternatively, BKI-1369, another inhibitor of CpCDPK1, shows its efficacy as a primary agent in combating Cryptosporidium infections in animals [126]. Specifically, it has shown effectiveness in treating neonatal calves infected with *C. parvum* [128]. However, these compounds cause cardiotoxicity and long QT syndrome in humans; thereby, more research efforts are needed to obtain better and safer derivatives of BKIs. Another potential anti-cryptosporidium drug molecule can be pyrazolopyrimidine derivative KDU731, which inhibits cryptosporidial lipid kinase PI (4)K (phosphatidylinositol-4-OH kinase) enzymatic activity [129].

The compound MMV665917, a piperazine derivative, showed inhibitory activity against both *C. parvum* and *C. hominis in vitro* as well as in mouse models [130]. A study conducted on the gnotobiotic piglet model strongly indicated that the use of MMV665917 resulted in the presence of *C. hominis* parasites in fecal matter, as well as a decrease in the shedding of oocysts, intestinal damage, and the severity of diarrhea [131]. However, like BKIs, MMV665917 also shows partial hERG inhibition and cardiotoxicity in humans [26]. Hence, further studies and research are needed to establish this molecule as an anti-cryptosporidial agent. The 6-carboxamide benzoxaborole AN7973 is also capable of inhibiting the growth of cryptosporidium and is termed safe and stable with good pharmacokinetic characteristics, but its mechanism of action and molecular targets in the parasite have not yet been identified [132]. The drugs under investigation against cryptosporidiosis are highlighted in **Figure 2B**.

6. Conclusions

In recent times, intestinal protozoan diseases, which were traditionally considered as tropical problems, are not restricted to tropical countries anymore. Although the understanding of genomes and the complex and diverse life cycles of these pathogens has considerably improved, no significant progress is achieved in finding new drugs for the treatment. The currently available drugs are inadequate due to limited numbers and limited chemical class diversity. Moreover, the available treatment options are not completely effective, and drug resistance is emerging. Very few drugs are currently in clinical trials. These lacunae highlight stringent need to pay renewed attention towords the drug discovery to combat these neglected pathogens. In light of modern "omics" based technologies, fundamental research and development efforts must be encouraged in order to have a deeper understanding of the molecular pathways orchestrating the myriad of novel functions within these pathogens. Lastly, the host-pathogen interactions can be another area which can be explored further to strenghten drug discovery efforts.

Acknowledgements

Sarika Thakur acknowledges the Department of Biotechnology (DBT) for financial assistance. Alka Sharma and Reena Negi acknowledge the University Non-NET fellowship from the Central University of Haryana, Mahendragarh – We thank Dr. Namrata Dhaka from Central University of Haryana for the valuable comments and editing.

Conflict of interest

The authors declare no conflict of interest.

Author details

Sarika Thakur, Alka Sharma, Reena Negi, Ram Gopal Nitharwal and Inderjeet Kaur*
Department of Biotechnology, Central University of Haryana,
Mahendragarh, Haryana, India

*Address all correspondence to: inderjeet@cuh.ac.in

References

[1] Ryan U, Paparini A, Oskam C. New technologies for detection of enteric parasites. Trends in Parasitology. 2017;**33**(7):532-546

[2] Fletcher SM, Stark D, Harkness J, Ellis J. Enteric protozoa in the developed world: A public health perspective. Clinical Microbiology Reviews. 2012;**25**(3):420-449

[3] Torgerson PR et al. The global burden of foodborne parasitic diseases: An update. Trends in Parasitology. 2014;**30**(1):20-26

[4] Chacon-Cruz E, Mitchell D. Intestinal protozoal diseases. Medicine Journal. 2003;**3**(5):1-11

[5] Tegen D, Damtie D, Hailegebriel T. Prevalence and associated risk factors of human intestinal protozoan parasitic infections in Ethiopia: A systematic review and meta-analysis. Journal of Parasitology Research. 2020;**2020**:8884064

[6] Giangaspero A, Gasser RB. Human cyclosporiasis. The Lancet Infectious Diseases. 2019;**19**(7):e226-e236

[7] Cacciò SM, Thompson RCA, McLauchlin J, Smith HV. Unravelling cryptosporidium and giardia epidemiology. Trends in Parasitology. 2005;**21**(9):430-437

[8] Haapanen S, Angeli A, Tolvanen M, Emameh RZ, Supuran CT, Parkkila S. Cloning, characterization, and inhibition of the novel β-carbonic anhydrase from parasitic blood fluke, Schistosoma mansoni. Journal of Enzyme Inhibition and Medicinal Chemistry. 2023;**38**(1):2184299

[9] Capela R, Moreira R, Lopes F. An overview of drug resistance in protozoal diseases. International Journal of Molecular Sciences. 2019;**20**(22):5748

[10] Lane S, Lloyd D. Current trends in research into the waterborne parasite giardia. Critical Reviews in Microbiology. 2002;**28**(2):123-147

[11] Kulakova L et al. Discovery of novel antigiardiasis drug candidates. Antimicrobial Agents and Chemotherapy. 2014;**58**(12):7303-7311

[12] Benchimol M, de Souza W. Observation of Giardia sp. in the termite gut of Heterotermes tenuis. Parasitology Research. 2021;**120**(3):1131-1135

[13] Rendtorff RC. The experimental transmission of human intestinal protozoan parasites. II. Giardia lamblia cysts given in capsules. American Journal of Hygiene. 1954;**59**(2):209-220

[14] Luján HD, Mowatt MR, Nash TE. Mechanisms of Giardia lamblia differentiation into cysts. Microbiology and Molecular Biology Reviews. 1997;**61**(3):294-304

[15] Cosar C, Julou L. The activity of 1-(2-hydroxyethyl)-2-methyl-5-nitroimidazole (R. P. 8823) against experimental Trichomonas vaginalis infections]. Ann Inst Pasteur (Paris). 1959;**96**(2):238-241

[16] Darbon A, Portal A, Girier L, Pantin J, Leclaire C. Treatment of giardiasis (lambliasis) with metronidazole. Apropos of 100 cases. Presse Médicale. 1962;**70**:15-16

[17] Escobedo AA, Cimerman S. Giardiasis: A pharmacotherapy review. Expert Opinion on Pharmacotherapy. 2007;**8**(12):1885-1902

[18] Gardner TB, Hill DR. Treatment of giardiasis. Clinical Microbiology Reviews. 2001;**14**(1):114-128

[19] Samuelson J. Why metronidazole is active against both bacteria and parasites. Antimicrobial Agents and Chemotherapy. 1999;**43**(7):1533-1541

[20] Ordoñez-Quiroz A, Ortega-Pierres MG, Bazán-Tejeda ML, Bermúdez-Cruz RM. DNA damage induced by metronidazole in Giardia duodenalis triggers a DNA homologous recombination response. Experimental Parasitology. 2018;**194**:24-31

[21] Ansell BRE et al. Transcriptomics indicates active and passive metronidazole resistance mechanisms in three seminal Giardia lines. Frontiers in Microbiology. 2017;**8**:398

[22] Campanati L, Holloschi A, Troster H, Spring H, de Souza W, Monteiro-Leal LH. Video-microscopy observations of fast dynamic processes in the protozoon Giardia lamblia. Cell Motility and the Cytoskeleton. 2002;**51**(4):213-224

[23] Uzlikova M, Nohynkova E. The effect of metronidazole on the cell cycle and DNA in metronidazole-susceptible and-resistant Giardia cell lines. Molecular and Biochemical Parasitology. 2014;**198**(2):75-81

[24] Oxberry ME, Thompson RCA, Reynoldson JA. Evaluation of the effects of albendazole and metronidazole on the ultrastructure of Giardia duodenalis, Trichomonas vaginalis and Spironucleus muris using transmission electron microscopy. International Journal for Parasitology. 1994;**24**(5):695-703

[25] Müller J, Sterk M, Hemphill A, Müller N. Characterization of Giardia lamblia WB C6 clones resistant to nitazoxanide and to metronidazole. Journal of Antimicrobial Chemotherapy. 2007;**60**(2):280-287

[26] Khan SM, Witola WH. Past, current, and potential treatments for cryptosporidiosis in humans and farm animals: A comprehensive review. Frontiers in Cellular and Infection Microbiology. 2023;**13**:1115522

[27] Checkley W et al. Asymptomatic and symptomatic cryptosporidiosis: Their acute effect on weight gain in Peruvian children. American Journal of Epidemiology. 1997;**145**(2):156-163

[28] Sullam PM, Slutkin G, Gottlieb AB, Mills J. Paromomycin therapy of endemic amebiasis in homosexual men. Sexually Transmitted Diseases. 1986;**13**(3):151-155

[29] Riches A, Hart CJS, Trenholme KR, Skinner-Adams TS. Anti-Giardia drug discovery: Current status and gut feelings. Journal of Medicinal Chemistry. 2020;**63**(22):13330-13354

[30] Hoge CW et al. Placebo-controlled trial co-trimoxazole for cyclospora infections among travellers and foreign residents in Nepal. The Lancet. 1995;**345**(8951):691-693

[31] Madico G, McDonald J, Gilman RH, Cabrera L, Sterling CR. Epidemiology and treatment of Cyclospora cayetanensis infection in Peruvian children. Clinical Infectious Diseases. 1997;**24**(5):977-981

[32] Goldberg E, Bishara J. Contemporary unconventional clinical use of co-trimoxazole. Clinical Microbiology and Infection. 2012;**18**(1):8-17

[33] Verdier R-I, Fitzgerald DW, Johnson WD Jr, Pape JW. Trimethoprim–sulfamethoxazole compared with ciprofloxacin for treatment and

prophylaxis of Isospora belli and Cyclospora cayetanensis infection in HIV-infected patients: A randomized, controlled trial. Annals of Internal Medicine. 2000;**132**(11):885-888

[34] U.S. Department of Health and Human Services. 14th Report on Carcinogens. 2016. pp. 1-8

[35] Chavez B, Gonzalezmariscal L, Cedillorivera R, Martinezpalomo A. Giardia lamblia: in vitro cytopathic effect of human isolates. Experimental Parasitology. 1995;**80**(1):133-138

[36] Pech-Santiago EO et al. Giardia duodenalis: Flavohemoglobin is involved in drug biotransformation and resistance to albendazole. PLoS Pathogens. 2022;**18**(9):e1010840

[37] Katiyar SK, Gordon VR, McLaughlin GL, Edlind TD. Antiprotozoal activities of benzimidazoles and correlations with beta-tubulin sequence. Antimicrobial Agents and Chemotherapy. 1994;**38**(9):2086-2090

[38] Tatsumi K, Yamada H, Yoshimura H, Kawazoe Y. Metabolism of furazolidone by milk xanthine oxidase and rat liver 9000g supernatant: Formation of a unique nitrofuran metabolite and an aminofuran derivative. Archives of Biochemistry and Biophysics. 1981;**208**(1):167-174

[39] Leitsch D. Drug resistance in the microaerophilic parasite Giardia lamblia. Current Tropical Medicine Reports. 2015;**2**:128-135

[40] Edlind TD. Susceptibility of Giardia lamblia to aminoglycoside protein synthesis inhibitors: Correlation with rRNA structure. Antimicrobial Agents and Chemotherapy. 1989;**33**(4):484-488

[41] Hemphill A, Mueller J, Esposito M. Nitazoxanide, a broad-spectrum thiazolide anti-infective agent for the treatment of gastrointestinal infections. Expert Opinion on Pharmacotherapy. 2006;**7**(7):953-964

[42] Saghaug CS et al. Genetic diversity in the metronidazole metabolism genes nitroreductases and pyruvate ferredoxin oxidoreductases in susceptible and refractory clinical samples of Giardia lamblia. International Journal for Parasitology: Drugs and Drug Resistance. 2023;**21**:51-60

[43] Brown DM, Upcroft JA, Upcroft P. A H2O-producing NADH oxidase from the protozoan parasite giardia duodenalis. European Journal of Biochemistry. 1996;**241**(1):155-161

[44] Lalle M, Hanevik K. Treatment-refractory giardiasis: Challenges and solutions. Infection and Drug Resistance. 2018;**11**:1921-1933

[45] Lopez-Velez R, Batlle C, Jiménez C, Navarro M, Norman F, Perez-Molina J. Short course combination therapy for giardiasis after nitroimidazole failure. The American Journal of Tropical Medicine and Hygiene. 2010;**83**(1):171

[46] Nabarro LEB, Lever RA, Armstrong M, Chiodini PL. Increased incidence of nitroimidazole-refractory giardiasis at the Hospital for Tropical Diseases, London: 2008-2013. Clinical Microbiology and Infection. 2015;**21**(8):791-796

[47] Yadav P, Tak V, Mirdha BR, Makharia GK. Refractory giardiasis: A molecular appraisal from a tertiary care Centre in India. Indian Journal of Medical Microbiology. 2014;**32**(4):378-382

[48] Morrison HG et al. Genomic minimalism in the early diverging intestinal parasite Giardia lamblia. Science (1979). 2007;**317**(5846):1921-1926

[49] Kourbeli V, Chontzopoulou E, Moschovou K, Pavlos D, Mavromoustakos T, Papanastasiou IP. An overview on target-based drug design against kinetoplastid protozoan infections: Human African trypanosomiasis, Chagas disease and leishmaniases. Molecules. 2021;**26**(15):4629

[50] Hahn J et al. High sensitivity of Giardia duodenalis to tetrahydrolipstatin (orlistat) in vitro. PLoS One. 2013;**8**(8):e71597

[51] Stevens AJ et al. Antigiardial activity of novel guanidine compounds. ChemMedChem. 2022;**17**(21):e202200341

[52] Krakovka S, Ranjbarian F, Luján LA, et al. Giardia intestinalis thymidine kinase is a high-affinity enzyme crucial for DNA synthesis and an exploitable target for drug discovery. Journal of Biological Chemistry. 2022;**298**(6):102028

[53] Custodio MM, Sparks J, Long TE. Disulfiram: A repurposed drug in preclinical and clinical development for the treatment of infectious diseases. Antiinfect Agents. 2022;**20**(3):e040122199856

[54] Michaels SA et al. Repurposing the kinase inhibitor Mavelertinib for Giardiasis therapy. Antimicrobial Agents and Chemotherapy. 2022;**66**(7):e00017-e00022

[55] Lagunas-Rangel FA, Bazán- Tejeda ML, García-Villa E, Bermúdez-Cruz RM. Nicotinamide induces G2 cell cycle arrest in Giardia duodenalis trophozoites and promotes changes in sirtuins transcriptional expression. Experimental Parasitology. 2020;**209**:107822

[56] Oliveira RVF, de Souza W, Vögerl K, Bracher F, Benchimol M, Gadelha APR. In vitro effects of the 4-[(10H-phenothiazin-10-yl) methyl]-N-hydroxybenzamide on Giardia intestinalis trophozoites. Acta Tropica. 2022;**232**:106484

[57] Maia-Brigagão C, Gadelha APR, De Souza W. New associated structures of the anterior flagella of Giardia duodenalis. Microscopy and Microanalysis. 2013;**19**(5):1374-1376

[58] Han J, Collins LJ. Reconstruction of sugar metabolic pathways of Giardia lamblia. International Journal of Proteomics. 2012;**2012**:980829

[59] Hennessey KM et al. Identification and validation of small-gatekeeper kinases as drug targets in Giardia lamblia. PLoS Neglected Tropical Diseases. 2016;**10**(11):e0005107

[60] Park E-A, Kim J, Shin MY, Park S-J. A polo-like kinase modulates cytokinesis and flagella biogenesis in Giardia lamblia. Parasites & Vectors. 2021;**14**:1-20

[61] Islas-Morales PF, Cárdenas A, Mosqueira MJ, Jiménez-García LF, Voolstra CR. Ultrastructural and proteomic evidence for the presence of a putative nucleolus in an Archaeon. Frontiers in Microbiology. 2023;**14**:1075071

[62] Best AA, Morrison HG, McArthur AG, Sogin ML, Olsen GJ. Evolution of eukaryotic transcription: Insights from the genome of Giardia lamblia. Genome Research. 2004;**14**(8):1537-1547

[63] Machado M, Dinis AM, Salgueiro L, Cavaleiro C, Custódio JBA, Sousa M d C. Anti-giardia activity of phenolic-rich essential oils: Effects of Thymbra capitata, Origanum virens, thymus zygis subsp. sylvestris, and Lippia graveolens on trophozoites growth, viability, adherence, and

ultrastructure. Parasitology Research. 2010;**106**:1205-1215

[64] Chakraborti S et al. Curcumin recognizes a unique binding site of tubulin. Journal of Medicinal Chemistry. 2011;**54**(18):6183-6196

[65] Cui Z, Li J, Chen Y, Zhang L. Molecular epidemiology, evolution, and phylogeny of Entamoeba spp. Infection, Genetics and Evolution. 2019;**75**:104018

[66] Fotedar R, Stark D, Beebe N, Marriott D, Ellis J, Harkness J. Laboratory diagnostic techniques for Entamoeba species. Clinical Microbiology Reviews. 2007;**20**(3):511-532

[67] Ouattara M, N'guéssan NA, Yapi A, N'goran EK. Prevalence and spatial distribution of Entamoeba histolytica/dispar and Giardia lamblia among schoolchildren in Agboville area (Côte d'Ivoire). PLoS Neglected Tropical Diseases. 2010;**4**(1):e574

[68] Samie A, Obi LC, Bessong PO, Stroup S, Houpt E, Guerrant RL. Prevalence and species distribution of E. histolytica and E. dispar in the Venda region, Limpopo, South Africa. American Journal of Tropical Medicine and Hygiene. 2006;**75**(3):565-571

[69] Samie A, ElBakri A, AbuOdeh R. Amoebiasis in the tropics: Epidemiology and pathogenesis. Current Topics in Tropical Medicine. 2012:201-226

[70] Nasrallah J et al. Updates on the worldwide burden of amoebiasis: A case series and literature review. Journal of Infection and Public Health. 2022;**15**(10):1134-1141

[71] Faust DM, Guillen N. Virulence and virulence factors in Entamoeba histolytica, the agent of human amoebiasis. Microbes and Infection. 2012;**14**:1428-1441

[72] Morán P et al. Amoebiasis: Advances in diagnosis, treatment, immunology features and the interaction with the intestinal ecosystem. International Journal of Molecular Sciences. 2023;**24**(14):11755

[73] Betanzos A et al. The EhCPADH112 complex of Entamoeba histolytica interacts with tight junction proteins occludin and claudin-1 to produce epithelial damage. PLoS One. 2013;**8**(6):e65100

[74] Shahi P, Moreau F, Chadee K. Entamoeba histolytica cyclooxygenase-like protein regulates cysteine protease expression and virulence. Frontiers in Cellular and Infection Microbiology. 2019;**8**:447

[75] Haque R, Huston CD, Hughes M, Houpt E, Petri WA Jr. Amebiasis. New England Journal of Medicine. 2003;**348**(16):1565-1573

[76] Kantor M, Abrantes A, Estevez A, et al. Entamoeba histolytica: Updates in clinical manifestation, pathogenesis, and vaccine development. Canadian Journal of Gastroenterology & Hepatology. 2018;**2018**:4601420

[77] Soedin K, Syukran OK, Fadillah A, Sidabutar P. Comparison between the efficacy of a single dose of secnidazole with a 5-day course of tetracycline and clioquinol in the treatment of acute intestinal amoebiasis. Pharmatherapeutica. 1985;**4**(4):251-254

[78] Rossignol J-F, Kabil SM, El-Gohary Y, Younis AM. Nitazoxanide in the treatment of amoebiasis. Transactions of the Royal Society of Tropical Medicine and Hygiene. 2007;**101**(10):1025-1031

[79] García CG, Marchat LA, López-Cánovas L, Ishiwara DGP,

Rodríguez MA, Orozco E. Drug resistance mechanisms in Entamoeba histolytica, Giardia lamblia, Trichomonas vaginalis, and opportunistic anaerobic protozoa. Antimicrobial Drug Resistance: Mechanisms of Drug Resistance. 2017;**1**:613-628

[80] Bansal D, Sehgal R, Chawla Y, Malla N, Mahajan RC. Multidrug resistance in amoebiasis patients. Indian Journal of Medical Research. 2006;**124**(2):189-194

[81] Debnath A et al. A high-throughput drug screen for Entamoeba histolytica identifies a new lead and target. Nature Medicine. 2012;**18**(6):956-960

[82] Ghosh S et al. COP9 signalosome is an essential and druggable parasite target that regulates protein degradation. PLoS Pathogens. 2020;**16**(9):e1008952

[83] Kangussu-Marcolino MM, Singh U. Ponatinib, lestaurtinib, and mTOR/PI3K inhibitors are promising repurposing candidates against Entamoeba histolytica. Antimicrobial Agents and Chemotherapy. 2022;**66**(2):e01207-e01221

[84] Burkey BF, Hoglen NC, Inskeep P, Wyman M, Hughes TE, Vath JE. Preclinical efficacy and safety of the novel antidiabetic, antiobesity MetAP2 inhibitor ZGN-1061. Journal of Pharmacology and Experimental Therapeutics. 2018;**365**(2):301-313

[85] Shrivastav MT, Malik Z, Somlata. Revisiting drug development against the neglected tropical disease, amebiasis. Frontiers in Cellular and Infection Microbiology. 2021;**10**:628257

[86] Eberhard ML, da Silva AJ, Lilley BG, Pieniazek NJ. Morphologic and molecular characterization of new Cyclospora species from Ethiopian monkeys: C. cercopitheci sp. n., C. colobi sp. n., and C. papionis sp. n. Emerging Infectious Diseases. 1999;**5**(5):651

[87] Marangi M et al. Detection of Cyclospora in captive chimpanzees and macaques by a quantitative PCR-based mutation scanning approach. Parasites & Vectors. 2015;**8**:1-5

[88] Ortega YR, Sanchez R. Update on Cyclospora cayetanensis, a food-borne and waterborne parasite. Clinical Microbiology Reviews. 2010;**23**(1):218-234

[89] Chacin-Bonilla L, Santin M. Cyclospora cayetanensis infection in developed countries: Potential endemic foci? Microorganisms. 2023;**11**(3):540

[90] Almeria S, Cinar HN, Dubey JP. Cyclospora cayetanensis and cyclosporiasis: An update. Microorganisms. 2019;**7**(9):317

[91] Sarfo FS et al. The clinical features and immunological signature of cyclospora cayetanensis co-infection among people living with HIV in Ghana. Microorganisms. 2022;**10**(7):1407

[92] Visvesvara GS et al. Concurrent parasitic infections in a renal transplant patient. Emerging Infectious Diseases. 2013;**19**(12):2044

[93] Mathison BA, Pritt BS. Cyclosporiasis—Updates on clinical presentation, pathology, clinical diagnosis, and treatment. Microorganisms. 2021;**9**(9):1863

[94] Almeria S, Chacin-Bonilla L, Maloney JG, Santin M. Cyclospora cayetanensis: A perspective (2020-2023) with emphasis on epidemiology and detection methods. Microorganisms. 2023;**11**(9):2171

[95] Li J, Cui Z, Qi M, Zhang L. Advances in cyclosporiasis diagnosis

and therapeutic intervention. Frontiers in Cellular and Infection Microbiology. 2020;**10**:43

[96] Sircar S, Rayan M, Okonoboh P. TMP-SMX induced type 4 hypersensitivity with multi-organ involvement. IDCases. 2023;**34**:e01917

[97] Shimizu Y, Hirai T, Ogawa Y, Yamada C, Kobayashi E. Characteristics of risk factors for acute kidney injury among inpatients administered sulfamethoxazole/trimethoprim: A retrospective observational study. Journal of Pharmaceutical Health Care and Sciences. 2022;**8**(1):20

[98] Hagras NA, Makled S, Sheta E, El-Hawary MA, Mogahed NMFH. Potent efficiency of the novel nitazoxanide-loaded nanostructured lipid carriers against experimental cyclosporiasis. PLoS Neglected Tropical Diseases. 2023;**17**(12):e0011845

[99] Zimmer SM, Schuetz AN, Franco-Paredes C. Efficacy of nitazoxanide for cyclosporiasis in patients with sulfa allergy. Clinical Infectious Diseases. 2007;**44**(3):466-467

[100] Shakya A, Bhat HR, Ghosh SK. Update on nitazoxanide: A multifunctional chemotherapeutic agent. Current Drug Discovery Technologies. 2018;**15**(3):201-213

[101] Hagras, Nancy Abd-elkader, et al. Potent efficiency of the novel nitazoxanide-loaded nanostructured lipid carriers against experimental cyclosporiasis. PLoS Neglected Tropical Diseases. 2023;**17**(12):e0011845

[102] Mogahed N, Gaafar M, Shalaby T, Sheta E, Arafa F. Potential efficacy of curcumin and curcumin nanoemulsion against experimental cyclosporiasis. Parasitologists United Journal. 2023;**16**(3):197-207

[103] Hussein EM et al. Antiprotozoal activity of magnesium oxide (MgO) nanoparticles against Cyclospora cayetanensis oocysts. Parasitology International. 2018;**67**(6):666-674

[104] Cinar HN et al. Comparative sequence analysis of Cyclospora cayetanensis apicoplast genomes originating from diverse geographical regions. Parasites & Vectors. 2016;**9**:1-14

[105] Seeber F, Aliverti A, Zanetti G. The plant-type ferredoxin-NADP+ reductase/ferredoxin redox system as a possible drug target against apicomplexan human parasites. Current Pharmaceutical Design. 2005;**11**(24):3159-3172

[106] Liu S, Wang L, Zheng H, et al. Comparative genomics reveals cyclospora cayetanensis possesses coccidia-like metabolism and invasion components but unique surface antigens. BMC Genomics. 2016;**17**:316

[107] Innes EA, Chalmers RM, Wells B, Pawlowic MC. A one health approach to tackle cryptosporidiosis. Trends in Parasitology. 2020;**36**(3):290-303

[108] Tyzzer EE. A sporozoan found in the peptic glands of the common mouse. Proceedings of the Society for Experimental Biology and Medicine. 1907;**5**(1):12-13

[109] Corso PS, Kramer MH, Blair KA, Addiss DG, Davis JP, Haddix AC. Costs of illness in the 1993 waterborne Cryptosporidium outbreak, Milwaukee, Wisconsin. Emerging Infectious Diseases. 2003;**9**(4):426

[110] Efstratiou A, Ongerth JE, Karanis P. Waterborne transmission of protozoan parasites: Review of worldwide

outbreaks-an update 2011-2016. Water Research. 2017;**114**:14-22

[111] Fayer R, Xiao L, editors. Cryptosporidium and Cryptosporidiosis. 2nd ed. Boca Raton: CRC Press; 2007. pp. 1-42

[112] Gharpure R, Perez A, Miller AD, Wikswo ME, Silver R, Hlavsa MC. Cryptosporidiosis outbreaks—United States, 2009-2017. American Journal of Transplantation. 2019;**19**(9):2650-2654

[113] Current WL, Reese NC. A comparison of endogenous development of three isolates of cryptosporidium in suckling mice 1. The Journal of Protozoology. 1986;**33**(1):98-108

[114] Lendner M, Daugschies A. Cryptosporidium infections: Molecular advances. Parasitology. 2014;**141**(11):1511-1532

[115] Checkley W et al. A review of the global burden, novel diagnostics, therapeutics, and vaccine targets for cryptosporidium. The Lancet Infectious Diseases. 2015;**15**(1):85-94

[116] Hussien SMM et al. Comparative study between the effect of nitazoxanide and paromomycine in treatment of cryptosporidiosis in hospitalized children. Journal of the Egyptian Society of Parasitology. 2013;**43**(2):463-470

[117] Zulu I et al. Albendazole chemotherapy for AIDS-related diarrhoea in Zambia—Clinical, parasitological and mucosal responses. Alimentary Pharmacology & Therapeutics. 2002;**16**(3):595-601

[118] Uip DE, Lima AL, Amato VS, Boulos M, Neto VA, Bem David D. Roxithromycin treatment for diarrhoea caused by cryptosporidium spp. in patients with AIDS. The Journal of Antimicrobial Chemotherapy. 1998;**41**(suppl. 2):93-97

[119] Hartmann G, Honikel KO, Knüsel F, Nüesch J. The specific inhibition of the DNA-directed RNA synthesis by rifamycin. Biochimica et Biophysica Acta (BBA)-Nucleic Acids and Protein Synthesis. 1967;**145**(3):843-844

[120] Fichtenbaum CJ, Zackin R, Feinberg J, Benson C, Griffiths JK, et al. Rifabutin but not clarithromycin prevents cryptosporidiosis in persons with advanced HIV infection. AIDS. 2000;**14**(18):2889-2893

[121] Blanshard C, Shanson DC, Gazzard BG. Pilot studies of azithromycin, letrazuril and paromomycin in the treatment of cryptosporidiosis. International Journal of STD & AIDS. 1997;**8**(2):124-129

[122] Smith NH, Cron S, Valdez LM, Chappell CL, White AC Jr. Combination drug therapy for cryptosporidiosis in AIDS. Journal of Infectious Diseases. 1998;**178**(3):900-903

[123] Dupuy F, Valot S, Dalle F, Sterin A, L'ollivier C. Disseminated Cryptosporidium infection in an infant with CD40L deficiency. IDCases. 2021;**24**:e01115

[124] Tomczak E, McDougal AN, White AC Jr. Resolution of cryptosporidiosis in transplant recipients: Review of the literature and presentation of a renal transplant patient treated with nitazoxanide, azithromycin, and rifaximin. Open Forum Infectious Diseases. 2021;**9**(1):ofab610

[125] Love MS, Choy RKM. Emerging treatment options for cryptosporidiosis. Current Opinion in Infectious Diseases. 2021;**34**(5):455-462

[126] Van Voorhis WC et al. One health therapeutics: Target-based drug development for cryptosporidiosis and other apicomplexa diseases. Veterinary Parasitology. 2021;**289**:109336

[127] Schaefer DA et al. Novel bumped kinase inhibitors are safe and effective therapeutics in the calf clinical model for cryptosporidiosis. The Journal of Infectious Diseases. 2016;**214**(12):1856-1864

[128] Lee S et al. Therapeutic efficacy of bumped kinase inhibitor 1369 in a pig model of acute diarrhea caused by Cryptosporidium hominis. Antimicrobial Agents and Chemotherapy. 2018;**62**(7):10-1128

[129] Manjunatha UH et al. A Cryptosporidium PI (4) K inhibitor is a drug candidate for cryptosporidiosis. Nature. 2017;**546**(7658):376-380

[130] Jumani RS et al. A novel piperazine-based drug lead for cryptosporidiosis from the medicines for malaria venture open-access malaria box. Antimicrobial Agents and Chemotherapy. 2018;**62**(4):10-1128

[131] Lee S et al. Piperazine-derivative MMV665917: An effective drug in the diarrheic piglet model of Cryptosporidium hominis. The Journal of Infectious Diseases. 2019;**220**(2):285-293

[132] Lunde CS et al. Identification of a potent benzoxaborole drug candidate for treating cryptosporidiosis. Nature Communications. 2019;**10**(1):2816